Advances in Veterinary Research

Advances in Veterinary Research

Edited by Dalton Higgins

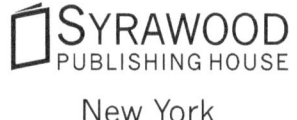
SYRAWOOD
PUBLISHING HOUSE

New York

Published by Syrawood Publishing House,
750 Third Avenue, 9th Floor,
New York, NY 10017, USA
www.syrawoodpublishinghouse.com

Advances in Veterinary Research
Edited by Dalton Higgins

© 2019 Syrawood Publishing House

International Standard Book Number: 978-1-68286-748-8 (Hardback)

Cataloging-in-Publication Data

Advances in veterinary research / edited by Dalton Higgins.
    p. cm.
Includes bibliographical references and index.
ISBN 978-1-68286-748-8
1. Veterinary medicine--Research. 2. Veterinary medicine. 3. Animals--Diseases.
4. Animal health. I. Higgins, Dalton.
SF756.3 .A38 2019
636.089--dc23

TABLE OF CONTENTS

Permissions

List of Contributors

Index

PREFACE

Veterinary medicine is a branch of medicine that is involved in the prevention, diagnosis and treatment of animal diseases, disorders and injuries. Some animal diseases can be transmitted to humans. Such diseases are called zoonotic diseases. They are caused by pathogens like viruses, fungi, parasites and bacteria. Some examples of zoonotic diseases are rabies, influenza, Ebola virus disease, salmonellosis, etc. The monitoring and control of such diseases is also under the domain of this discipline. Veterinary medicine extends to all domesticated and wild animals, however, specializations may also exist for applications for a specific group of animals such as zoo animals, livestock, laboratory animals or pets. Other specializations in this field include veterinary surgery, internal medicine, dermatology and laboratory animal medicine. This book discusses the fundamentals as well as modern approaches of veterinary science. It aims to shed light on some of the unexplored aspects and the recent researches in this field. As this field is emerging at a rapid pace, the contents of this book will help the readers understand the modern concepts and applications of the subject.

The researches compiled throughout the book are authentic and of high quality, combining several disciplines and from very diverse regions from around the world. Drawing on the contributions of many researchers from diverse countries, the book's objective is to provide the readers with the latest achievements in the area of research. This book will surely be a source of knowledge to all interested and researching the field.

In the end, I would like to express my deep sense of gratitude to all the authors for meeting the set deadlines in completing and submitting their research chapters. I would also like to thank the publisher for the support offered to us throughout the course of the book. Finally, I extend my sincere thanks to my family for being a constant source of inspiration and encouragement.

Editor

Historical analysis of Newfoundland dog fur colour genetics

J. Bondeson*

Department of Rheumatology, School of Medicine, Cardiff University, Cardiff, CF14 4XN, UK

Abstract

This article makes use of digitized historic newspapers to analyze Newfoundland dog fur colour genetics, and fur colour variations over time. The results indicate that contrary to the accepted view, the 'Solid' gene was introduced into the British population of Newfoundland dogs in the 1840s. Prior to that time, the dogs were white and black (Landseer) or white and brown, and thus spotted/spotted homozygotes. Due to 'Solid' being dominant over 'spotted', and selective breeding, today the majority of Newfoundland dogs are solid black. Whereas small white marks on the chest and/or paw appears to be a random event, the historical data supports the existence of an 'Irish spotted' fur colour pattern, with white head blaze, breast, paws and tail tip, in spotted/spotted homozygotes.

Keywords: Fur colour genetics, Irish spotting, Landseer Newfoundland, MITF, Newfoundland dog.

Introduction

The Newfoundland is one of the most majestic and distinctive breeds of dog (Waters, 2006; Bondeson, 2012). Originating in Newfoundland, these dogs were exported, mainly to Britain, as early as the 1730s, for use as ship's dogs. By the 1780s, the Newfoundland dogs had become fashionable as pets, and Britain had a considerable population of them (Bondeson, 2012). According to recent breed monographs, the original Newfoundland dogs were solid black (Fig. 1). These publications also allege that the white and black spotted Newfoundland dogs became popular for a while in the 1820s and 1830s, after being portrayed by Sir Edwin Landseer, who had a great liking for these animals, but they then sank back into obscurity (Booth Chern, 1975; Drury, 1978; Barlowe, 2001; Kosloff, 2006). Since the 1880s, these white and black dogs have been known as 'Landseer Newfoundlands', a name coined not by any kennel club or dog breeding association, but by the eccentric Victorian dog fancier Dr William Gordon Stables (Stables, 1875,1880).

Sir Edwin Landseer was one of many British or continental European painters from the first half of the nineteenth century to have depicted white and black spotted Newfoundland dogs; his production does not include any solid black, or solid brown, specimens (Fig. 2). Landseer portrayed many solid black dogs of other breeds, and it is not conceivable that a painter of his talent would be unable to depict a black Newfoundland, if these dogs had been common in his time (Mellencamp, 1976, 1978; Waters, 2006). Inventories of Newfoundland dog iconography demonstrate that from the 1740s until the 1840s, there were many paintings and drawings of white and black [and also some white and brown] Newfoundland dogs, but no convincing illustrations to support the existence of solid black [or brown] dogs at the time, in Britain or on the European continent (Conlon, 1989; Matenaar, 1989; Waters, 2006; Bondeson, 2011, 2012).

The accepted facts of Newfoundland dog fur colour genetics are that the basic colour of a Newfoundland dog is determined by what is known as the B locus, with 'Black' colour being dominant over 'brown'. Thus, the BB homozygotes will be black, as will the Bb heterozygotes; only the bb homozygotes will be brown. Then there is the D locus, with 'Non Dilute' dominant over 'dilute'. The DD and Dd dogs will be black, whereas the dd homozygotes will be grey, or diluted black. There are some grey Newfoundland dogs in the United States, but very few elsewhere. The regulation of solid colour versus spotting in Newfoundland dogs is controlled by the S locus, where 'Solid' colouring is dominant over 'spotted'. Thus the SS homozygotes and the Ss heterozygotes will be solid black (or brown), whereas the ss homozygotes will be spotted. In Newfoundlands, there are several different patterns of spotting, ranging from dogs that are white with a few black spots, to dogs that are black with white feet, chest and tail tip. Dr Charles Little constructed a model with an allelic series where S is Solid, s^i is 'Irish spotting' with white head blaze, breast, paws and tail tip, s^p piebald spotting with coloured plates, separated or confluent, and s^w extreme-white piebald spotting. He discussed the possibility of plus and minus modifiers affecting the type of spotting, and also the putative existence of a 'pseudo-Irish' spotting pattern that might occur in Solid/spotted heterozygotes in some breeds of dogs (Little, 1957). Dr Øjwind Winge preferred a simpler model with two alleles at the locus for white mottled: T for solid coloured or nearly so, and t for white mottled (Winge, 1950). The various loci discussed above are of course not proper genes,

*Corresponding Author:** Jan Bondeson. Department of Rheumatology, School of Medicine, Cardiff University, Cardiff, CF14 4XN, UK. E-mail: *BondesonJ@cf.ac.uk*

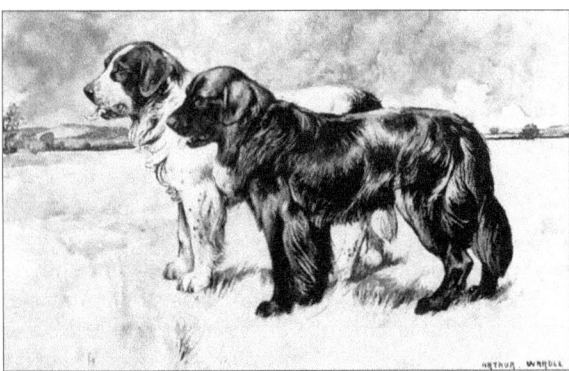

Fig. 1. A solid black Newfoundland and a Landseer, from Rawdon Lee's *History and Description of the Modern Dogs of Great Britain and Ireland.*

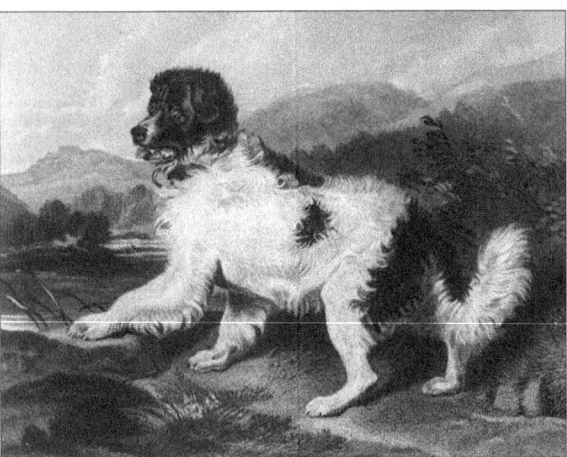

Fig. 2. A print of Landseer's painting of the Newfoundland dog Lion.

resulting from genotyping or genomic sequencing, but rather interpretations of breeding results.

Later, a model of polygenic inheritance was applied to the piebald spotting patterns in Landseer Newfoundland dogs and Holstein-Friesian cattle (Pape, 1990). The Landseers were divided into three classes: the dark dogs with white legs, chest, tail and head blaze (Mantel), the white and black spotted dogs with white legs and tail (Medium), and the nearly all white dogs with a black face-mask and a few black sports on the body (Light). It was postulated that the recessive major spotting gene worked with at least two modifiers, which he termed s_2 and s_3. Dogs that were S_3S_3 homozygotes, and either S_2S_2 homozygotes or S_2s_2 heterozygotes, were dark (Mantel). Dogs that were s_2s_2 homozygotes, and either s_3s_3 homozygotes or S_3s_3 heterozygotes, were nearly all white (Light). All other combinations resulted in the traditional white and black spotted dogs (Medium). This model was tested in large populations of cattle (n=1118), and a much smaller population of dogs (n=110), and proved to work quite well, according to

a combined sum and Fisher test (Pape, 1990), it would have been interesting to see it evaluated in a larger population of dogs.

The same paper also addressed the problem of the inheritance of small white marks in Newfoundland dogs (Pape, 1990). Although most Solid/spotted heterozygotes were solid black or brown, it was presumed that modifier genes might again be playing a part in the 'pseudo-Irish' spotting, as well as in the inheritance of other patterns of small white markings. In Pape's classification system, there were solid-coloured dogs without white marks (Class I), solid-coloured dogs with some white on the chest (Class IIA), dogs with small white marks on the chest and one or more paws (Class IIB), and 'Irish spotted' dogs with white on the head, chest, belly, paws and tail tip (Class III). Again, a model of two modifiers determining these spotting patterns was constructed, and tested using a database of stud book material. This theory worked reasonably well, with the exception that the number of 'Irish spotted' pups was underestimated when dogs from Class I were mated either with each other, or with dogs from Class II. When dogs from Class I were mated together, the expected values of Class I, II and III pups were 1740, 250 and 9, respectively; the observed values were 1765, 234 and 0, respectively, quite possibly indicating that solid-coloured dogs do not have 'Irish spotted' pups. In matings with dogs from Class I with dogs from Class II, the expected values of Class I, II and III pups were 641, 293 and 16, respectively; the observed values were 627, 320 and 3, respectively. Again the underestimation of the number of 'Irish spotted' pups casts some doubt on the validity of this inheritance model.

In 2007, the gene 'Microphtalmia associated transcription factor' (MITF) was recognized as causing one or more spotting patterns in dogs, including Landseer Newfoundlands. The insertion of a short interspersed nucleotide element (SINE) in the MITF start codon was linked with random spotting in many dog breeds (Karlsson *et al.*, 2007). A later population study indicated that dogs homozygous for the SINE had white markings comparative to those in Pape's three classes of Landseer Newfoundlands. In most breeds, dogs heterozygous to the SINE insertion were either solid coloured or had minimal white markings, but in certain breeds, the dogs had the 'pseudo-Irish' pattern discussed by Little (Schmutz *et al.*, 2009).

Results and Discussion

To investigate the historical variation of Newfoundland dog fur colour, the 'Times Digital Archive' (Gale Databases) database of the advertisements for lost or stolen dogs in the *Times* newspaper was used. For these advertisements to be useful, they needed to contain a good description of the animal in question, thus helping to eliminate the potential bias due to carelessness or journalistic license. Many of the descriptions of the dogs are sufficiently detailed, such as this one from 1785:

"LOST on Saturday last, May 28th, a large Black Newfoundland Dog, has White Feet, a little White in the Forehead, the end of his Tail White, answers to the Name of Lyon".

Advertisements that did not describe the fur colour of the dogs in question, or that concerned mongrels were excluded, resulting in a total of 134 advertisements to recover lost or stolen Newfoundland dogs from 1785 until 1890. Further excluding a grey Newfoundland advertised for in 1814, and a white and yellow 'Newfoundland' dog advertised for in 1839, the remaining 132 dogs belonged to the fur colour patterns that are recognized today (Table 1). Prior to the year 1840, there was not a single advertisement describing a solid black (or brown) Newfoundland, but 15 dogs that were obvious white and black (or brown) spotted. Most of these Landseers belonged to the 'Medium' and 'Light' subgroups. Between 1840 and 1850, solid black dogs begin appearing in the *Times* advertisements, and in the time period 1850-1859, they were nearly as frequently described as the other fur colour variations. In the time period 1860-1890, solid black dogs were in the majority. Thus it appears as if solid black Newfoundland dogs were very scarce in Britain prior to 1840, before ultimately becoming the most common fur colour variant.

Using Pape's classification system (Pape, 1990), it was clear that the 'III' pattern of fur colour was represented in many early (pre-1840) dogs. The 'IIA' and 'IIB' dogs were all post-1850, however, and thus appeared after the 'Solid' gene had been introduced. This supports the hypothesis that small white marks on the chest and paws are a random event rather than the result of a specific allele. During embryogenesis, the melanocytes, the cells producing pigment, migrate down from the spinal column. But not all the dogs complete this process by birth or thereafter, and this incomplete migration results in a white toe or a white spot on the chest in an otherwise solid-coloured animal (the 'IIB' and 'IIA' classes, respectively). Table 1 provides no support for the existence of a 'pseudo-Irish' spotting phenomenon in Newfoundland dogs, but instead supports Little's original hypothesis of an 'Irish spotting' allele. Since 8 Newfoundland dogs with the 'III' fur colour pattern were described in the time period 1785-1839 (Table 1), before the 'Solid' gene had been introduced, this would indicate that the 'III' for colour pattern occurs in spotted/spotted homozygotes. The role of modifiers in regulating this fur colour pattern remains unclear.

It was also possible to use a second online newspaper database, the 'Nineteenth Century British Library Newspapers' (Gale Databases). This database covers a large number of historic London and provincial UK papers, although it was a concern that the descriptions of the dogs (for sale, for auction, and lost or found) were often much less detailed than those in the Times Digital Archive. Since advertisement quality seemed to decline over time, it was not possible to continue past 1839. It should be noted that where the dogs have been pointed out to be solid black, rather than just 'black', they have been put in a special 'solid black' category. Out of a total of 149 advertisements in the British Library database, there were two solid white dogs and one red and white dog; the remainder fitted into the present-day classification system (Table 2). The tallied results were much the same as for the Times Digital Archive, although the British Library database indicates that there were a few solid black dogs in Britain prior to 1840. This discrepancy in solid black dog may be a result of a lack of cynological sophistication in the provincial newspapers of the time. Not only was the definition of a Newfoundland dog somewhat vague in Georgian times, but a brief advertisement such as 'For sale by auction, a black Newfoundland dog' does not rule out that the animal had some white markings. Still, a few of the advertisements for solid black 'Newfoundlands' appear bona fide, perhaps indicating that although the larger, white and black or white and brown spotted Newfoundland dogs were preferred by the dog fanciers, a few of the smaller, solid-coloured, retriever-like black dogs were imported from Newfoundland at the time. However, these dogs would not appear to have been interbred with the spotted Newfoundland dogs to any extent prior to the 1840s, when solid black dogs became fashionable.

In late Victorian times, there was much interest in dogs and their doings: kennel clubs were founded, breed standards established, and large dog shows held. The late Victorian dog fancy sometimes rewrote the history of their favourite breeds: for example, the original purpose of the Bulldog as a bull-baiting dog was conveniently 'forgotten', and emphasis was instead put on its pure and ancient English stock, and its friendly and affectionate nature (Ritvo, 1986).

Table 1. Fur colour variation in Newfoundland dogs over time, from the 'Times Digital Archive' database, 1785-1890.

Time period	Landseer	White/ Brown	IIA	IIB	III	Black	Brown
1785-1799	1	1	0	0	1	0	0
1800-1819	2	1	0	0	2	0	0
1820-1839	8	2	0	0	5	0	0
1840-1849	9	1	0	0	6	4	1
1850-1859	10	1	4	3	4	17	1
1860-1869	6	0	5	2	5	20	1
1870-1890	1	0	2	0	0	6	0

Table 2. Fur colour variation in Newfoundland dogs over time, from the 'Nineteenth Century British Library Newspapers' database, 1760-1839.

Time period	Landseer	White/Brown	IIA	IIB	III	Solid Black	Black	Brown
1760-1769	1	2	0	0	0	0	1	0
1770-1779	20	2	0	0	9	1	2	0
1780-1789	10	4	0	0	3	0	3	0
1790-1799	12	2	0	0	1	0	0	1
1800-1809	14	1	0	0	4	0	0	1
1810-1819	12	0	0	0	4	0	1	0
1820-1829	14	1	0	0	1	0	1	0
1830-1839	16	0	0	0	2	1	0	0

A prime mover in the late Victorian Newfoundland dog fancy was Dr William Gordon Stables, a former naval surgeon who had left medical practice and established himself as a writer of juvenile fiction (Fig. 3). He wrote at least a hundred novels, as well as countless articles for the *Boy's Own Paper* and other periodicals (Graham, 2006; Bondeson, 2012). He also wrote a number of books on animals, including *Our Friend the Dog* that went through a number of editions. Although having no academic education in the fields of zoology and veterinary medicine, and possessing only an outdated medical degree, Dr Stables fancied himself as an expert on all canine matters. He considered the Newfoundland to be the most sagacious of all dog breeds, and himself kept a number of these dogs over the years; an irresponsible dog owner, he was fond of watching dog fights involving his own animals, and on occasion even set his dogs on human beings. For some reason or other, possibly that his own favourite Newfoundland champion 'Theodore Nero' had been solid black, Dr Stables made up his mind that the solid black variety was the original breed of the Newfoundland dog. The white and black spotted dogs had briefly been fashionable in the time of Sir Edwin Landseer, who liked to paint them, but now they were again in a decline (Fig. 4). When interviewed in 1875, Dr Stables said that the white and black Newfoundland dog should be called the Landseer, since they had so often been included in his paintings (Stables, 1875). In an 1880 article, Dr Stables proclaimed that "The black-and-white breed is now generally called the 'Landseer Newfoundland', a name the writer originated a few years ago" (Stables, 1880). The denomination 'Landseer Newfoundland' thus does not originate with any dog breeding association, or knowledgeable expert on dogs, but with a Victorian eccentric who wrote silly children's books, and who liked to scatter German marching bands with his mischievous Newfoundland dog. The views of Dr Stables on Newfoundland fur colour were also widely regurgitated at the time, and are still quoted with approval today.

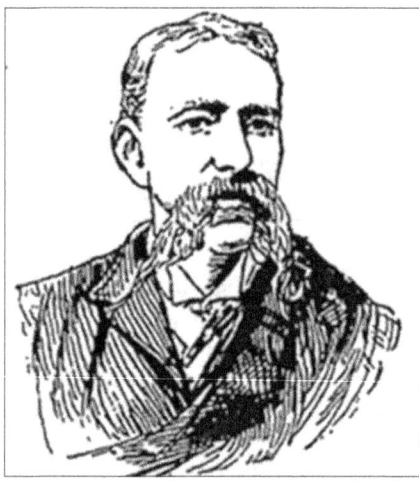

Fig. 3. Dr William Gordon Stables, from the *Penny Illustrated Paper*, March 19, 1892.

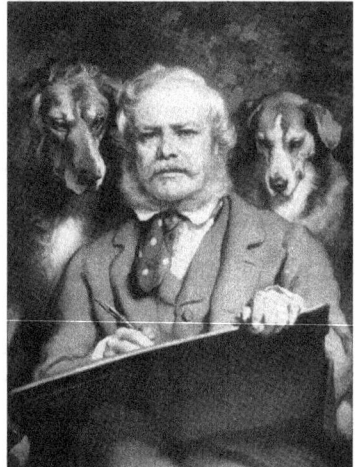

Fig. 4. An 1865 print of Landseer's 'The Connoisseurs': a self-portrait with two of his dogs.

The best way of studying dog colour genetics is by way of recording breeding histories, but prior to the late Victorian dog fancy, there was very little interest in recording the breeding of dogs. Thus the historical study of Newfoundland dog fur colour genetics would have to rely on contemporary descriptions of lost or stolen dogs, or dogs for sale or for auction. Based on the data described above, and the art history studies of fur colour variation in Newfoundlands, it is reasonable to suggest that the 'Solid' gene was introduced into the British population of Newfoundland dogs in the 1840s, quite possibly through importation of smaller, solid black dogs from parts of Newfoundland. Certain dog fanciers may have used these imported dogs in breeding experiments to produce solid black Newfoundland dogs with the same size and general phenotype as the finest white and black spotted specimens. Being dominant over 'spotted', the 'Solid' gene soon impacted on the Newfoundland dog phenotype, particularly since the solid black dogs became highly fashionable in late Victorian times. When Dr William Gordon Stables and other Victorian dog fanciers rewrote the history of the Newfoundland dog, they wrongly claimed that Landseer had a preternatural liking for white and black dogs, and that the solid black dogs were the original breed (Bondeson, 2012). This statement would appear to have originated in the good doctor's imagination rather than in factual observations, however, and it is time that the breed monograph 'accepted truth' about Newfoundland dog history is challenged.

References
Barlowe, A. 2001. Newfoundland. Dorking UK: Interpet Publishing, pp: 2-9.

Bondeson, J. 2011. Amazing Dogs. Ithaca NY: Cornell University Press, pp: 162-188.

Bondeson, J. 2012. Those Amazing Newfoundland Dogs. Bideford UK: CFZ Press.

Booth Chern, M. 1975. The New Complete Newfoundland. New York: Howell Book House, pp: 38.

Conlon, D. 1989. Sir Edwin Landseer (1803-1873) and the Landser Dog. In: Zuchtbuch Nr. 2 of the Deutscher Landseer Club, Pfungstad: DLC, pp: 14-55.

Drury, K.M. 1978. This is the Newfoundland. Neptune City NJ: T.F.C. Publications, pp: 45-58.

Graham, S. 2006. An Introduction to William Gordon Stables 1837-1910. Twyford UK: Twyford and Ruscombe Local History Society.

Karlsson, E.K., Baranowska, I., Wade, C.M., Salmon Hillbertz, N.H., Zody, M.C., Anderson, N., Biagi, T.M., Patterson, N., Pielberg, G.R., Kulbokas, EJ. 3rd., Comstock, K.E., Keller, E.T., Mesirov, J.P., von Euler, H., Kämpe, O., Hedhammar, A., Lander, E.S., Andersson, G., Andersson, L. and Lindblad-Toh, K. 2007. Efficient mapping of mendelian traits in dogs through genome-wide association. Nature Genetics 39, 1321-1328.

Kosloff, J. 2006. Newfoundlands. New York: Barron's Educational Series, pp: 5-11.

Little, C.C. 1957. The Inheritance of Coat Colour in Dogs. New York: Howell Book House.

Matenaar, C. 1989. Frühe Zeugnisse für den 'Newfoundland dog' in England und auf dem Kontinent. In: Zuchtbuch Nr. 2 of the Deutscher Landseer Club, Pfungstad: DLC, pp: 57-200.

Mellencamp, E.H. 1976. What color is a Newfoundland and when? Newf. Tide. 7(4), 9-11.

Mellencamp, E.H. 1978. A tale of black beauties. Newf. Tide. 9(1), 16-19.

Pape, H. 1990. The inheritance of the piebald spotting pattern and its variation in Holstein-Friesian cattle and in Landseer-Newfoundland dogs. Genetica 80, 115-128.

Ritvo, H. 1986. Pride and pedigree: The evolution of the Victorian dog fancy. Victorian Studies 29, 227-253.

Schmutz, S.M., Berryere, T.G. and Dreger, D.L. 2009. MITF and white spotting in dogs: A population study. J. Hered. 100, S66-S74.

Stables, W.G. 1875. The Newfoundland. Fancier's Gazette March 25, 1875.

Stables, W.G. 1880. Boys' dogs, and all about them. Boy's Own Paper May 1, 1880.

Waters, N. 2006. The Newfoundland in Heritage and Art. the Hague: BB Press.

Winge, Ø. 1950. Inheritance in Dogs with Special Reference to the Hunting Breeds. Ithaca, NY: Cornell University Press.

Automated tru-cut imaging-guided core needle biopsy of canine orbital neoplasia: A prospective feasibility study

A. Cirla[1,*], M. Rondena[2] and G. Bertolini[1]

[1]San Marco Veterinary Clinic, via Sorio 114/c – 35141 Padova, Italy
[2]San Marco Veterinary Laboratory, via Sorio 114/c – 35141 Padova, Italy

Abstract

The purpose of this study was to evaluate the diagnostic value of imaging-guided core needle biopsy for canine orbital mass diagnosis. A second excisional biopsy obtained during surgery or necropsy was used as the reference standard. A prospective feasibility study was conducted in 23 canine orbital masses at a single centre. A complete ophthalmic examination was always followed by orbital ultrasound and computed tomography (CT) examination of the head. All masses were sampled with the patient still on the CT table using ultrasound (US) guided automatic tru-cut device. The most suitable sampling approach to the orbit was chosen each time based on the CT image analysis. One of the following different approaches was used: trans-orbital, trans-conjunctival or trans-masseteric. In all cases, the imaging-guided biopsy provided a sufficient amount of tissue for the histopathological diagnosis, which concurred with the biopsies obtained using the excisional technique. CT examination was essential for morphological diagnosis and provided detailed topographic information that allowed us to choose the safest orbital approach for the biopsy. US guided automatic tru-cut biopsy based on CT images, performed with patient still on the CT table, resulted in a minimally invasive, relatively easy, and accurate diagnostic procedure in dogs with orbital masses.
Keywords: Computed tomography, Core-needle biopsy, Dogs, Orbital mass, Ultrasound.

Introduction

A number of neoplasias have been reported to affect the orbit or retrobulbar space in dogs (Hendrix and Gelatt, 2000; Kato et al., 2012; Spiess and Pot, 2013). These neoplasias can be primary or secondary tumors reaching the orbital region via either metastasis or extension from adjacent sites (Attali-Soussay et al., 2001; Van der Woerdt, 2008). Orbital neoplasia can be easily detected on advanced imaging examinations in many circumstances. It may be found incidentally on computed tomography (CT) or magnetic resonance imaging (MRI) examinations of the skull, performed for other non-ophthalmological diseases (Armour et al., 2011; Boland et al., 2013). More often, however, the lesion may be looked for directly with imaging in those patients with ophthalmological signs suspected for an orbital lesion. With few exceptions, the majority of orbital diseases are space-occupying lesions leading to characteristic clinical signs such as exophthalmos and orbital or periorbital pain (Featherstone and Heinrich, 2013). Orbital neoplasia should be differentiated from inflammatory conditions such as orbital abscess or orbital cellulitis. Orbital CT has been reported as a highly specific imaging test for differentiating inflammatory and neoplastic conditions in small animals (Boroffka et al., 2007; Wang et al., 2009; Armour et al., 2011; Lederer et al., 2015).

Given the wide variety of diseases that can be encountered, advanced imaging modalities play a major role in the diagnostic and staging assessment of the lesion, guiding therapeutic decisions and monitoring or follow-up of treatment (Penninck et al., 2001; Collins et al., 2013). CT, MRI (Boroffka and Voorhout, 1999; Armour et al., 2011; Lederer et al., 2015) and ultrasound (US) have been demonstrated to be accurate in evaluating orbital disease (Mason et al., 2001; Boroffka et al., 2007). In addition, US has been demonstrated to be particularly useful in guiding interventional procedures throughout the body both in veterinary and in human patients (Phillips and Schneider, 1981; Gupta et al., 1999; Constantin et al., 2010; Orlandi et al., 2013; Spiess and Pot, 2013). However, imaging alone is not sufficient for a definitive diagnosis (Boroffka and Voorhout, 1999; Boroffka et al., 2007). To determine the nature of the mass and choose an appropriate treatment, pathological investigations remain necessary (Hendrix and Gelatt, 2000; Attali-Soussay et al., 2001). Invasive diagnostic modalities in orbital neoplasia include excisional and incisional biopsy (open biopsy). While these methods provide sufficient histological tissue, they require high morbidity surgical intervention (Slatter and Abdelbaki, 1979; Gilger et al., 1994; Boston, 2010; Hakannsson and Hakannsson, 2010; Gelatt and Withley, 2011; Spiess and Pot, 2013). In contrast, fine needle aspiration biopsy is effective and sometimes may be acceptable in ocular oncology (Tani et al., 2006; Agrawi et al., 2013; Nair and Sankar, 2014). Imaging-guided core needle biopsy is often performed in oncology, and unlike fine needle aspiration biopsy, it can provide sufficient tissue sample for histology (Ballo and Sneige, 1996; Yarovoy et al., 2013). To be effective, an imaging-guided core needle biopsy technique requires precise localization and documentation of the needle inside the target lesion, especially in cases of deep retrobulbar lesions.

To date, few articles in veterinary literature describe a US-CT multimodality approach for orbital mass sampling for morphologic examination (LeCouteur et al., 1982; Boroffka and Voorhout, 1999; Boroffka et al., 2007; Lederer et al., 2015). In this study, we investigate the feasibility and accuracy of imaging-guided core needle biopsy in a population of dogs with orbital masses, using a US-CT combined system and different biopsy approaches.

Material and Methods

Animals

Subjects for this prospective feasibility study were enrolled from dogs referred to the ophthalmology service of the San Marco Veterinary Clinic during a 2-year period, from April 2012 through April 2014. Dogs were included in the study based on a presumptive clinical and imaging diagnosis of orbital neoplasia in at least one orbit.

Ophthalmic examination

Each patient received physical and complete ophthalmic examinations. All the ophthalmic examinations were performed by the same ophthalmologist (AC). Complete ophthalmic examination included neuro-ophthalmic examination, slit-lamp biomicroscopy (SL-15, Kowa Company Ltd, Tokyo, Japan), and indirect ophthalmoscopy (Heine Omega 500 and Heine 30D lens; Heine Optotechnik Inc, Herrsching, Germany). Schirmer tear test I (Schirmer Tear Test, Schering-Plough Animal Health, Union, NJ), retention of corneal sodium fluorescin dye (HS Haag-Streit International fluorescein, Switzerland) and intraocular pressure estimation (TonoPen Vet, Reichert Inc., Depew, NY) were performed.

The orbital mass was suspected during ophthalmic examination and confirmation was obtained by orbital ultrasound. To further characterize the mass, staging, and therapeutic planning, all dogs underwent 16-multidetector-row CT (16-MDCT, Lightspeed 16, GE Healthcare, Milan, Italy) or 128-dual source CT (SOMATOM Definition Flash, Siemens Healthcare, Forchheim, Germany). Owner consent allowed sedation and anesthesia for CT and CT-US combined biopsy procedures. Complete hemato-biochemical work-up (complete blood count, biochemical profile, serum protein electrophoresis, and coagulation tests), and urinalysis were performed for all patients prior to the procedures.

MDCT scanning protocol

Food and water were withheld from dogs overnight prior to CT procedures. A 14–16 GA intravenous catheter was placed in the right or left cephalic vein for fluid administration throughout the anaesthetic period. All patients were premedicated using methadone (0.2 mg/kg IM; Semfortan, Dechra Pharmaceuticals) and dexmedetomidine (2 mg/kg IM; Dexdomitor, Orino Pharma). General anesthesia was inducted with propofol (5 mg/kg IV; Vetofol, Esteve), and mantained with isoflurane (IsoFlo; Halocarbon Laboratories) in oxygen. Multidetector CT scans of the head were obtained with patient in sternal recumbency on the CT table with open mouth. Acquisition parameters were as follow: helical modality, detector configuration 16x0.625, pitch 0.562:1, and 0.7 s gantry rotation. Dose parameters were 120 kVp and 210 mAs. Images were reconstructed using both bone and standard algorithm (non-enhancing–non-smoothing reconstruction algorithm) with 512x512 matrix size and 50% overlap section thickness. Non-contrast and contrast scans were always obtained. For enhanced scans, iodixanol (320 mg I/mL), an iodinated, non-ionic, iso-osmolar contrast medium, was injected at 37°C into a cephalic vein (640 mg I/kg) through the intravenous catheter. A uniphasic injection (3–5 mL/s) of the contrast medium was made, followed by a saline flush at same injection rate via a dual-syringe injector system (Medrad, Stellant CT Injection System). Multidetector CT data were reviewed directly at the CT-console (GB). Multiplanar reformation (MPR) post-processing techniques of both unenhanced and enhanced series were used to analyse site, shape, and appearance of the mass. Based on previously established imaging criteria (Boroffka et al., 2007; Lederer et al., 2015), orbital masses showing CT characteristics consistent with abscess or post-traumatic orbital hematoma were not sampled by tru-cut and instead excluded from this study.

Technique, safety and diagnostic assessment of orbital biopsies

The safest biopsy approach was based on the topography of the mass, as seen on orthogonal and multi-oblique CT-planes (Fig. 1). Care was taken to preserve neurovascular structures and regional nerves, in order to avoid fluid-suprafluid areas of the mass, interpretable as necrotic or hemorrhagic in nature. The cutting-needle US-guided procedure was performed immediately after the CT scan with the patient still under general anesthesia on the CT exam table. All biopsies were performed with use of a real time US system (Logiq C5 Premium, GE Healthcare, Milan, Italy) with a 10 or 12-Mhz transducer. US guidance was obtained using either a linear or mini-convex probe according to the lesion location. Based on CT characteristics, one of the following three approaches was performed: trans-orbital, trans-conjunctival or trans-masseteric (Fig. 2). The path of the needle was monitored by means of continuous US visualization. By

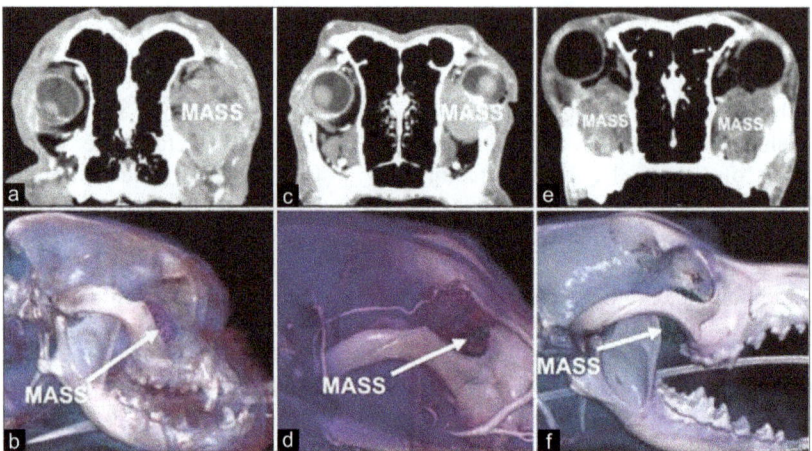

Fig. 1. Images from MDCT examinations of the skull of three different dogs with orbital masses. (a and b) Transverse and 3D volume rendered (right lateral view of the skull) images of a Boxer (case 4) having a sarcoma in the left orbit, postero-inferior to the globe. (c and d) are transverse and right lateral views of 3D volumes rendered images respectively in an American Cocker Spaniel (case 11) with a left-sided orbital rhabdomyosarcoma located anterior to the globe. (e and f) are transverse and right-lateral 3D volume rendered images of a Border Collie (case 3) with bilateral orbital masses located postero-ventrally the eyeballs (B-cell lymphoma).

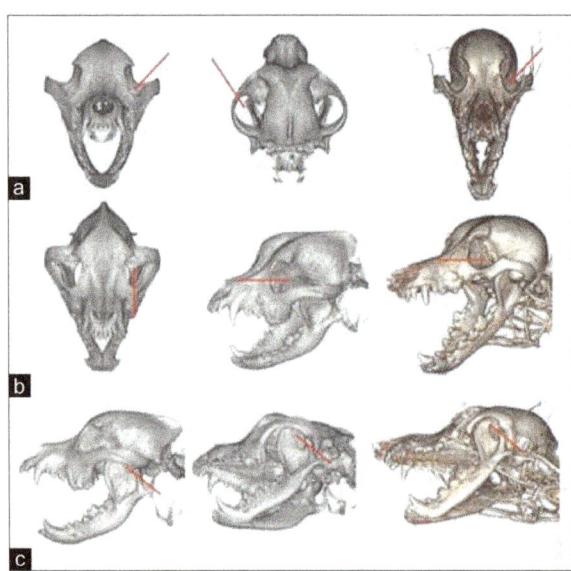

Fig. 2. (a) Trans-orbital approach to the posterior orbital space (supero and infero-lateral). With the patient in sternal recumbency, the biopsy needle is inserted just dorsal to the zygomatic arch and guided in a 45° oblique ventral direction. (b) Trans-conjunctival approach to the anterior orbital space (ventro-lateral and medial). With the patient in sternal recumbency, the biopsy needle is placed on the edge of the lacrimal bone. (c) Trans-masseteric approach to the posterior orbital space and to its floor. With the patient in lateral recumbency with open mouth, the biopsy needle is positioned in the space between the mandibular coronoid process and the zygomatic temporal process.

using an aseptic technique, all the masses were sampled with an automatic high-speed core biopsy system (Bard MagnumBiopsy System, Bard Peripheral Vascular, Inc., Tempe, AZ) with sterile disposable needle (14G, 16G), and a depth of penetration ranging from 15 to 22 mm. An adequate sterile field around the affected eye was set and, if necessary, a 2 mm skin incision was made to facilitate the core needle insertion. The needle was inserted into the orbit slowly during puncture while controlling the resistance and observing the eye globe condition. The orbital mass was punctured one time. After the procedure, the puncture site was manually compressed for 2-5 minutes and a compressive bandage and ice were applied over the relevant eye when needed. All the patients were kept under observation for 1 hour, an Elizabethan collar prevented self-trauma at the biopsy site. Carprofen was given the first 24 hours post procedure (2 mg\Kg IV; Rimadyl, Pfizer Animal Health) to address pain and inflammation.

Methods that were used for determining safety of the procedure included: 1) biopsy site monitoring by CT scan immediately after the procedure 2) orbital US monitoring 1 and 2 hours, post-biopsy and prior to the discharge. 3) a 3 and 6-day clinical recheck.

Presence or absence of complications related to the biopsy procedure were recorded each time stated 1-3.

To assess the diagnostic performance of the tru-cut samples, an excisional biopsy was obtained from 11/17 patients during surgical procedures and 6/17 patients from necropsy representing the reference standard. The main reason for open biopsy after imaging-guided core needle biopsy was the surgical treatment. In case of necropsy, written informed consent was obtained from each owner. All the biopsy specimens obtained were fixed in 10% buffered isotonic formalin dehydratated with automated histological processor (Shandon Excelsior ES, Thermo Scientific, Fremont, CA) and paraffin embedded. Four micrometer-thick microtomic sections were then obtained and hematoxylin eosin stained for histologic evaluation (Fig. 3).

Immunohistochemistry (IHC)

IHC was performed on lymphomas and rhabdomyosarcoma using ABC peroxidase method. Four micrometer-thick sections were rehydratated and endogenous peroxidase blocking were performed with immersing sections in H2O2-PBS solution for 45 minutes. Primary antibodies were applied for 18 hours at 4°C as reported in Table 1. Secondary biotilated antibody (Vector®) was applied for 30 minutes at room temperature (RT). ABC complex (Vector®) was then applied for 30 minutes at RT. Signal was stained with IMMPACT Nova RED (Vector SK-4805) and sections were counterstained with hematoxylin, dehydratated in serial alcohol and xylene, then coverslide was mounted.

Results

Seventeen dogs (7 Mongrels, 1 Dobermann, 1 Rottweiler, 1 Border Collie, 1 Boxer, 1 Golden Retriever, 1 Dachshund, 1 American Cocker Spaniel, 1 Belgian Shepherd, 1 Miniature Poodle, 1 German Shepherd), 9 males and 8 females met the inclusion criteria and were included in the study. The median age was 8.1 years (range from 1.1 to 13.8 years) and the median body weight was 17.7 kg (ranging from 6 to 48 kg) (Table 2). Eleven/17 dogs presented with unilateral orbital neoplasia (4 right eye, 7 left eye) and in 6/17 dogs the orbital disease was bilateral. A total of 23 orbital masses, having a maximum diameter between 25 and 38.5 mm were studied. Where bilateral both masses were sampled.

All the 23 core biopsies yielded adequate specimens for histologic analysis. Based on pathology results, 11 masses (monolateral) underwent to surgery and an excisional biopsy was obtained during the procedure. Twelve masses (bilateral) were not treated, due to poor prognosis. In such cases, upon owner request, the dogs were euthanatized and necropsy was performed. In all the tru-cut biopsies the histologic analysis concurred with the larger sample obtained through surgical

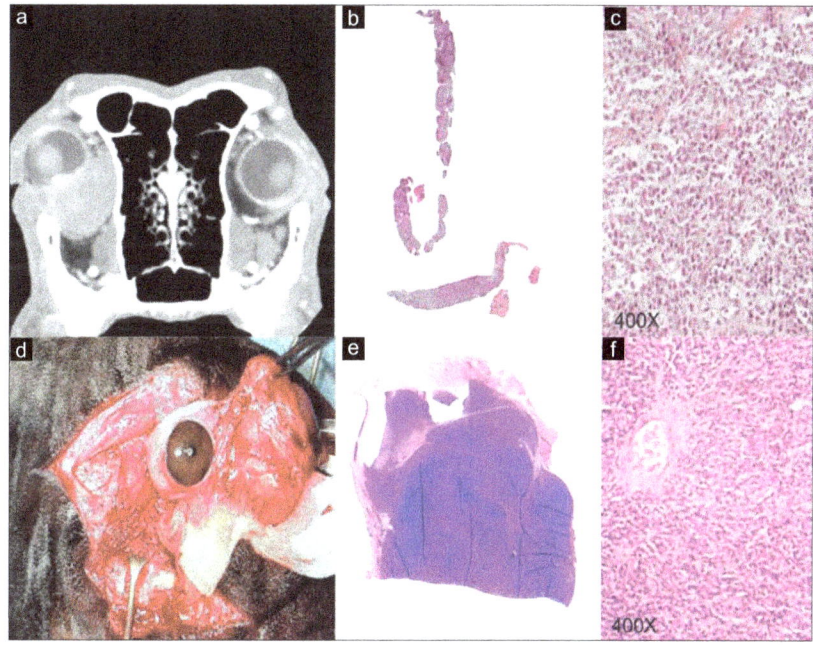

Fig. 3. Case 1. Dobermann. Anaplastic high grade STS in the right orbit anterior to the globe. (a) Transverse image from MDCT examination of the skull. (b and c) Tru-cut sample: subgross (b) and high magnification (c) of the histologically processed sample. (d) Intraoperative image of the same patient. (e and f) Surgical excisional biopsy: subgross (e) and high magnification (f) of the histologically processed sample. Note: similar quality in both sampling.

Table 1. IHC: Antibodies, source, dilution and antigen retrival.

Primary antibody	Source	Clone	Dilution	Antigen retrival
Anti CD3	Dako	Policlonal	1:1000	Pepsin Solution Digest-All 3 (Novex) 10 min, 37°C
Anti CD20	Thermo Scientific	Policlonal	1:1000	None
Anti Vimentin	Dako	V9	1:1000	High Temperature pH 6.0 20 min, 95°C
Anti Actin	Dako	HHF35	1:1000	High Temperature pH 6.0 20 min, 95°C
Anti Desmin	Dako	D33	1:200	High Temperature pH 6.0 20 min, 95°C
Anti Myoglobin	Dako	Policlonal	1:200	High Temperature pH 6.0 20 min, 95°C

Table 2. Signalment and histological diagnosis.

Case	Sex	Age (years)	Breed	Eye	Diagnosis
1	M	3	Dobermann	OD	Anaplastic high grade STS
2	MN	10	Rottweiler	OS	Metastatic melanoma
3	M	1.5	Border Collie	OU	B-cell lymphoma
4	MN	8	Boxer	OS	Anaplastic high grade STS
5	FS	13.3	Dachshund	OS	MTB
6	MN	5.5	Mongrel	OU	B-cell lymphoma
7	F	9.6	Golden Retriever	OD	Anaplastic high grade STS
8	FS	13.8	Mongrel	OS	Fibrosarcoma
9	FS	10	Mongrel	OU	B-cell lymphoma
10	MN	8.3	Mongrel	OD	Fibrosarcoma
11	M	1.1	American Cocker Spaniel	OS	Rhabdomyosarcoma
12	FS	11	Belgian Shepherd	OD	SCC
13	M	4.6	Mongrel	OU	Fibrosarcoma
14	F	7.5	Miniature Poodle	OS	Fibrosarcoma
15	M	9	German Shepherd	OS	MTB
16	FS	7.5	Mongrel	OU	B-cell lymphoma
17	FS	12	Mongrel	OU	B-cell lymphoma

F: Intact female, M: Intact male, SF: Spayed female, NM: Neutered male, OD: Right eye, OS: Left eye, OU: Both eyes, MTB: Multilobular tumor of bone, SCC: Squamous cell carcinoma, STS: Soft tissue sarcoma

excisional biopsy or during necropsy.

Twenty-three biopsies revealed a malignant process: anaplastic high grade soft tissue sarcoma ($n = 3$), fibrosarcoma ($n = 5$), rhabdomyosarcoma ($n = 1$), B-cell lymphoma ($n = 10$), metastatic melanoma ($n = 1$), squamous cell carcinoma ($n = 1$), multilobular tumor of bones ($n = 2$). One out of 17 patients (5.88%) developed a localized hematoma at the puncture site that subsided spontaneously. No other early or later complications occurred.

Discussion

Surgical biopsy of space-occupying lesions of the orbit, particularly of those retrobulbar in location, presents substantial technical difficulties (Attaly-Soussay et al., 2001; Spiess and Pot, 2013). Papers reporting the use of CT guidance to perform biopsy of orbital masses are limited (Hendrix and Gelatt, 2000; Boroffka et al., 2007; Héran et al., 2014). Boroffka et al. (2007) made a comparison between helical CT and US guidance in 43

dogs affected by neoplastic and non-neoplastic orbital masses, reporting similar diagnostic value for both imaging techniques (Boroffka et al., 2007). A major disadvantage of CT over ultrasound was the lack or real-time visualisation during needle placement and biopsy. Our results demonstrated that imaging-guided core needle biopsy combining the two imaging modalities is a feasible, safe and effective procedure to perform histological biopsies in such a critical area of the body like the orbit. The procedure to obtain tissue is simple, minimally invasive and generally well tolerated by the patient. In contrast to fine needle aspiration biopsy, which is cytological, the aim of imaging-guided core needle biopsy is to obtain adequate tissue sample for histological diagnosis. Core needle biopsies are widely used in many oncological subspecialties as an effective alternative to open biopsy (Ortiz et al., 1996; Boland et al., 2013; Finger, 2014; Héran et al., 2014). Many recent studies, in human literature, report advantages of core biopsy over fine needle aspiration biopsy as oncological diagnostic procedure (Woodcock and Morgan, 1998; Orlandi et al., 2013). The automated-loaded tru-cut biopsy needles used in our study allowed tissue samples to be taken without tissue damage, because of a rapid cutting action and narrow diameter (14 and 16 gauge). The needle sizes used for the study resulted to be adequate for tissue sampling and safe for the orbital structures at the same time.

We had no cases of eye globe, optic nerve or orbital wall damage of clinical significance.

To prevent major complications, this procedure must be carefully planned by means of high quality CT data. An experienced ophthalmologist-radiologist team should perform the procedure under constant US visual control. This increases the accuracy and safety of the bioptic procedure. In our series of orbital neoplasia, we reported no inadequate specimens and final diagnosis was reached by the pathologist in 100% of cases. Small subcutaneous haematoma experienced in one dog resolved spontaneously in less than 6 days. It is important to know, that retrobulbar haematoma could represent a major complication with potentially irreversible visual sequelae. However, prompt diagnosis and immediate pharmacological therapy may prevent such an occurrence. Needle-track tumor seeding after fine needle aspiration biopsy/core needle biopsy is another possible complication as with any other type of needle biopsy, although literature reports are controversial (Diaz et al., 1991; Nyland et al., 2002; Vignoli et al., 2007; Brenner and Gordon, 2011; Klopfleisch et al., 2011). In this small group of patients, we did not see any evidence of tumor spread or recurrence at the site of biopsy. Furthermore, only in one out of seventeen dogs developed a localized hematoma at puncture site that subsided spontaneously. Results from our study suggests that the tru-cut imaging guided biopsy technique is a safe procedure. However, studies with a larger population should be performed to delineate the risk of metastatic spread and potential complications using this technique. All lesions included in our series were of 25 mm or larger. Thus, feasibility and accuracy of such a procedure in smaller lesions are yet to be demonstrated. Our case series includes 23 biopsies revealed a malignant process: anaplastic high grade soft tissue sarcoma ($n = 3$), fibrosarcoma ($n = 5$), rhabdomyosarcoma ($n = 1$), B-cell lymphoma ($n = 10$), metastatic melanoma ($n = 1$), squamous cell carcinoma ($n = 1$), and multilobular tumor of bones ($n = 2$). All bilateral neoplasias were related to the same oncologic disease (fibrosarcoma and B-cell lymphoma). In all these cases upon owner request the dogs were euthanatized due to the advanced stage of the diseases and the poor prognosis.

In conclusion, semi-automated imaging-guided core needle biopsy of orbital masses is a useful diagnostic technique in dogs. It provides a sufficient amount of tissue for histopathological analysis. The complications reported in our experience are minor; this procedure can really reduce the number of open biopsies and can be a useful supplement or alternative to fine needle aspiration biopsy in selected cases.

Conflict of interest

The authors declare that there is no conflict of interest

References

Agrawi, P., Dey, P. and Lal, A. 2013. Fine-Needle Aspiration Cytology of orbital and Eyelid Lesions. Diagn. Cytopathol. 41, 1000-1011.

Armour, M.D., Broome, M., Dell'Anna, G., Blades, N.J. and Esson, D.W. 2011. A review of orbital and intracranial magnetic resonance imaging in 79 canine and 13 feline patients (2004-2010). Vet. Ophthalmol. 14, 215-226.

Attali-Soussay, K., Jegou, J.P. and Clerc, B. 2001. Retrobulbar tumors in dogs and cats: 25 cases. Vet. Ophthalmol. 4, 19-27.

Ballo, M.S. and Sneige, N. 1996. Can core needle biopsy replace fine-needle aspiration cytology in the diagnosis of palpable breast carcinoma: A comparative study of 124 women. Cancer 78, 773-777.

Boland, L., Gomes, E., Payen, G., Bouvy, B. and Poncet, C. 2013. Zygomatic salivary gland diseases in the dog: three cases diagnosed by MRI. J. Am. Anim. Hosp. Assoc. 49, 333-337.

Boroffka, S.A. and Voorhout, G. 1999. Direct and reconstructed multiplanar computed tomography of the orbits of healthy dogs. Am. J. Vet. Res. 60, 1500-1507.

Boroffka, S.A., Verbruggen, A.M., Grinwis, G.C.M., Voorhout, G. and Barthez, P.Y. 2007. Assessment of ultrasonography and computed tomography for the evaluation of unilateral orbital disease in dogs. J. Am. Vet. Med. Assoc. 230, 671-680.

Boston, S.E. 2010. Craniectomy and orbitectomy in dogs and cats. Can. Vet. J. 51, 537-540.

Brenner, R.J. and Gordon, L.M. 2011. Malignant seeding following percutaneous breast biopsy: documentation with comprehensive imaging and clinical implications. Breast J. 17, 651-656.

Collins, S.P., Matheson, J.S., Hamor, R.E., Mitchell, M.A., Labelle, A.L. and O'Brien, R.T. 2013. Comparison of the diagnostic quality of computed tomography images of normal ocular and orbital structures acquired with and without the use of general anesthesia in the cat. Vet. Ophthalmol. 16, 352-358.

Constantin, A., Brisson, M.L., Kwan, J. and Proulx, F. 2010. Percutaneous US-guided Renal Biopsy: A Retrospective Study Comparing the 16-gauge End-cut and 14-gauge Side-notch Needles. J. Vasc. Interv. Radiol. 21, 357-361.

Diaz, L.K., Wiley, E.L. and Venta, L.A. 1991. Are malignant cells displaced by large-gauge needle core biopsy of the breast?. Am. J. Roentgenol. 173, 1303-1313.

Featherstone, H.J. and Heinrich, C.L. 2013. Ophthalmic examination and diagnostics, part 1: the eye examination and diagnostic procedures. In Veterinary Ophthalmology, Eds., Gelatt K.N., Gilger, B.C. and Kern, T.J., MI: Wiley-Blackwell, pp: 540-541.

Finger, P.T. 2014. Minimally invasive anterior orbitotomy biopsy: finger's aspiration cutter technique (FACT). Eur. Ophthalmol. 22, 309-315.

Gelatt, K.N. and Withley, R.D. 2011. Surgery of the orbit. In Veterinary Ophthalmic Surgery, Eds., Gelatt, K.N. and Gelatt, J.P., MI: Elsevier, pp: 51-88.

Gilger, B.C., Withley, R.D. and McLaughlin, S.A. 1994. Modified lateral orbitotomy for removal of orbital neoplasms in two dogs. Vet. Surg. 23, 53-58.

Gupta, S., Sood, B., Gulati, M., Takhtani, D., Bapuraj, R., Khandelwal, N., Singh, U., Rajwanshi, A., Gupta, S. and Suri, S. 1999. Orbital mass lesions: US-guided fine-needle aspiration biopsy-experience in 37 patients. Radiol. 213, 568-572.

Hakannsson, N.W. and Hakannsson, B.W. 2010. Transfrontal orbitotomy in the dog: an adaptable three-step approach to the orbit. Vet. Ophthalmol. 13, 377-383.

Hendrix, D.V. and Gelatt, K.N. 2000. Diagnosis, treatment and outcome of orbital neoplasia in dogs: a retrospective study of 44 cases. J. Small. Anim. Pract. 41, 105-108.

Héran, F., Bergès, O., Blustajn, J., Boucenna, M., Charbonneau, F., Koskas, F., Lafitte, F., Nau, E., Roux, P., Sadik, J.C., Savatovsky, J. and

Williams, M. 2014. Tumor pathology of the orbit. Diagn. Interv. Imaging 95, 933-944.

Kato, Y., Notake, H., Kimura, J., Murakami, M., Hirata, A., Saki, H. and Yanai, T. 2012. Orbital embryonal rhabdomyosarcoma with metastasis in a young dog. J. Comp. Pathol. 147, 191-194.

Klopfleisch, R., Sperling, C., Kershaw, O. and Gruber, A.D. 2011. Does the taking of biopsies affect the metastatic potential of tumours? A systematic review of reports on veterinary and human cases and animal models. Vet. J. 190, 31-42.

LeCouteur, R.A., Fike, J.R., Scagliotti, R.H. and Cann, C.E. 1982. Computed tomography of orbital tumors in the dog. J. Am. Vet. Med. Assoc. 180, 910-913.

Lederer, K., Ludewig, E., Hechinger, H., Parry, A.T., Lamb, C.R. and Kneissl, S. 2015. Differentiation between inflammatory and neoplastic orbital conditions based on computed tomographic signs. Vet. Ophthalmol. 18, 271-275.

Mason, D.R., Lamb, C.R. and McLellan, G.J. 2001. Ultrasonographic findings in 50 dogs with retrobulbar disease. J. Am. Anim. Hosp. Assoc. 37, 557-562.

Nair, L.K. and Sankar, S. 2014. Role of fine needle aspiration cytology in the diagnosis of orbital masses: a study of 41 cases. J. Cytol. 31, 87-90.

Nyland, T.G., Wallack, S.T. and Wisner, E.R. 2002. Needle-tract implantation following US-guided fine-needle aspiration biopsy of transitional cell carcinoma of the bladder, urethra, and prostate. Vet. Radiol. Ultrasound 43, 50-53.

Orlandi, D., Sconfienza, L.M., Lacelli, F., Bertolotto, M., Sola, S., Mauri, G., Savarino, E. and Serafini, G. 2013. Ultrasound-guided core-needle biopsy of extra-ocular orbital lesions. Europ. Radiol. 23, 1919-1924.

Ortiz, O., Bastug, D. and Ellis, B. 1996. CT-Guided Percutaneous Lateral Suprazygomatic Approach for Posterior Orbital Wall Biopsy. Skull Base Surg. 6, 249-251.

Penninck, D., Daniel, G.B., Brawer, R. and Tidwell, A.S. 2001. Cross-sectional imaging techniques in veterinary ophthalmology. Clin. Tech. Small Anim. Pract.16, 22-39.

Phillips, G. and Schneider, M. 1981. Ultrasonically guided percutaneous fine needle aspiration biopsy of solid masses. Cardiovasc. Intervent. Radiol. 4, 33-38.

Slatter, D.H. and Abdelbaki, Y. 1979. Lateral orbitotomy by zygomatic arch resection in the dog. J. Am. Vet. Med. Assoc. 175, 1179-1182.

Spiess, B.M. and Pot, S.A. 2013. Diseases and surgery of the canine orbit. In Veterinary Ophthalmology, Eds., Gelatt K.N., Gilger, B.C. and Kern, T.J., MI: Wiley-Blackwell, pp: 793-831.

Tani, E., Seregard, S., Rupp, G., Soderlind, V. and Skoog, L. 2006. Fine-needle aspiration cytology and immunocytochemistry of orbital masses. Diagn. Cytopathol. 34, 1-5.

Van der Woerdt, A. 2008. Orbital inflammatory disease and pseudotumor in dogs and cats. Vet. Clin. North. Am. Small Anim. Pract. 38, 389-401.

Vignoli, M., Rossi, F., Chierici, C., Terragni, R., De Lorenzi, D., Stanga, M. and Olivero, D. 2007. Needle tract implantation after fine needle aspiration biopsy (FNAB) of transitional cell carcinoma of the urinary bladder and adenocarcinoma of the lung. Schweiz Arch. Tierheilkd. 149, 314-318.

Wang, A.L., Ledbetter, E.C. and Kern, T.J. 2009. Orbital abscess bacterial isolates and in vitro antimicrobial susceptibility patterns in dogs and cats. Vet. Ophthalmol. 12, 91-96.

Woodcock, M.B. and Morgan, M.R.C. 1998. Ultrasound-guided Tru-cut biopsy of the breast. Ann. R. Coll. Surg. Engl. 80, 253-256.

Yarovoy, A., Bulgakova, E.S., Shatskikh, A.V., Uzunyan, D.G., Kleyankina, S.S. and Golubeva, O.V. 2013. CORE needle biopsy of orbital tumors. Graefe's Arch. Clin. Exp. Ophthalmol. 251, 2057-2061.

3

Metastatic anal sac carcinoma with hypercalcaemia and associated hypertrophic osteopathy in a dog

A. Giuliano*, R. Salgüero and J. Dobson

Queen's Veterinary School Hospital, University of Cambridge, Madingley Road, Cambridge, CB3 0ES, United Kingdom

Abstract

A seven-year-old male neutered Irish setter was treated for a metastatic anal sac adenocarcinoma (ASAC) and hypercalcaemia by complete surgical excision of the primary tumour and partial excision of the sublumbar lymph nodes. Further enlargement of the sublumbar lymph nodes was linked to recurrent hypercalcaemia 3 months after surgical treatment. Medical treatment with Toceranib and Clodronate showed modest results in the treatment of the tumour and the hypercalcaemia. Radiotherapy of the sublumbar lymph nodes and later concurrent carboplatin chemotherapy resulted in partial tumour remission with marked reduction in size of the lymph nodes and normalization of the calcaemia. Unfortunately, concurrently with subsequent relapse of the hypercalaemia, the dog developed hypertrophic osteopathy (HO) and lumbar spinal metastasis and the dog was euthanized. To the authors' knowledge, this is the second case of metastatic apocrine gland carcinoma of the anal sac associated with HO and the first case that describe the development of HO late in the stage of the disease.

Keywords: Anal sac carcinoma, Hypercalcaemia, Hypertrophic osteopathy.

Introduction

Anal sac carcinoma is a relatively uncommon neoplasia in dogs that originates from the apocrine glands of the anal sac (Withrow, 2001). Anal sac carcinoma is an aggressive tumour with a tendency to metastasise to sublumbar lymph node and later to liver and lungs. Paraneoplastic hypercalcaemia is relatively common occurring in 25-53% of cases, often complicating the clinical management of the affected patients (Ross *et al.*, 1991; Bennett *et al.*, 2002; Williams *et al.*, 2003).

Hypertrophic osteopathy (HO) is characterized by the deposition of periosteal new bone mainly in the distal appendicular skeleton. In people, HO is mainly associated with pulmonary diseases, usually cancer (Carroll and Doyle, 1974). In dogs, HO has been described in both neoplastic and non-neoplastic conditions affecting mainly the thoracic cavity. However it has also been described in association with tumours of the bladder, liver esophagus and non-neoplastic conditions (Mather and Low, 1953; Brodey, 1971; Halliwell and Ackerman, 1974; Hesselink and van den Tweel, 1990; Wylie *et al.*, 1993; Watrous and Blumenfeld, 2002; Makungu *et al.*, 2007; Lee *et al.*, 2012; Salyusarenko *et al.*, 2013; Withers *et al.*, 2013). In a recent review of HO in dogs it was found that all the patients had pulmonary nodules in the lungs, two were primary pulmonary tumours and 28 were metastasis. The most common histological type of metastatic tumour was osteosarcoma, but other tumour types were present in particular; bladder transitional cell carcinoma, prostatic carcinoma, renal carcinoma, renal adenocarcinoma with osteosarcomatous differentiation, chondrosarcoma, fibrosarcoma and leiomyosarcoma (Withers *et al.*, 2013).

The pathogenesis of HO is not completely understood; but was thought to be an increase in the peripheral vascular supply to the periosteum due to stimulation of nerve fibers that innervate vascular tissue directly related to the pharyngeal and vagus nerves (Carroll and Doyle, 1974). More recently, it has been proposed that the release of vascular endothelial growth factor (VEGF) and platelet-derived growth factor (PDGF) from platelets, due to abnormal platelet circulation could be involved in HO (Dickinson and Martin, 1987; Martinez-Lavin, 2007).

Case Details

A seven-year-old male neutered Irish setter was presented for severe polyuria and polydipsia and the suspicion of an anal sac tumour on the left side. Physical examination revealed a mass in the left anal gland. Haematology was unremarkable and biochemistry revealed moderate increase in total calcium, 3.94 mmol/L (ref range 2.15-2.72). The rest of the biochemistry was unremarkable.

Thoracic radiographs were performed which revealed two small pulmonary nodules (1 and 0.66 cm in size) that were suspicious of metastatic spread. Abdominal radiographs showed a marked sublumbar soft tissue opacity. Abdominal ultrasound revealed marked left sublumbar (most likely medial iliac) lymphadenopathy. Haematology was unremarkable and biochemistry

*Corresponding Author: Antonio Giuliano. Queen's Veterinary School Hospital, University of Cambridge, Madingley Road, Cambridge, CB3 0ES, United Kingdom. Email: *ag847@cam.ac.uk*

showed severe hypercalcaemia with an ionised calcium of 2.08 mmol/L (reference range, 1.18-1.4) with no other significant abnormalities detected. Fine needle aspirate of the left anal sac mass was not performed in view of the very typical presentation for an anal sac tumour. After saline (0.9%) fluid therapy at four times maintenance rate, oral clodronate 400 mg and a single subcutaneous injection of 6 mg dexamethasone, the hypercalcaemia almost resolved, (ionized calcium= 1.48mmol/L) and surgery was performed. The left anal sac mass and ipsilateral medial iliac lymph node were removed resulting in post-operative normocalcaemia. Histopathology of the mass confirmed anal sac carcinoma with metastatic spread to the lymph node. The decision was made to monitor the patient and re-examine in the following three months. In the meantime, total calcium levels were checked monthly by the referring veterinary surgeon.

Three months after surgery, the dog presented with polyuria and polydipsia. An abdominal ultrasound confirmed the recurrence of metastatic carcinoma with marked sublumbar lymphadenopathy. Ionised calcium was elevated again. Treatment with toceranib 2.5 mg/kg every other day and clodronate 11 mg/kg twice a day was initiated. The dog achieved partial remission with reduction in size of the sublumbar lymph nodes and normocalcaemia. Toceranib was well tolerated with only mild neutropenia as side effect, which was controlled by reducing the dose of toceranib to every third day.

Unfortunately, the patient developed hypercalcaemia again after two months and thoracic and abdominal radiographs showed marked enlargement of the sublumbar lymph nodes. The two pulmonary nodules that were seen in previous examination were similar in size (Fig. 1a). Abdominal ultrasound revealed marked enlargement of the sublumbar lymph nodes, the rest of the abdomen was unremarkable and the dog had no other lymphadenopathy to suggest an alternative diagnosis of lymphoma. After discussion with the owner the decision was made to irradiate the sublumbar lymph nodes as a palliative treatment in the attempt to reduce hypercalcaemia and to restore a good quality of life. Two coarse fractions of 800 centigrays (cGys) radiation were administered 7 days apart via a parallel opposed beam configuration (400 cGys from right and left portals). Clodronate treatment was continued and toceranib was stopped. The radiotherapy resulted in reduction in size of the sublumbar lymph nodes and normocalcaemia. Hypercalcaemia was noticed again one month later in combination with further enlargement of the sublumbar lymph nodes. Another two fractions of radiotherapy were administered in combination with carboplatin 300 mg/m² every three weeks. The chemo- and radiotherapy resulted again in reduction in size of the sublumbar lymph nodes and

restoration of normocalcaemia without clodronate treatment.

Two months later, the patient again developed hypercalcaemia with severe increase in size of the sublumbar lymph nodes. On physical examination, the dog was lame in all four limbs and reluctant to stand up. All four distal limbs were swollen and painful on palpation. Thoracic and abdominal radiographs, abdominal ultrasound and radiographs of the appendicular long bones were performed. Previous pulmonary nodules had mildly increased in size to 2 and 1.6 cm and a few small new nodules were present as well (Fig. 1b). Radiographs and ultrasound of the caudal abdomen revealed marked sublumbar lymphadenopathy and local invasion of the lumbar vertebrae. No other abdominal abnormalities were found (Fig. 2a and b). Radiographs of the distal long bones had a palisading periosteal reaction, with the typical appearance of HO (Fig. 3a and b). Due to the extension, the lack of control of the disease and the development of HO, the patient was euthanized.

Discussion

In many ways this case is typical of anal sac adenocarcinoma (ASAC), a tumour that classically metastasizes early in the course of the disease with 79% of cases having sublumbar metastases at time of presentation and frequently associated with paraneoplastic hypercalcaemia in 25-53% of cases (Ross et al., 1991; Bennett et al., 2002; Williams et al., 2003). The unusual feature of this case is the development of HO, relatively late in the course of the disease, without a significant radiographically detectable progression of the existing pulmonary pathology. The pulmonary nodules were initially assumed to be metastases from the ASAC, as the dog had no history or evidence of concurrent malignant disease. The slow progression of the nodules were considered to be consistent with the documented behaviour of this ASAC (Jeffery et al., 2000; Polton and Brearley, 2007) but a post mortem examination was not performed to confirm this to be the case.

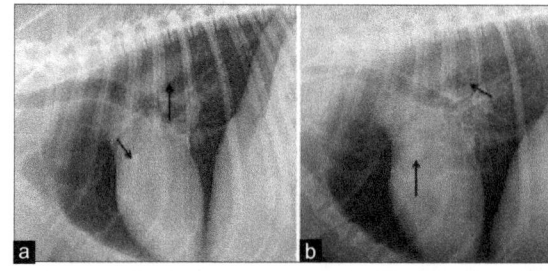

Fig. 1. Lateral chest radiographs. (a) Shows two small rounded soft tissue opacities in the lung fields (black arrows) at first presentation. (b) Shows a more diffuse nodular interstitial pattern, with nodules of different sizes consistent with metastases at third presentation. Increased in size of nodules seen in image a (black arrow).

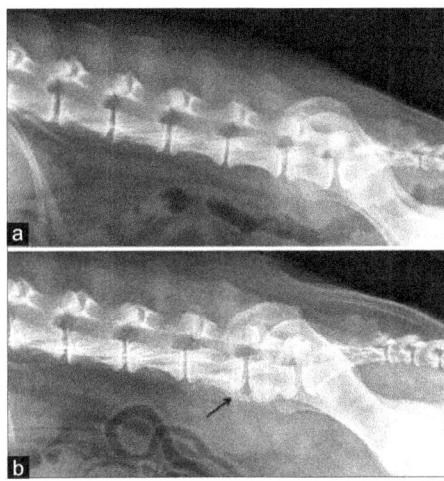

Fig. 2. Caudal abdominal radiographs at first (a) and 3rd examination (b). (a) Soft tissue opacity ventral to lumbar vertebrae 6 and 7 displacing the colon ventrally consistent with moderate sublumbar lymph node enlargement. (b) Large multilobulated soft tissue opacity ventral to L6, L7, displacing the colon ventrally, and concurrent moth eaten lysis and new bone at L6 and L6-L7 (black arrow), consistent with lymph node and vertebral metastases.

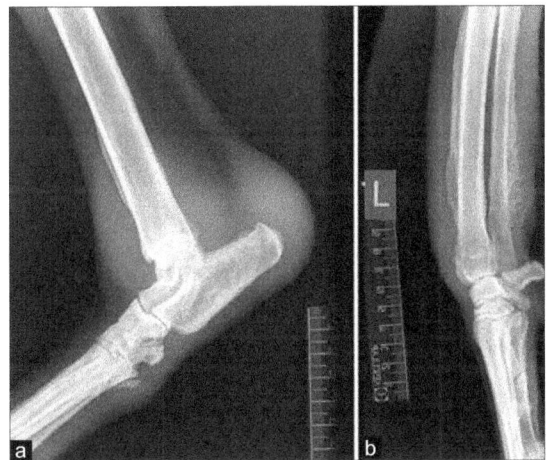

Fig. 3. (a) Medio-lateral view of the right hock shows marked soft tissue swelling, lamellar periosteal reaction on distal tibia, dorsal and plantar aspect of the tuber calcis and dorsally on the metatarsal bones. (b) Medio-lateral view of the left antebrachium shows marked soft tissue swelling, diffuse lamellar periosteal reaction on the cranial aspect of the radius and lamellar and palisading periosteal reaction on the distal ulna diaphysis.

The main challenge in the management of this case was the recurrence of the metastases in the sublumbar lymph nodes with a concomitant hypercalcaemia. Control of the tumour and the nodal metastases resulted in normalization of the calcaemia. Oral bisphosphonate (clodronate) was preferred to injectable biphosphonate in this case due to the good clinical condition of the dog and the resolution of the hypercalcaemia after tumour

control. Surgical resection is the treatment of choice for ASAC and as shown in this case, surgical resection of metastatic sublumbar nodes is possible and can restore normocalaemia. The value of adjunctive treatment is debatable with some patients achieving long term survival with only surgery (Hobson *et al.*, 2006). Post-operative RT may be used at primary site where completeness of excision is uncertain, although the proximity to anus can lead to potential complications. The value of chemotherapy in prevention and management of metastatic disease is less well defined, but treatment with both carboplatin and mitoxantrone have been reported (Polton and Brearley, 2007), as has melphalan (Emms, 2005). More recently, toceranib has been reported to achieve clinical benefit in 28/32 dogs with ASAC (London *et al.*, 2012).

HO has been described in numerous reports mainly associated with an extensive mass in the chest, or diffuse cancerous or non-cancerous pathology affecting the lungs; this is only the second report of HO in a dog with anal sac carcinoma (Hammond *et al.*, 2009).

This case is of interest due to the fact that the dog did not have extensive pulmonary pathology, or any respiratory signs. The two small nodules present on initial presentation did not cause initially any signs of HO and the few small new nodules visible on the last thoracic radiograph were considered unlikely to be the cause of the HO. The dog had also suffered from significant and recurrent sublumbar lymphadenopathy, during the course of his treatment, so this also seems unlikely to be the cause or trigger of HO. No other abdominal lesions were noted on ultrasound examination. It has been reported that there is no consistent radiografhical finding regarding location, number and size of the pulmonary nodules (Withers *et al.*, 2013). Therefore, it was reasonable to think that a mild increase in number and size of the nodules in the chest would not be, although possible, a reasonable explanation of the HO. It is interesting to note that the HO developed three months after toceranib was stopped. This drug is a selective inhibitor of VEGF and PDGF receptors. Recent publications have proposed a connection between increases these two growth factors in the periosteum and HO (Dickinson and Martin, 1987; Martinez-Lavin, 2007). The administration of toceranib could have bound the VEGF and PDGF receptors in this case, causing a delay in the appearance of the HO which only became evident after withdrawal of the drug.

In conclusion, this is the second reported case of metastatic apocrine gland carcinoma of the anal sac associated with HO and unusually describe the development of HO very late in the stage of the disease.

References

Bennett, P.F., DeNicola, D.B., Bonney, P., Glickman, N.W. and Knapp, D.W. 2002. Canine anal sac adenocarcinomas: Clinical presentation and response to therapy. J. Vet. Intern. Med. 16, 100-104.

Brodey, R. 1971. Hypertrophic osteoarthropathy in the dog: A clinicopathologic study of 60 cases. J. Am. Vet. Med. Assoc. 159, 1242.

Carroll, K.B., and Doyle, L. 1974. A common factor in hypertrophic osteoarthropathy. Thorax. 29(2), 262-264.

Dickinson, C.J. and Martin, J.F. 1987. Megakaryocytes and platelet clumps as the cause of finger clubbing. Lancet. 2, 1434-1435.

Emms, S.G. 2005. Anal sac tumours of the dog and their response to cytoreductive surgery and chemotherapy. Aust. Vet. J. 83, 340-343.

Halliwell, W.H. and Ackerman, N. 1974. Botryoid rhabdomyosarcoma of the urinary bladder and hyperosteoarthropathy in a young dog. J. Am. Vet. Med. Assoc. 165, 911-913.

Hammond, T.N., Turek, M.M. and Regan, J. 2009. What is your diagnosis? Metastatic anal sac adenocarcinoma with paraneoplastic hypertrophic osteopathy. J. Am. Vet. Med. Assoc. 235(3), 267-268.

Hesselink, J.W. and van den Tweel, J.G. 1990. Hypertrophicosteopathy in a dog with a chronic lung abscess. J. Am. Vet. Med. Assoc. 196, 760-762.

Hobson, H.P., Brown, M.R. and Rogers, K.S. 2006. Surgery of Metastatic Anal Sac Adenocarcinoma in Five Dogs. Vet. Surg. 35, 267-270.

Jeffery, N., Phillips, S.M. and Brearley, M.J. 2000. Surgical management of metastases from anal sac apocrine gland adenocarcinoma of dogs. J. Small Anim. Pract. 41, 390.

Lee, J.H., Lee, J.H., Yoon, H.Y., Kim, N.H., Sur, J.H. and Jeong, S.W. 2012. Hypertrophic osteopathy associated with pulmonary adenosquamous carcinoma in a dog. J. Vet. Med. Sci. 74(5), 667-672.

London, C., Mathie, T., Stingle, N., Clifford, C., Haney, S., Klein, M.K., Beaver, L., Vickery, K., Vail, D.M., Hershey, B., Ettinger, S., Vaughan, A., Alvarez, F., Hillman, L., Kiselow, M., Thamm, D., Higginbotham, M.L., Gauthier, M., Krick, E., Phillips, B., Ladue, T., Jones, P., Bryan, J., Gill, V., Novosad, A., Fulton, L., Carreras, J., McNeill, C., Henry, C. and Gillings, S. 2012. Preliminary evidence for biologic

activity of toceranib phosphate (Palladia (®)) in solid tumours. Vet. Comp. Oncol. 10(3), 194-205.

Makungu, M., Malago, J., Muhairwa, A.P., Mpanduji, D.G. and Mgasa, M.N. 2007. Hypertrophic osteopathy secondary to esophageal foreign body in a dog - a case report. Vet. Arhiv. 77, 463-467.

Martinez-Lavin, M. 2007. Exploring the cause of the most ancient clinical sign of medicine: Finger clubbing. Semin. Arthritis Rheum. 36, 380-385.

Mather, G. and Low, D. 1953. Chronic pulmonary osteoarthropathy in the dog. J. Am. Vet. Med. Assoc. 122, 167-171.

Polton, G.A. and Brearley, M.J. 2007. Clinical stage, therapy, and prognosis in canine anal sac gland carcinoma. J. Vet. Intern. Med. 21(2), 274-280.

Ross, J.T., Scavelli, T.D., Matthiesen, D.T. and Patnaik, A. 1991. Adenocarcinoma of the apocrine glands of the anal sac in dogs: A review of 32 cases. J. Am. Anim. Hosp. Assoc. 27, 349-355.

Salyusarenko, M., Peeri, D., Bibring, U., Ranen, E., Bdolah-Abram, T., Aroch, I. 2013. Hypertrophic Osteopathy: A Retrospective Case Control Study of 30 Dogs. Israel J. Vet. Med. 68, 209-217.

Watrous, B.J. and Blumenfeld, B. 2002. Congenital megaesophagus with hypertrophic osteopathy in a 6-year-old dog. Vet. Radiol. Ultrasound 43, 545-549.

Williams, L.E., Gliatto, G.M., Dodge, R.K., Johnson, J.L., Gamblin, R.M., Thamm, D.H., Lana, S.E., Szymkowski, M. and Moore, A.S. 2003. Carcinoma of the apocrine glands of the anal sac in dogs: 113 cases (1985-1995). J. Am. Vet. Med. Assoc. 223(6), 825-831.

Withers, S.S., Johnson, E.G., Culp, W.T., Rodriguez, C.O., Skorupski, K.A. and Rebhun, R.B. 2013. Paraneoplastic hypertrophic osteopathy in 30 dogs. Vet. Comp. Oncol. doi: 10.1111/vco.12026.

Withrow, S.J. 2001. Perianal tumors. In: Withrow SJ, MacEwen EG, eds. Small Animal Clinical Oncology, 3rd ed. Philadelphia, PA: WB Saunders. pp: 346-353.

Wylie, K.B., Lewis, D.D., Pechman, R.D., Cho, D.Y. and Roy, A. 1993. Hypertrophic osteopathy associated with Mycobacterium fortuitum pneumonia in a dog. J. Am. Vet. Med. Assoc. 202, 1986-1988.

4

The effect of renal diet in association with enalapril or benazepril on proteinuria in dogs with proteinuric chronic kidney disease

A. Zatelli[1,*], X. Roura[2], P. D'Ippolito[1], M. Berlanda[3] and E. Zini[3,4,5]

[1]Medical Consultancy Services, G. Calì Street 60, TBX1424 TàXbiex, Malta

[2]Hospital Clínic Veterinari, Universitat Autònoma de Barcelona, Spain

[3]Department of Animal Medicine, Production and Health, viale dell'Università 16, 35020 Legnaro (PD), University of Padova, Italy

[4]Clinic for Small Animal Internal Medicine, Vetsuisse Faculty, University of Zurich, Winterthurerstrasse 260, 8057 Zurich, Switzerland

[5]Istituto Veterinario di Novara, Strada Provinciale 9, 28060 Granozzo con Monticello (NO), Italy

Abstract

Treating proteinuria in dogs reduces the progression of chronic kidney disease (CKD); renal diets and angiotensin-converting enzyme (ACE)-inhibitors are cornerstones of treatment. Whether different ACE-inhibitors have distinct kidney protective effects is unknown; it is therefore hypothesized that renal diets and enalapril or benazepril have different beneficial effects in proteinuric CKD dogs. Forty-four dogs with proteinuric CKD (IRIS stages 1-4) were enrolled in the study and were fed renal diet for 30 days. Thereafter, they were randomly assigned to one of 2 groups. Dogs in group A (n=22) received enalapril (0.5 mg/kg, q12h) and in group B (n=22) benazepril (0.5 mg/kg, q24h); in both groups, dogs were fed the same renal diet. After randomization, dogs were monitored for 120 days. Body weight and body condition score (BCS), serum concentrations of creatinine, blood urea nitrogen (BUN), albumin and total proteins, and urine protein-to-creatinine (UPC) ratio were compared at different time-points. After 30 days of renal diet, creatinine, BUN and UPC ratio decreased significantly (p<0.0001). Compared to randomization, body weight, BCS, albumin, total proteins, creatinine and BUN did not vary during follow-up in the 44 dogs and differences between group A and B were not observed. However, the UPC ratio of group A at day 60, 90 and 150 was significantly lower than in group B and compared to randomization (p<0.05). In group B it did not vary overtime. It is concluded that the renal diet is beneficial to decrease creatinine, BUN and UPC ratio in proteinuric CKD dogs. Enalapril further ameliorates proteinuria if administered along with renal diet.

Keywords: ACE-I, CKD, Diet, Proteinuria.

Introduction

Proteinuria has a high prevalence in dogs with chronic kidney disease (CKD) and several studies have shown its role in promoting the progression of renal disorders (Jacob et al., 2002; D'Amico and Bazzi, 2003). In endemic areas for vector-borne diseases, such as leishmaniosis, the prevalence of proteinuric CKD has been reported to vary between 30.2% and 52.7% (Cortadellas et al., 2006). Among dogs at risk for developing proteinuric CKD, other than those living or having lived in endemic areas for vector-borne disease, there are also some breeds that are genetically predisposed to develop proteinuric glomerulonephritis (Chew et al., 2011; Harley and Langston, 2012). Early identification and treatment of proteinuria is important in dogs, not only because of the high prevalence of proteinuric CKD, but also because its management allows to slow the progression of CKD, thus leading to decrease the risk of uremic crisis, and kidney-related mortality (Jacob et al., 2002; Jacob et al., 2005; Brown et al., 2013). Angiotensin-converting enzyme (ACE)-inhibitors and dietary intervention are the major cornerstones of treatment in proteinuric CKD dogs; they have been shown to minimize clinical signs of uremia and, at least for the latter, to maintain optimal body conditions (Grauer et al., 2000; Tenhündfeld et al., 2009; Brown et al., 2013; Cortadellas et al., 2014). In order to limit the accumulation of nitrogenous waste products and to slow the progression of CKD, dietary protein restriction has been recommended for CKD dogs in International Renal Interest Society (IRIS) stages 1 with urine protein-to-creatinine ratio (UPC) >0.5 (IRIS substage P) and in any case in IRIS stages 2, 3 and 4 (Jacob et al., 2002; Brown et al., 2013; Cortadellas et al., 2014; IRIS Guidelines). Nonetheless, in some dogs, anti-proteinuric treatments (renal diet administered along with ACE-inhibitors) do not provide substantial reduction of proteinuria (Brown et al., 2013; Bugbee et al., 2014). Previously published study (Cortadellas et al., 2014) demonstrated a doubtful antiproteinuric efficacy of some ACE-inhibitors. Whether different ACE-inhibitors have distinct antiproteinuric and kidney protective effects is unknown; it is possible that renal diets and enalapril or

*Corresponding Author: Andrea Zatelli. Medical Consultancy Services, G. Calì Street 60, XBX1424 TàXbiex, Malta.
E-mail: andreazatelli1@gmail.com

benazepril provide different advantages in proteinuric CKD dogs. Moreover, in dogs with severe proteinuric glomerulonephritis (unresponsive to anti-proteinuric treatment) renal diets may not adequately meet protein requirements, thus leading to malnutrition and hypoalbuminemia, both frequent in dogs with proteinuric CKD. Furthermore, malnutrition and hypoalbuminemia have been associated with increased morbidity and risk of mortality (Remillard et al., 2001; Cave, 2010; Parker and Freeman, 2011).

In light of these premises, proteinuric CKD dogs were included to investigate the short-term effect of renal diet given alone and the medium-term effect of the same renal diet combined with the administration of the ACE-inhibitors enalapril or benazepril; their efficacy on body weight and BCS, on serum concentrations of creatinine, blood urea nitrogen (BUN), albumin and total proteins, and on the UPC ratio was assessed.

Materials and Methods

Animals and inclusion criteria

Dogs of any age and sexual status were considered for the present study if affected by naturally occurring CKD in IRIS stages 1, 2, 3 and 4 and if proteinuria was documented (UPC ratio >0.5; IRIS substage P) (IRIS Guidelines). The database at admission consisted of history, physical examination including body weight and body condition score (BCS; based on a 1 to 5 scale with 3 being optimal) (Thatcher et al., 2010), hematologic and serum biochemical profile, urinalysis, UPC ratio, immunofluorescence antibody titer (IFAT) for Leishmania infantum, Ehrlichia canis and Anaplasma phagocytophilum, and non-invasive determination of systolic arterial pressure.

Dogs presenting inflammatory diseases of the genitourinary tract, cardiac disease, neoplasia or endocrinopathies, severe hypertension (≥180 mmHg) (IRIS Guidelines) or anemia with hematocrit <25% and/or hemoglobin <10.0 g/dL, and seropositive for Leishmania infantum, Ehrlichia canis or Anaplasma phagocytophilum with associated clinical or laboratory signs other than UPC ratio >0.5 were excluded. Dogs that had received ACE-inhibitors, angiotensin II receptor blockers, or corticosteroids during the 12 weeks previous to admission were also excluded. Furthermore, to be enrolled, dogs had to show stable renal function, as defined by serum creatinine concentrations that did not increase or decreased by more than 15% within 4 weeks from admission; a maximum variation of 0.4 mg/dL have been considered indicative of stable renal function (Jacob et al., 2002; IRIS Guidelines). Dogs were recruited if an informed consent form to participate in the study was signed by the owners.

Study design

Following admission, all dogs initially included were fed a renal diet (Prescription Diet Canine k/D, Hill's Pet Nutrition, Topeka, KS) for 30 days. After 30 days, dogs were re-evaluated and allocated to one of the two following groups: group A receiving oral enalapril (Enacard, Merial, Milan, Italy) at 0.5 mg/kg, q12h, plus renal diet, and group B receiving oral benazepril (Fortekor, Novartis Animal Health, Milan, Italy) at 0.5 mg/kg, q24h, plus the same renal diet. Randomization was achieved with a software (MedCalc®, Version 11.3.0.0 (http://www.medcalc.com/)). Either enalapril or benazepril were administered using the recommended dosages of their commercial claims. At the time of the study, both drugs were registered for use in proteinuric CKD dogs in the country where the study was performed (Italy). Every dog included in the study was examined at day 0 (admission), at day 30 (randomization) and at days 45, 60, 90 and 150. The list of exams performed during each evaluation is reported in Table 1. The listed exams were used to evaluate the effect of treatment and to rule-out laboratory abnormalities caused by one of the infectious diseases stated above.

Blood samples

Venous blood samples (5.0 mL each) were collected in overnight fasted dogs and every sample was placed in tubes containing K3-EDTA (1.5 mL) and in tubes without anticoagulant (3.5 mL). Serum was obtained within 30 minutes from collection and stored along with samples in K3-EDTA tubes at 4°C. Hematologic and serum biochemical profiles were determined within 24 hours with standard methods (BC-2800Vet, MINDRAY, Mindray Co., Shenzhen, China; Cobas

Table 1. Time schedule and exams performed at each evaluation in all dogs.

Exams	Time point (days)					
	0	30	45	60	90	150
Body weight	X	X		X	X	X
Body condition score	X	X		X	X	X
Systolic arterial pressure	X	X		X	X	X
Hematology*	X				X	X
Biochemical profile 1**	X				X	X
Biochemical profile 2***		X	X	X		
Serology†	X					X
Urinalysis‡	X	X	X	X	X	X

*: Including erythrocyte, leukocytes and platelet counts, hematocrit, hemoglobin, **: Including creatinine, BUN, alanine aminotransferase, alkaline phosphatase, bilirubin, cholesterol, albumin, total proteins, albumin to globulin ratio, serum electrophoresis, ionized and total calcium, phosphorus, sodium, potassium, and chloride, ***: Including creatinine, BUN, albumin, total proteins, albumin to globulin ratio, ionized and total calcium, phosphorus, sodium, potassium, chloride, †: Including IFAT for Leishmania infantum, Ehrlichia canis and Anaplasma phagocytophilum, ‡: Including chemical-physical and sediment examination, and UPC ratio

Mira, Roche Diagnostic, Basel, Switzerland). Regarding the biochemical profile, based on the reference range for serum albumin at our laboratory (2.8-3.8 g/dL), severe hypoalbuminemia was arbitrarily considered if the concentration was <2.0 g/dL. Dogs with severe hypoalbuminemia received oral acetylsalicylic acid at 2.0 mg/kg, q24h, to prevent thrombosis (Brown *et al.*, 2013; Dudley *et al.*, 2013).

Urine samples

To collect urines, ultrasound-guided cystocentesis were performed in every dog using a 5.0 mL syringe connected to a 23-gauge needle. Before analysis, urine samples were placed in a 10.0 mL, sterile, evacuated collection tube. Urines were stored at room temperature and examined within 4 hours from collection. Urine sediment was obtained by centrifugation (10 minutes at $900 \times g$) of 5.0 mL of urine, followed by removal of 4.5 mL of supernatant, and resuspension of the remaining 0.5 mL of urine. A sample of 12 µL of the resuspended sediment was microscopically assessed. Erythrocytes and leukocytes were expressed as mean number of cells/10 high-power fields (hpf, 40× magnification). Urine sediment with bacteriuria, and/or >5 erythrocytes/hpf or leukocytes/hpf, was considered indicative of inflammation (active sediment) and excluded for the UPC ratio measurement (Beatrice *et al.*, 2010). The supernatant was transferred into separate tubes and stored at –20°C to determine urine protein and creatinine concentrations within 7 days. To calculate the UPC ratio, protein concentration (mg/dL) was measured with pyrogallol red and creatinine (mg/dL) using the Jaffé method (Real Time Diagnostic System); measurements were performed with an automated spectrophotometer (Cobas Mira, Roche Diagnostic, Basel, Switzerland). Based on a previous study (Rossi *et al.*, 2012), according with laboratory standard operating procedures (SOP), urine samples were manually diluted 1 to 20 with distilled water to fit linearity of the method. Occasionally, particularly concentrated urine samples were further diluted to 1:100 to fit the linearity of the method. Quality control was performed before any work session with two levels (normal and high) of control serums (Normal Control Serum and Pathological Control Serum) for creatinine. For urinary protein a specific control with bovine albumin (100 mg/dL) was used.

Statistical analysis

To study the effect of the renal diet on serum concentrations of creatinine and BUN, and on the UPC ratio, values were compared between admission and after 30 days with the Wilcoxon matched pairs test. To verify whether characteristics of the two groups were similar at randomization (i.e. after 30 days of renal diet and before introduction of ACE-inhibitors), age, body weight, serum concentrations of albumin, total proteins, creatinine and BUN, and the UPC ratio were compared with the Mann-Whitney test followed by Bonferroni post hoc test. Sex distribution and BCS were compared between groups with Fisher's exact test. To study the effect of enalapril or benazepril administered along with the renal diet, on serum concentrations of albumin, total proteins, creatinine and BUN, and on the UPC ratio data were analyzed using an unequally spaced repeated measures model (Littell *et al.*, 1998), assuming as covariance structure a spatial power law on the repeated individual values at different times (day 30, 45, 60, 90 and 150) with baseline values as covariates. The model included the fixed effects of treatment (group A vs. B), time and their interaction; the dog was the repeated random factor. For statistical differences showed by time and time × treatment effects, all pairwise contrasts were also calculated and corrected with Bonferroni post hoc test. Normality of residuals was evaluated by Shapiro-Wilk test and values ≥0.9 were considered as normal. Independence of residuals was graphically checked. Statistical significance was considered for $p<0.05$. Data were analyzed with softwares (GraphPad QuickCalcs calculator (2002-2005) by GraphPad Software, San Diego, CA; SAS 9.3, SAS Institute, Cary, NC).

Results

Animals

Forty-four dogs were included in the study. Median age at admission was 5 years (range: 1-19 years), median body weight was 26 kg (range: 3.8-69), and the median BCS was 3 (range: 2-4). Twenty-one dogs were intact males, 13 were spayed females, 6 were intact females and 4 were castrated males. Eight dogs were cross-breed and 36 were pure-breed, including 9 Boxers, 4 Yorkshire Terriers, 3 Cocker Spaniels and Golden Retrievers, 2 Bernese Mountain dogs and Rottweilers and, one each of American Staffordshire, Beagle, Bolognese, Italian Bracco, Bull Terrier, Czechoslovakian Wolfdog, Dachshund, Fox Terrier, German Shepherd, Irish Setter, Scottish Terrier, Samoyed and Weimaraner.

Effects of renal diet

After 30 days of renal diet, serum creatinine and BUN, and UPC ratio decreased (Fig. 1). In particular, median creatinine at admission was 2.4 mg/dL (range: 1.0-9.1) and after 30 days it was 2.2 mg/dL (range: 0.6-7.5) ($p<0.0001$); creatinine decreased in 38 dogs (86.4%) and increased in the remaining 6 (13.6%). Median BUN at admission was 56 mg/dL (range: 18-148) and after 30 days it was 47 mg/dL (range: 10-108) ($p<0.0001$); BUN decreased in 41 dogs (93.2%) and increased in the remaining 3 (6.8%). Median UPC ratio at admission was 2.9 (range: 0.8-19.8) and after 30 days it was 2.2 (range: 0.6-14.4) ($p<0.0001$); UPC ratio decreased in 42 dogs (95.5%) and increased in the remaining 2 (4.5%).

Effects of enalapril or benazepril associated with renal diet

Randomization performed after 30 days of renal diet and before introduction of ACE-inhibitors showed

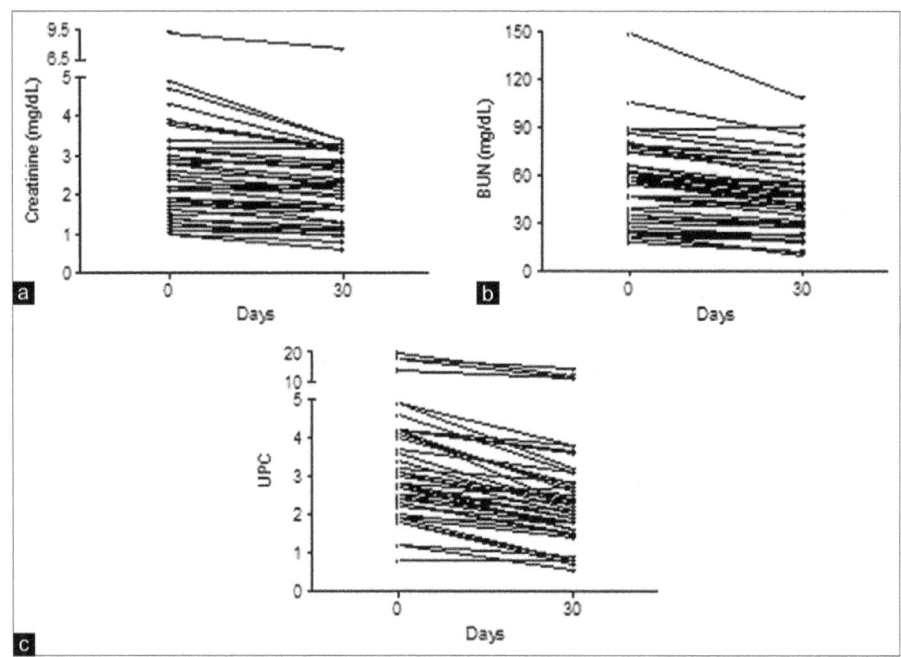

Fig. 1. Serum concentrations of creatinine (a) and BUN (b), and UPC ratio (c) in all dogs before any treatment (day 0) and after one month of renal diet (day 30).

that age, body weight, BCS, serum concentrations of albumin, total proteins, creatinine and BUN, and the UPC ratio did not differ between dogs allocated to group A or B (Table 2).

Twenty-two dogs were initially included into group A and received enalapril. Twenty-two were included into group B and received benazepril. Both groups were fed the same renal diet. In group A, 3 of the 22 dogs (13.6%) died during the study period; 2 of them died between 60 and 90 days following the start of the study and 1 between 90 and 150 days. In the group B, 2 of the 22 dogs (9.1%) died, 1 between 60 and 90 days and 1 between 90 and 150 days following the start of the study. In all 5 dogs, death was due to the progressive worsening of CKD; of the same dogs, after 30 days of renal diet, 5 had a decrease of creatinine, 4 of BUN and 5 of the UPC ratio. Furthermore, 3 dogs (13.6%) in group B were missed at follow-up visits, 2 between 60 and 90 days and 1 between 90 and 150 days after the start of the study.

Serum concentrations of albumin, total proteins, creatinine and BUN, and UPC ratio of dogs in groups A and B at randomization and during follow-up are reported in Table 3. Serum concentrations of albumin, total proteins, creatinine and BUN did not vary during the follow-up period to any significant degree in the 44 dogs grouped together, as compared to randomization (day 30). Furthermore, for the same parameters, differences between groups A and B were not observed during treatment. Dogs in group A had significantly lower UPC ratio at day 60 (p<0.05), day 90 (p<0.01)

Table 2. Comparison of variables used to assess adequacy of matching of dog groups. Values are reported as median and range or as number of dogs and frequency.

Variable	Group A	Group B	p-value
Age (years)	6 (2-12)	4 (1-19)	0.916
Sex			1.000
Female	3 (13.6%)	3 (13.6%)	
Spayed female	7 (31.9%)	6 (27.3%)	
Male	9 (40.9%)	12 (54.5%)	
Castrated male	3 (13.6%)	1 (4.6%)	
Body weight (kg)	25.9 (4.2-57)	27 (3.8-69)	0.916
BCS			1.000
2	6 (27.3%)	8 (36.4%)	
3	15 (68.2%)	12 (54.5%)	
4	1 (4.5%)	2 (9.1%)	
Albumin (g/dL)	2.7 (1.7-3.5)	2.9 (1.6-4.0)	0.350*
Total proteins (g/dL)	5.7 (4.8-7.0)	6.4 (4.9-8.5)	0.084*
Creatinine (mg/dL)	1.8 (0.6-3.4)	2.3 (1.0-3.3)	0.117
BUN (mg/dL)	42 (12-72)	49 (10-108)	0.110
UPC ratio	2.3 (0.7-11.5)	2.0 (0.6-14.4)	0.404

*: p-value corrected with Bonferroni's post hoc test

and day 150 (p<0.05) as compared to randomization (Table 3), whereas dogs in group B had not different UPC

Table 3. Serum concentrations of albumin, total proteins, creatinine and BUN, and UPC ratio of dogs in groups A and B at randomization (30 days) and follow-up evaluations. Median and range are reported.

Variable	Time point (days)				
	30	45	60	90	150
Albumin (g/dL)					
Group A	2.6 (1.7-3.5)	2.7 (1.6-3.4)	2.6 (1.9-3.4)	2.7 (1.9-3.5)	2.7 (2.1-3.4)
Group B	2.9 (1.6-4.0)	2.8 (1.7-3.6)	2.8 (1.8-3.6)	2.8 (2.0-3.3)	2.8 (1.8-3.1)
Total proteins (g/dL)					
Group A	5.7 (4.8-7.0)	5.8 (4.8-6.7)	5.8 (5.0-6.8)	5.9 (5.2-6.8)	5.8 (5.1-7.0)
Group B	6.4 (4.9-8.5)	6.3 (4.8-7.9)	6.3 (5.0-7.7)	6.0 (5.2-7.7)	6.2 (5.1-6.9)
Creatinine (mg/dL)					
Group A	1.8 (0.6-3.4)	1.8 (0.7-3.7)	1.6 (0.8-3.9)	1.6 (0.9-4.3)	1.5 (0.9-3.4)
Group B	2.3 (1.0-3.3)	2.4 (1.0-5.0)	2.3 (0.8-5.5)	2.3 (0.9-7.5)	2.4 (0.9-5.0)
BUN (mg/dL)					
Group A	42 (12-72)	42 (17-66)	40 (13-89)	37 (15-89)	36 (16-67)
Group B	49 (10-108)	49 (19-112)	50 (16-143)	50 (20-100)	50 (20-85)
UPC					
Group A	2.3 (0.7-11.5)	2.3 (0.8-8.0)	1.6 (0.4-5.6)*	1.2 (0.3-8.9)†	1.2 (0.5-4.5)*
Group B	2.0 (0.6-14.4)	2.2 (0.6-9.2)	2.2 (0.5-9.8)	1.8 (0.6-9.0)	1.9 (0.6-9.2)

Significant differences between follow-up evaluations and randomization within groups: *: $p<0.05$; †: $p<0.01$

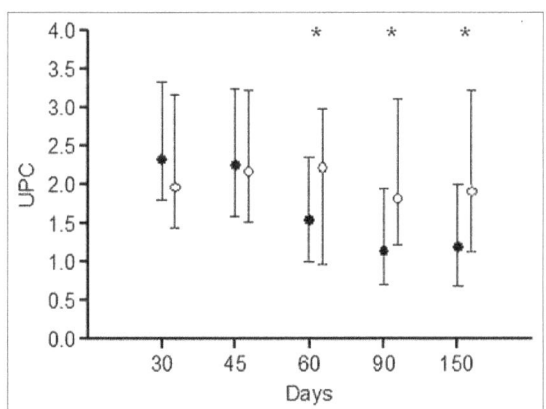

Fig. 2. UPC ratio in dogs receiving enalapril and renal diet (group A, black dots) or benazepril and renal diet (group B, white dots) at randomization (day 30) and follow-up. Median values and interquartile ranges are shown. Significant differences between group A and B are depicted with asterisks ($p<0.05$).

ratio at each time point during follow-up compared to randomization. Dogs in group A had significantly lower UPC ratio than dogs in group B at day 60 ($p<0.05$), 90 ($p<0.05$) and 150 ($p<0.05$) (Fig. 2).

Discussion

Because persistent renal proteinuria in dogs has been associated with a poorer prognosis (Harley and Langston, 2012) its treatment is recommended in order to improve quality of life and survival time. For this

purpose, the potential beneficial effects of renal diet and of the ACE-inhibitors enalapril and benazepril in dogs with proteinuric CKD were assessed in the present study. With regard to dietary management, we substantiated the beneficial effect of using renal diet in proteinuric CKD dogs. Indeed, during the first 30 days of the trial, the enrolled dogs were managed with the renal diet but did not receive any medication and a significant improvement of serum concentrations of creatinine and BUN, as well as the UPC ratio was observed compared to baseline. Main characteristics of the selected diet, which are the key points of the dietary management (Roudebush *et al.*, 2010; Polzin, 2013) are protein restriction with high biological value, phosphorus and sodium reduction and supplementation with ω-3 polyunsaturated fatty acids (PUFAs). Among them, content and quality of proteins as well as phosphorus and sodium restriction seem to be the most important aspects to consider in proteinuric CKD dogs, whereas the effect of PUFAs is yet not fully known and deserves further investigation (Roudebush *et al.*, 2010; Brown *et al.*, 2013).

For the present trial, the ACE-inhibitors enalapril and benazepril were administered using the recommended dosages of their commercial claims. The group treated with enalapril showed a significant reduction of the UPC ratio after 30 days of treatment (60 days from the beginning of the study); however, the group treated with benazepril did not show ameliorations of the UPC ratio, at any time. One recent study showed that benazepril might not be effective in reducing renal proteinuria in dogs (Cortadellas *et al.*, 2014). However, as proposed by the same authors, the lack of efficacy of benazepril in their investigation might have been due to the drug dosage used (Cortadellas *et al.*, 2014). Indeed, based on studies in humans, increasing the dosage of ACE-inhibitors can improve the antiproteinuric effect, possibly suggesting that higher dosages of benazepril might also be beneficial to decrease proteinuria in CKD dogs (Weinberg *et al.*, 2001; Tylicki *et al.*, 2012). On the other hand, another investigation in dogs showed a reduction of the UPC ratio associated with the administration of benazepril (Tenhündfeld *et al.*, 2009). However, comparison between our results and those of Tenhündfeld *et al.* (2009) is difficult because they had three different groups of only 10 dogs, treated with placebo, benazepril and benazepril plus heparin, which were not homogeneous for UPC ratio at the time treatment was started. Furthermore, they observed a beneficial effect on UPC ratio only by day 180 for dogs in the benazepril group and by day 90 for dogs in the benazepril plus heparin group. Therefore, if an effect of benazepril exists on proteinuria, it would likely be delayed compared to that achieved with enalapril, questioning the real benefit of benazepril to treat proteinuric CKD dogs based on the current recommended dosages.

In the present study, the significant reduction of UPC ratio in the group treated with enalapril was evident by 30 days of therapy, whereas no significant amelioration was observed if tested after only 15 days of treatment with the ACE-inhibitor. This result may provide useful information for the monitoring of proteinuric CKD dogs in clinical practice. To assess the potential favorable effect of enalapril to control proteinuria in dogs, the UPC ratio should be evaluated after 30 days of treatment; therefore, absence of improvement at 15 days should not be regarded as indicative of lack of efficacy.

During the study period, none of the dogs developed severe hypertension and thus needed to receive amlodipine or other anti-hypertensive treatments. The fact that blood pressure did not increase throughout the study may be due to the limited duration of the trial, or to the administration of ACE-inhibitors.

Some limitations of the study need to be mentioned, including the relative small sample size, the lack of blinding and of renal biopsies. The risk associated with lack of masking was minimized by randomization and by excluding statistical differences between the groups at the time the ACE-inhibitors were started. Absence of renal histology did not allow excluding that, in some dogs, proteinuria was primarily due to tubular or tubulointerstitial damage, rather than being of glomerular origin. However, if this was the case, it is likely that dogs with tubular or tubulointerstitial damage were

evenly distributed between groups. In addition, dogs with severe hypoalbuminemia (<2 g/dL) received oral acetylsalicylic acid. As hypothesized by some authors (Grauer *et al.*, 2000; Cortadellas *et al.*, 2014), low dosages of acetylsalicylic acid have a beneficial effect on proteinuria in dogs with glomerulonephritis and, therefore, its use might have partly biased the results of the study. Nonetheless, the potential beneficial effect of acetylsalicylic acid was likely similar between groups as the frequency of dogs with severe hypoalbuminemia that received it did not differ.

In conclusion, the administration of renal diet ameliorates serum creatinine, BUN and UPC ratio, and adding enalapril decreases the UPC ratio further in dogs with proteinuric CKD. Using benazepril, at the present dosage and for 120 days, was not beneficial compared with enalapril. Future studies are needed to verify the effect of benazepril over longer periods or at higher dosages in dogs with proteinuric CKD, or that of angiotensin II receptor blockers or PUFAs, administered along with renal diet.

Conflict of interest

The Authors declares that there is no conflict of interest.

Acknowledgment

The study is partly supported by Merial Italy. The authors are grateful to Dr. Barbara Contiero for her statistical advice.

References

Beatrice, L., Nizi, F., Callegari, D., Paltrinieri, S., Zini, E., D'Ippolito, P. and Zatelli, A. 2010. Comparison of urine protein-to-creatinine ratio in urine samples collected by cystocentesis versus free catch in dogs. J. Am. Vet. Med. Assoc. 236, 1221-1224.

Brown, S., Elliott, J., Francey, T., Francey, T., Polzin, D. and Vaden, S. 2013. Consensus recommendations for standard therapy of glomerular disease in dogs. J. Vet. Intern. Med. 27(Suppl 1), S27-43.

Bugbee, A.C., Coleman, A.E., Wang, A., Woolcock, A.D. and Brown, S.A. 2014. Telmisartan treatment of refractory proteinuria in a dog. J. Vet. Intern. Med. 28, 1871-1874.

Cave, N. 2010. Immunology and nutrition. In: Ettinger SJ, Feldman EC, eds. Textbook of veterinary internal medicine. 7th ed. St. Louis: Saunders Elsevier, pp: 638-642.

Chew, D.J., DiBartola, S.P. and Schenck, P.A. 2011. Familial renal diseases of dogs and cats. In: Chew DJ, DiBartola SP, Schenck PA, eds. Canine and feline nephrology and urology 2nd ed. St. Louis, Missouri, Elsevier Saunders, pp: 197-211.

Cortadellas, O., Fernández del Palacio, M.J., Bayón, A., Albert, A. and Talavera, J. 2006. Systemic hypertension in dogs with leishmaniasis: prevalence and clinical consequences. J. Vet. Intern. Med. 20, 941-947.

Cortadellas, O., Talavera, J. and Fernández del Palacio, M.J. 2014. Evaluation of the effects of a therapeutic renal diet to control proteinuria in proteinuric non-azotemic dogs treated with benazepril. J. Vet. Intern. Med. 28, 30-37.

D'Amico, G. and Bazzi, C. 2003. Pathophysiology of proteinuria. Kidney Int. 63, 809-825.

Dudley, A., Thomason, J., Fritz, S., Grady, J., Stokes, J., Wills, R., Pinchuk, L., Mackin, A. and Lunsford, K. 2013. Cyclooxygenase expression and platelet function in healthy dogs receiving low-dose aspirin. J. Vet. Intern. Med. 27, 141-149.

Grauer, G.F., Greco, D.S., Getzy, D.M., Cowgill, L.D., Vaden, S.L., Chew, D.J., Polzin, D.J. and Barsanti, J.A. 2000. Effects of enalapril versus placebo as a treatment for canine Idiopathic glomerulonephritis. J. Vet. Intern. Med. 14, 526-533.

Harley, L. and Langston, C. 2012. Proteinuria in dogs and cats. Can. Vet. J. 53, 631-638.

IRIS Guidelines. International Renal Interest Society. Available at: http://www.iris-kidney.com/guidelines.

Jacob, F., Polzin, D.J., Osborne, C.A., Allen, T.A., Kirk, C.A., Neaton, J.D., Lekcharoensuk, C. and Swanson, L.L. 2002. Clinical evaluation of dietary modification for treatment of spontaneous chronic renal failure in dogs. J. Am. Vet. Med. Assoc. 220, 1163-1170.

Jacob, F., Polzin, D.J., Osborne, C.A., Neaton, J.D., Kirk, C.A., Allen, T.A. and Swanson, L.L. 2005. Evaluation of the association between initial proteinuria and morbidity rate or death in dogs with naturally occurring chronic renal failure. J. Am. Vet. Med. Assoc. 226, 393-400.

Littell, R.C., Henry, P.R. and Ammerman, C.B. 1998. Statistical analysis of repeated measures data using SAS procedures. J. Anim. Sci. 76, 1216-1231.

Parker, V.J. and Freeman, L.M. 2011. Association between body condition and survival in dogs with acquired chronic kidney disease. J. Vet. Intern. Med. 25, 1306-1311.

Polzin, D.J. 2013. Evidence-based step-wise approach to managing chronic kidney disease in dogs and cats. J. Vet. Emerg. Crit. Care (San Antonio) 23, 205-215.

Remillard, R.L., Darden, D.E., Michel, K.E., Marks, S.L., Buffington, C.A. and Bunnell, P.R. 2001. An investigation of the relationship between caloric intake and outcome in hospitalized dogs. Vet. Ther. 2, 301-310.

Roudebush, P., Polzin, D.J., Adams, L.G., Towell, T.L. and Forrester, S.D. 2010. An evidence-based review of therapies for canine chronic kidney disease. J. Small Anim. Pract. 51, 244-252.

Tenhündfeld, J., Wefstaedt, P. and Nolte, I.J. 2009. A randomized controlled clinical trial of the use of benazepril and heparin for the treatment of chronic kidney disease in dogs. J. Am. Vet. Med. Assoc. 234, 1031-1037.

Thatcher, C.D., Hand, M.S. and Remillard, R.L. 2010. Small animal clinical nutrition: an iterative process. In: Hand, M.S., Thatcher, C.D., Remillard, R.L., Roudebush, P. and Novotny, B.J., eds. Small animal clinical nutrition. 5th ed. Topeka, Kansas: Mark Morris Institute, pp: 3-21.

Tylicki, L., Lizakowski, S. and Rutkowski, B. 2012. Renin-angiotensin-aldosterone system blockade for nephroprotection: current evidence and future directions. J. Nephrol. 25, 900-910.

Weinberg, M., Weinberg, A., Cord, R. and Zappe, D. 2001. The effect of high-dose angiotensin II receptor blockade beyond maximal recommended doses in reducing urinary protein excretion. J. Renin Angiotensin Aldosterone Syst. 2(Suppl 1), 196-198.

5

Changes in intraocular pressure and horizontal pupil diameter during use of topical mydriatics in the canine eye

Liga Kovalcuka[1,*], Agris Ilgazs[1], Dace Bandere[2] and David L. Williams[3]

[1]*Latvia University of Agriculture, Faculty of Veterinary Medicine, Clinical Institute, K. Helmaņa iela 8, Jelgava, LV-3004, Latvia*
[2]*Riga Stradiņš University, Faculty of Pharmacy, Department of Pharmaceutical Chemistry, Dzirciema iela 16, Rīga, LV-1007, Latvia*
[3]*University of Cambridge, Department of Veterinary medicine, United Kingdom*

Abstract

The objective of this study was to determine the effects of topical 0.5% tropicamide, 1% atropine sulphate and 10% phenylephrine hydrochloride ophthalmic solutions on intraocular pressure (IOP) and horizontal pupil diameter (HPD) in the dog during the first hour after treatment. Forty clinically and ophthalmologically normal canine patients (between the ages of 2 and 6 years) of varying breed and sex were used in this study. Animals were randomly divided into four groups of ten and given one drop of tropicamide, atropine, phenylephrine or saline into one eye. IOP and HPD were measured in both eyes every 5 minutes for 60 minutes. Tropicamide increased IOP by 8.8±4.0 mmHg 35 minutes post-treatment compared to pre-treatment (P<0.01) only in treated eye. IOP in the contralateral eye did not increase. With atropine the maximum increase in IOP was 2.6±2.8 mmHg at 20 minutes post treatment in the treated eye (P<0.01). IOP in the contralateral eye did not increase. Phenylephrine increased IOP by 2.3±2.1 mmHg (P<0.05) 10 minutes after treatment. Also in the untreated eye IOP increased by 2.3±2.1 mmHg, 20 minutes post-treatment. Maximum HPD in eyes treated with tropicamide occurred at 55 minutes and with atropine at 60 minutes. There were no HPD changes in the contralateral, untreated eye. Topical 10% phenylephrine showed maximal pupil dilation 60 minutes after treatment, but the HPD of the – untreated eye slightly decreased at 15 minutes, but this change only reached statistical significance at 40 min post- treatment (P<0.05). Normal saline showed no influence on IOP or HPD. The drugs investigated here show a significant increase in IOP after mydriatics.
Keywords: Atropine sulphate, Horizontal pupil diameter, Intraocular pressure, Phenylephrine, Tropicamide.

Introduction

In ophthalmology mydriatics – specifically tropicamide hydrochloride and atropine sulphate – are employed to provide pupil dilation: during examination of the posterior segment of the eye (tropicamide) and as therapeutic agents for treatment of uveitis (atropine) by relieving ciliary spasm through cycloplegia and preventing formation of synechiae through mydriasis. The phenylephrine is used to localize the site of sympathetic denervation in Horner's syndrome, producing mydriasis as part of sympathomimetic action (Smith and Raynard 1992; Ward, 1998).

In humans an increase of intraocular pressure (IOP) has been observed after use of topical mydriatics such as atropine (Gartner and Billet, 1957), tropicamide and phenylephrine (Harris 1968; Harris and Galin, 1969; Rengstorff and Doughty, 1982) both in normal subjects and in patients with narrow filtration angle glaucoma (Harris and Galin, 1969) and with primary open angle glaucoma (Shaw and Lewis, 1986; Marchini *et al.*, 2003). Latest report in five years old girl presented to the hospital for a routine retina check-u, after pupil

dilation with 1 % tropicamide and 10 % phenylephrine for retinal examination, showed an acute elevation of intraocular pressure (Wu *et al.*, 2015).

Effects of topical 1% atropine, 0.5% tropicamide, 1% homatropine, 10% phenylephrine, and 2% ibopamine on IOP and pupil diameter has been investigated in sheep. Topical atropine, tropicamide, and homatropine induced pupil dilation but did not change IOP in eyes of healthy sheep, but phenylephrine did not change any of the parameters evaluated (Ribeiro *et al.*, 2014). Hacker and Farver (1988) investigated whether use of mydriatics could cause an increase in intraocular pressure in dogs and reported negative findings. However, these researchers measured the IOP before drug administration and at maximal pupil dilation but never during the process of pupil dilation, but Grozdanic *et al.* (2010) showed increase of IOP in dogs with closed angle glaucoma.

The parasympatholytic agent tropicamide is a cholinergic antagonist used in animals for pupil dilation because of its rapid action and short duration (Marchini *et al.*, 2003). In several studies with dogs neither

---

*Corresponding Author: Liga Kovalcuka. Latvia University of Agriculture, Faculty of Veterinary Medicine, Clinical Institute, K. Helmaņa iela 8, Jelgava, LV-3004, Latvia. Email: *kovalcuka@gmail.com*

unilateral nor bilateral application of 1% tropicamide was shown to cause significant changes of IOP measured after maximal pupil dilation (Hacker and Farver 1988; Molleda et al., 1988; Wallin-Hakanson and Wallin-Hakanson, 2001), although one group of researchers noticed that Siberian Huskies had a greater IOP variability after dilation (Taylor et al., 2007). A study focused on the effects of 0.5% topical tropicamide in Spanish Water Hounds reported no significant changes in IOP after unilateral application (Molleda et al., 1988) but again, changes in IOP were not measured during dilation.

A previous study in cats showed IOP increases in both eyes 30 min after unilateral treatment of 0.5% tropicamide in the right eye. However, 60 min after treatment the IOP increase of the right eye was significantly greater than the left (Stadtbaumer et al., 2002). In a more recent study by the same author the effects of topical 1% atropine and 10% phenylephrine in cats demonstrated a significant IOP increase after atropine, but no effect after phenylephrine. The highest IOP was measured in the treated eye between 5 and 28 h after treatment and these differences were statistically significant at 1, 3, 6, 12 and 16 h post-treatment (Stadtbaumer et al., 2006). In study with normal cats and cats with inherited primary glaucoma, topical 0.5% tropicamide increased IOP in normal cats those with primary inherited glaucoma (Gomes et al., 2011).

Contradictory findings regarding the effects of atropine on the dynamics of aqueous humour outflow have been reported (Green and Elijah, 1981; Miichi and Nagataki, 1982). Some authors suggested that atropine could change aqueous outflow through cycloplegic actions (Harris, 1968; Valle, 1974); others suggested that mechanical obstruction of iridocorneal angle might be the possible cause of IOP increase (Stadtbaumer et al., 2006). However, these researchers observed that the maximum dilation of the pupil lasted longer than the statistically significant increase of the IOP in cats, arguing against mechanical obstruction of iridocorneal angle (Stadtbaumer et al., 2006).

Few data exist in literature concerning the effects of phenylephrine on the IOP in animals. In monkeys there were no significant changes in the IOP two hours after a single unilateral application of 5% phenylephrine, but in the same study in human patients IOP was found to have increased significantly (Takayama et al., 2004). In another study with human subjects, 10% phenylephrine did not cause significant increase in IOP after treatment (Marchini et al., 2003).

Regarding the effects of tropicamide on horizontal pupil diameter (HPD) in dogs, the small amount of data in the literature shows significant HPD increase after topical 0.5% tropicamide application in both eyes (Wallin-Hakanson and Wallin-Hakanson, 2001). Maximal pupil dilation in cats was observed 2h after topical 0.5% tropicamide (Stadtbaumer et al., 2002). Tropicamide causes significant mydriasis in dogs with and without Therapeutic soft contact lenses (Hatzav et al., 2016). With regard to atropine, maximal pupil dilation was obtained 30-60 min after topical application in dogs, cats and cattle (Gelatt et al., 1973, 1995; Gelatt and MacKey, 1998). In one feline study, HPD started to decrease 24 hours after the topical atropine was administered and after 96 hours the pupil returned to pre-treatment size (Stadtbaumer et al., 2006).

There are contradictory findings in the literature about the effect of phenylephrine on HPD. In cats there is a poor mydriatic effect after application of 10% phenylephrine (Stadtbaumer et al., 2006). In Rhesus monkeys the maximal pupil dilation occurred 15 minutes after application of two doses of 10% phenylephrine, although the pupils remained dilated more than 65 minutes (Marchini et al., 2003; Ostin and Glasser, 2004). Rubin and Wolfes (1962), tested phenylephrine in dogs and found maximal dilation at approximately 2 hours.

In the most studies researchers have looked at the IOP at the time of maximal pupil dilation, therefore, our goal in this study was to determine the IOP in the eye immediately after administration of topical mydriatics and in five minutes intervals during the first hour after treatment. The purpose of this study was to determine the effects of topical mydriatics - 0.5% tropicamide, 1% atropine sulphate, and 10% phenylephrine on the IOP and the HPD in the canine eye during the first hour after treatment.

Materials and Methods

Data

All animals examined were outpatients at Clinical Institute of the Faculty of Veterinary Medicine at the Latvia University of Agriculture and at the Queen's Veterinary School Hospital, University of Cambridge. This study was approved by the Committee for Animal Protection and Ethical use of Latvian State Food and Veterinary Service and by the Ethics Committee of the Department of Veterinary Medicine, University of Cambridge. In all cases informed consent was obtained from the pet owners for the study.

All animals included in this study were examined by the same person clinically and ophthalmologically, to ensure they were both systemically and ophthalmologically healthy. The clinical examination included signalment (animal breed, age and sex were recorded), general appearance, vital signs (body weight, temperature, heart/pulse rate, respiratory rate), physical examination (systems approach). The ocular examination included direct and indirect ophthalmoscopy (Keeler Practitioner, Windsor, UK), monocular ophthalmoscopy with the Pan Optic ophthalmoscope (Welch Alynn, Romford, UK) and slit lamp biomicroscopy (Kowa SL15, Nagoya, Aichi, Japan). Tonometry with the Tonovet tonometer (TonoVet®, Tiolat Ltd. Finland) was a part of the initial examination. Four groups, each containing 10 healthy, randomly assigned dogs of different sexes and breeds were used.

The first group all animals received one drop of 0.5% tropicamide (Alcon – Couvreur, Belgium) in the right eye, in the second group one drop of 1% atropine sulphate (Martindale Pharmaceuticals Ltd. UK) in the right eye. In the third group one drop of 10% phenylephrine hydrochloride was used in the right eye. In the fourth control group, one drop of normal saline was used in the right. The effects of mydriatics on the IOP and the HPD were determined in all groups.

In all treatment groups the first IOP and HPD measurement was taken before treatment (T_0). After treatment, IOP and HPD were recorded every five minutes in both eyes (T_5; T_{10}; …$T_{60/65}$). During all measurements, the animals were handled gently to avoid any tension on the animal's neck which might influence IOP neck (Pauli *et al.*, 2006).

All tonometric measurements were performed by the same person employing rebound tonometry with the Tonovet tonometer (TonoVet®, Tiolat Ltd. Finland), using values that were less than a 5% standard deviation among six measurements. Use of topical anaesthesia is not required for this tonometer. Horizontal pupil diameter was measured with *Jameson* calipers under fixed light conditions every five minutes as described above. All measurements were done at approximately same time of day (9.00-11.00 am) because of the effects of light conditions at different times of day on the IOP and the HPD (Gelatt *et al.*, 1981; Giannetto *et al.*, 2009).

Statistical method
To determine the effect of topical tropicamide, atropine and phenylephrine, the arithmetic mean values (X) and standard deviation (SD) of the IOP and the HPD were calculated for each eye separately. Changes in the IOP and the HPD between eyes and over time period were evaluated using a paired two-sample repeated measures T-test. P values less than 0.05 were considered to be statistically significant.

Results
No signs of ocular irritation or pain were detected in animals during the study.
Group 1 (tropicamide)
Initial pre-treatment IOP are shown in Table 1. Mean IOP values before topical tropicamide application between right and left eye were not significantly different (P=0.27). The IOP increased from the first post-treatment measurement in the treated eye and at T35 time point IOP had increased from the pre-treatment value of mean 8.8±4.0 mmHg in reaching a

maximum 21.6±4.1 mmHg (P=0.002) (Fig. 1.). From this time forward IOP continually decreased until at 60 minutes after treatment the IOP had returned to a T0 values (P>0.05).

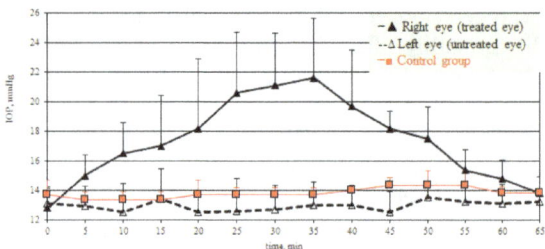

Fig. 1. Effect of unilateral application of 0.5% tropicamide on the intraocular pressure (mean values) in dogs.

The IOP in the contralateral eye did not significantly increase throughout the treatment period: the IOP values were between 12.5±1.4 mmHg and 13.5±1.1 mmHg (Table 1). The increase in IOP in the treated eye compared to the untreated eye was statistically significant (P=0.002) from the T5 of the measurement period.

Our results concerning the effects of tropicamide on the HPD are shown in Table 2. Before treatment there were no significant differences in the HPD between the eyes. HPD at T5 was increasing relatively to T0 and continued to increase, gaining a maximum mean value of 13.2±1.7 mm at T55. During the last five minutes the HPD decreased but still was significantly higher than pre-treatment values (P<0.05). The increase in pupil diameter from the T0 value until the end of the study was 6.6±1.2mm (Fig. 2).

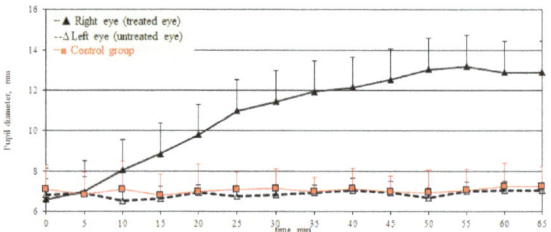

Fig. 2. Effect of 0.5% tropicamide on the horizontal pupil diameter (mean values) in dogs.

Differences in the HPD between the treated and untreated eye and control group were statistically significant (P<0.003).
Group 2 (atropine sulphate)
In the second group, there were no significant differences in IOP between the left and right eyes before application of 1% atropine sulphate (P>0.05) (Table 1).

The dynamics of IOP after topical application of 1% atropine sulphate are shown in Figure 3.

Table 1. Effect of mydriatics on intraocular pressure (mean values ± SD) in the dog's right and left eye.

Topical mydriatics	Right eye (treated eye)			Left eye (untreated eye)		
	Initial IOP (mean ± SD)	Maximal IOP (mean ± SD), time	% of IOP increase	Initial IOP (mean ± SD)	Maximal IOP (mean ± SD), time	% of IOP increase
Tropicamide	12.8 ± 1.4	21.6 ± 4.1 (35min)	68.8% **	13.1 ± 1.1	13.5 ± 1.1 (50 min)	3.1%
Atropine sulphate	17.7 ± 3.1	20.3 ± 3.1 (20 min)	14.7 %**	17.3 ± 2.8	18.1 ± 3.9 (15 min)	4.6 %
Phelylephrine hydrochloride	15.0 ± 3.3	17.3 ± 4.1 (10 min)	15.3%	14.0 ± 2.8	16.3 ± 2.3 (20 min)	16.4%
Saline	16.6 ± 2.0	17.3 ± 2.6 (15 min)	4.2 %	16.6 ± 2.0	17.3 ± 2.6 (15 min)	4.2 %

** $P < 0.01$

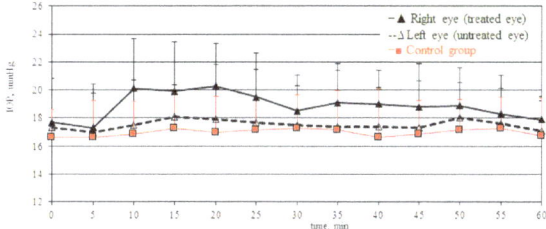

Fig. 3. Effect of unilateral application of 1% atropine sulphate on the intraocular pressure (mean values) in dogs.

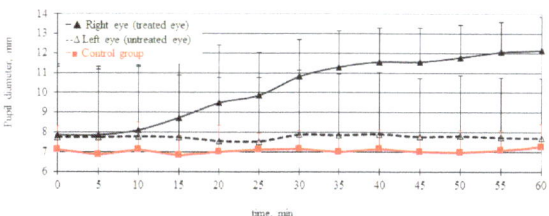

Fig. 4. Effect of 1% atropine sulphate on the horizontal pupil diameter (mean values) in dogs.

An increase in IOP was seen at T10 after treatment and continued until maximum of IOP at T20 when increase was 2.6±2.8 mmHg higher than at pre-treatment (P=0.008). The IOP started to decrease at T25 and continued to decrease until 60 minutes after treatment. The IOP did not significantly change during the last 25 minutes.

At the last measurement the IOP was higher than in the contralateral eye, but this difference was not statistically significant. Mean IOP in the treated eye compared to the untreated eye and the control group values were higher throughout the measurement period but only significantly (P<0.05) from 10 until 25 minutes after treatment (Fig. 3). In the contralateral eye, the IOP did not significantly increase throughout the treatment period, with IOP values varying from 17.0±3.2 mmHg to 18.1±3.9 mmHg.

Our results regarding the influence of topical 1% atropine on the horizontal pupil diameter show that there is no significant differences in the HPD between the eyes (P=0.17) before topical atropine (Table 2). The pupil was dilated at T10 after application of 1% atropine and continued to increase, gaining a maximum mean value of 12.1±1.7 mm at 60 minutes (P<0.003). HPD did not change in two last measurements (Fig. 4). The increase in pupil diameter from the pre-treatment value until the end of the study was 4.2±2.7 mm. Differences in the HPD between the treated and untreated eye were statistically significant (P<0.003) from 10 minutes after application of atropine until 60 minutes or the end of study period.

Group 3 (phenylephrine)
In the third group of dogs we investigated the effects of topical 10% phenylephrine on the IOP and the HPD. There were no significant differences in the IOP between the right eye and the left eye (Table 1) before topical application of phenylephrine (P>0.05).
The effect of topical 10% phenylephrine is shown in Figure 5.

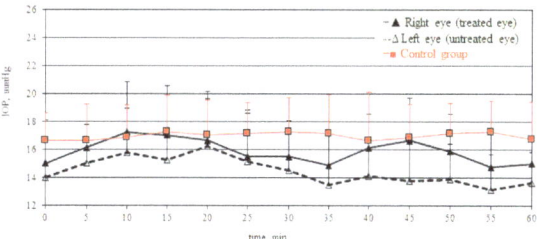

Fig. 5. Effect of unilateral application of 10% phenylephrine on the intraocular pressure (mean values) in dogs.

In the right eye IOP statistically significantly increased at T5 time point, compared to T0 values. The IOP continued to increase till T10 showing 17.3±4.1 mmHg, having increase of 2.3±2.1 mmHg compare to T0 (P<0.05) and by T35 the IOP had decreased to 14.9±2.3 mmHg. A second phase of IOP increase was recorded 45 minutes after treatment, with IOP rising to 16.6±4.1 mmHg; however, the second increase of IOP was not statistically significant (P>0.05). At T55 IOP decreased to 14.8±1.4 mmHg, (Fig. 5), not statistically different from pre-treatment values (P>0.05).

Table 2. Effect of mydriatics on horizontal pupil diameter (mean values ± SD) in the dog's right and left eye.

Topical mydriatics	Right eye (treated eye)			Left eye (untreated eye)		
	Initial HPD (mean ± SD)	Maximal HPD (mean ± SD), time	% of HPD increase	Initial HPD (mean ± SD)	Maximal HPD (mean ± SD), time	% of HPD increase
Tropicamide	6.6 ± 0.8	13.2 ±1.7 (55min)	100% **	6.8 ± 0.9	7.1 ± 0.6 (40min)	4.4
Atropine sulphate	7.9 ± 3.6	12.1 ± 1.7 (50 min)	53.2 %**	7.7 ± 3.6	7.9 ± 3.0 (60 min)	2.6 %
Phenylephrine hydrochlorid	7.9 ± 1.5	9.9 ± 2.0 (60 min)	25.3%	7.7 ± 1.3	6.5 ± 1.2 (60 min)	-15.6%
Saline	7.1 ± 1.2	7.3 ± 1.2 (60 min)	2.8%	7.1 ± 1.2	7.3 ± 1.2 (60 min)	2.8%

** P < 0.01

Importantly, in the left, untreated eye we noticed changes in the IOP (Fig. 5.). As in right eye, the IOP increased in the first five minutes after treatment. Statistically significant IOP increases in the untreated eye were observed 10 and 20 minutes after application of phenylephrine; respectively 15.8±3.3 mmHg and 16.3±2.3 mmHg (P<0.05), an increase of 1.8±2.1 mmHg and 2.3±2.1 mmHg compared to pre-treatment values. Between 35 and 60 minutes after treatment IOP returned to pre-treatment values (P>0.05). The mean IOP in the treated eye compared to the untreated eye was significantly higher (P<0.05) throughout the measurement period, except at 20 and 25 minutes after treatment (Fig. 5). The results regarding the effect of topical 10% phenylephrine on the HPD are shown in Table 2. The HPD was increased ten minutes after treatment in the right eye (Fig. 6.). Fifteen minutes after treatment it slightly decreased. Statistically significant increases of the HPD were obtained at T20 and T25 minutes after phenylephrine (P<0.05). At T30 and T35 minutes after treatment, the HPD decreased, but it was still significantly higher than the pre–treatment values (Fig. 6). The pupil diameter continued to enlarge 40 - 60 minutes after treatment, being widest at the time of the last measurement (9.9±2.0 mm).

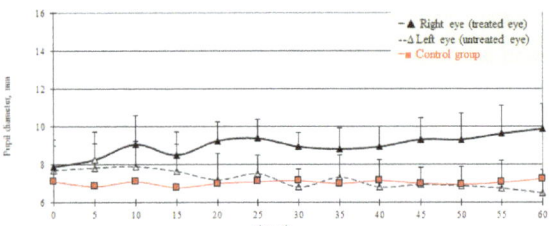

Fig. 6. Effect of 10% phenylephrine on the horizontal pupil diameter (mean values) in dogs.

In the left eye the HPD slightly decreased 15 minutes after treatment, and by 40 minutes had reached 6.5±1.2 mm (Fig. 6), which was statistically significantly lower than before the topical administration of phenylephrine (P<0.05).

Group 4 (saline)
In the fourth group of dogs we investigated the effects of topical saline on the IOP and the HPD. There were no significant differences in the IOP between right and left eye (16.6±2.0 mmHg) before topical application of saline (P>0.05). The mean IOP of the treated eye compared to the untreated eye did not change significantly throughout the measurement period; the IOP values varied from 16.6±2.0 mmHg – 17.3±2.0 mmHg. Our results regarding influence of topical saline on the HPD show that the mean HPD before application of saline in the right and the left eye was 7.1±1.2 mm; there were no significant differences in the HPD between eyes. Mean HPD in the treated eye compared to untreated eye did not significantly change throughout the measurement period (P>0.05).

Discussion
The IOP before drug administration in all dogs included in this study ranged from 12.8±1.8 mmHg to 17.7±3.1 mmHg. This is similar to previously reported values – 16.7±4.0 mmHg to 18.7±5.5 mmHg (Miller *et al.*, 1993; Gelatt and Mackay, 1998). In group 1 of this study we investigated the effects of topical 0.5% tropicamide on the IOP and the HPD during the first hour after treatment, to assess whether there is an increase in the IOP during diagnostic mydriasis. Contrary to the findings of Hacker and Farver (1988) where a significant increase in IOP was not observed after unilateral or bilateral tropicamide application, our research shows a significant increase in IOP immediately after unilateral application of 0.5% tropicamide while mydriasis was occurring. The IOP in the contralateral eye did not increase, showing no systemic influence. Importantly, the previous studies did not measure IOP throughout the period of mydriasis but merely at the point of maximal mydriasis (Hacker and Farver, 1988; Taylor *et al.*, 2007) while we show an increase during the phase of increasing pupil size, returning to normal at the point of maximal dilation. In similar research in cats, after unilateral application of tropicamide, the IOP significantly increased in the treated eye 1 and 1.5 h after treatment (Stadtbaumer *et*

al., 2006). Our findings showed that during the period of mydriasis in dogs, a statistically significant increase was occurred. In group 2 we determined the effects of the longer-acting parasympatholytic cholinergic blocking agent 1% atropine sulphate. In the treated eye the IOP increased significantly 10 minutes after application of topical atropine, retaining the maximal effect for 20 minutes. During the same period the IOP in the untreated eye did not change, suggesting that there are no systemic effects of 1% atropine sulphate after topical application in one eye.

Topical atropine increased the HPD, reaching a maximal pupil size maximum at 30 to 60 minutes after treatment, but without changing HPD in the contralateral eye. This data is similar to that published by Gelatt, demonstrating maximal pupil dilation in dogs, cats and cows at 30-60 min after administration of atropine (Gelatt *et al.*, 1973, 1995).

Latest research shows that 0.5% tropicamide and 1% atropine counteracted 0.005% latanoprost miotic effect, with atropine caused significantly larger mydriasis, but in this combination neither drug counteracted the hypotensive effect of latanoprost during this study period in healthy Labrador retrievers (Kahane *et al.*, 2016). Novel results were obtained with unilateral application of 10% phenylephrine. As well as increasing IOP in the treated eye, the contralateral eye also showed a significant increase in IOP, demonstrating that phenylephrine is absorbed into the circulation from the eye and has a profound systemic influence. This correlates with research by Pascoe *et al.* (1994) and Herring *et al.* (2004), where topical application of phenylephrine increase blood pressure and heart rate, indicating systemic absorption.

Studies regarding the influence of 10% phenylephrine on canine IOP have not been published in the literature until now, although studies in cats, monkeys and humans demonstrated no significant increase of IOP after topical application of phenylephrine in those species (Marchini *et al.*, 2003; Takayama *et al.*, 2004; Stadtbaumer *et al.*, 2006). Ten percent phenylephrine showed opposite effects on the HPD in the treated as compared to the un-treated eye: in treated eye HPD increased, but in the contralateral eye HPD decreased. These results are perplexing and show the need for further research on this drug.

In group 4, the control group, we investigated the effects of topical saline on the IOP and the HPD during the first hour after treatment. As we anticipated there were no changes in the IOP and the HPD in either eye during the full period of measurement.

Conclusion

In this study, contrary to previously published reports, we obtained an increase in the IOP in ophthalmically normal canine eyes undergoing mydriasis. The short period during which the IOP rises should not give rise

for concern for normal dog eyes, but where glaucoma is possible, as in dogs predisposed by breed to glaucoma, where the iridocorneal angle is already abnormal as shown by gonioscopy or where the contralateral eye already has glaucoma, caution should be taken in the mydriasis of the remaining sighted eye. We do not know whether mydriasis of eyes at risk of glaucoma might lead to a catastrophic permanent increase in IOP. However, we feel that the novel results here should be taken into consideration when performing ophthalmic examinations of dogs with breed or family history of glaucoma, or ones where gonioscopy has shown dysplastic changes in the iridocorneal angle. Further research is needed to define more completely the mechanism or mechanisms that can cause an increase of the IOP.

Conflict of interest

Authors declare that there was no conflict of interest.

Acknowledgments

The authors would like to thank assoc. prof. Ilze Matīse - VanHautan from Latvia University of Agriculture Faculty of Veterinary Medicine for her assistance and reviewing the manuscript.

References

Gartner, S. and Billet, E. 1957. Mydriatic glaucoma. Am. J. Ophthalmol. 43, 975-976.

Gelatt, K.N., Boggess, T.S. and Cure, T.H. 1973. Evaluation of mydriatics in the cat. J. Am. Anim. Hosp. Assoc. 9, 283-287.

Gelatt, K.N., Gum, G.G., Barrie, K.P. and Williams, L.W. 1981. Diurnal variations in intraocular pressure in normotensive and glaucomatous Beagles. Glaucoma 3, 121-124.

Gelatt, K.N., Gum, G.G. and Mackay, E.O. 1995. Evaluation of mydriatics in cattle. Vet. Comp. Ophthalmol. 5, 46-49.

Gelatt, K.N. and Mackay, E.O. 1998. Distribution of intraocular pressure in dogs. Vet. Ophthalmol. 1, 109-114.

Giannetto, C., Piccione, G. and Giudice, E. 2009. Daytime profile of the intraocular pressure and tear production in normal dog. Vet. Ophthalmol. 12(5), 302-305.

Gomes, F.E., Bentley, E., Lin, T.L. and McLellan, G.J. 2011. Effects of unilateral topical administration of 0.5% tropicamide on anterior segment morphology and intraocular pressure in normal cats and cats with primary congenital glaucoma. Vet. Ophthalmol. 14(Suppl. 1), 75-83.

Green, K. and Elijah, D. 1981. Drug effects on aqueous humor formation and pseudofacility in normal rabbit eyes. Exp. Eye Res. 33, 239-245.

Grozdanic, S.D., Kecova, H., Harper, M.M., Nilawera, W.M., Kuehn, M.H. and Kardon, R.H. 2010. Functional and structural changes in the canine model of hereditary primary angle-closure glaucoma. Invest. Ophthalmol. Vis. Sci. 51, 255-263.

Hacker, D.V. and Farver, T.B. 1988. Effects of tropicamide on intraocular pressure in normal dogs. J. Am. Anim. Hosp. Assoc. 24, 411-415.

Harris, L.S. 1968. Cycloplegia- induced intraocular pressure elevations a study of normal and open-angle glaucomatous eyes. Arch. Ophthalmol. 79(3), 242-246.

Harris, L.S. and Galin, M.A. 1969. Cycloplegic provocative testing. Arch. Ophthalmol. 81, 356-358.

Hatzav, M., Bdolah-Abram, T. and Ofri, R. 2016. Interaction with therapeutic soft contact lenses affects the intraocular efficacy of tropicamide and latanoprost in dogs. J. Vet. Pharmacol. Ther. 39(2), 138-143.

Herring, I.P., Jacobson, J.D. and Pickett, J.P. 2004. Cardiovascular effects of topical ophthalmic 10% phenylephrine in dogs. Vet. Ophthalmol. 7, 41-46.

Kahane, N., Raskansky, H., Bdolah-Abram, T. and Ofri, R. 2016. The effects of topical parasympatholytic drugs on pupil diameter and intraocular pressure in healthy dogs treated with 0.005% latanoprost. Vet. Ophthalmol. 19, 464-472.

Marchini, G., Babighian, S., Tosi, R., Perfetti, S. and Bonomi, L. 2003. Comparative study of the effects of 2% ibopamine, 10% phenylephrine, and 1% tropicamide on the anterior segment. Invest. Ophthalmol. Vis. Sci. 44, 281-289.

Miichi, H. and Nagataki, S. 1982. Effects of cholinergic drugs and adrenergic drugs on aqueous humor formation in the rabbit eye. Japanese J. Ophthalmol. 26, 425-436.

Miller, P.E., Pickett, J.P., Majors, L.J. and Kurzman, I.D. 1993. Clinical comparison of the Mackay-Marg and Tonopen applanation tonometers in the dog. Pro. Vet. Comp. Ophthalmol. 3, 67-73.

Molleda, J.M., Frau, M., Lopez, R., Bandrés, P. and Novales, M. 1988. Acción de los midriáticos sobre la presión intraocular en el perro. Med. Vet. 5, 29-32.

Ostin, L.A. and Glasser, A. 2004. The effects of phenylephrine on pupil diameter and accommodation in Rhesus monkeys. Invest. Ophthalmol. Vis. Sci. 45, 215-221.

Pascoe, P.J., Ilkiw, J.E., Stiles, J. and Smith, E.M. 1994. Arterial hypertension associated with topical ocular use of phenylephrine in dogs. J. Am. Vet. Med. Assoc. 205(11), 1562-1564.

Pauli, A.M., Bentley, E., Diehl, K.A. and Miller, P.E. 2006. Effects of the application of neck pressure by a collar or harness on intraocular pressure in dogs. J. Am. Anim. Hosp. Assoc. 42, 207-211.

Rengstorff, R.H. and Doughty, C.B. 1982. Mydriatic and cycloplegic drugs: a review of ocular and systemic complications. Am. J. Optom. Physiol. Opt. 59, 162-177.

Ribeiro, A.P., Crivelaro, R.M., Teixeira, P.P., Trujillo, D.Y., Guimarães, P.J., Vicente, W.R., Martins Bda, C. and Laus, J.L. 2014. Effects of different mydriatics on intraocular pressure, pupil diameter, and ruminal and intestinal motility in healthy sheep. Vet. Ophthalmol. 17(6), 397-402.

Rubin, L.F. and Wolfes, R.L. 1962. Mydriatics for veterinary ophthalmoscopy. J. Am. Vet. Med. Assoc. 140, 137-141.

Shaw, B.R. and Lewis, R.A. 1986. Intraocular pressure elevation after pupillary dilation in open-angle glaucoma. Arch. Ophthalmol. 104, 1185-1188.

Smith, C.M. and Reynard, A.M. 1992. Antimuscarinic Drugs. In Textbook of Pharmacology, Eds., Melsaac, R.J.: W.B. Saunders Company Philadelphia, pp: 108-115.

Stadtbaumer, K., Frommlet, F. and Nell, B. 2006. Effects of mydriatics on intraocular pressure and pupil size in the normal feline eye. Vet. Ophthalmol. 9, 233-237.

Stadtbaumer, K., Kostlin, R.G. and Zahn, K.J. 2002. Effects of topical 0.5% tropicamide on intraocular pressure in normal cats. Vet. Ophthalmol. 5, 107-112.

Takayama, J., Mishima, A. and Ishii, K. 2004. Effects of topical phenylephrine on blood flow in the posterior segment of monkey and aged human eyes. Japanese J. Ophthalmol. 3, 243-248.

Taylor, N.R., Zele, A.J., Vingrys, A.J. and Stanley, R.G. 2007. Variation in intraocular pressure following application of tropicamide in three different dog breeds. Vet. Ophthalmol. 10(Suppl. 1), 8-11.

Valle, O. 1974. Effect of cyclopentolate on the aqueous dynamics in incipient or suspected open-angle glaucoma. Acta Ophthalmol. Suppl. 123, 52-60.

Wallin-Hakanson, N. and Wallin-Hakanson, B. 2001. The effects of topical tropicamide and systemic medetomidine, followed by atipamezole reversal, on pupil size and intraocular pressure in normal dogs. Vet. Ophthalmol. 4, 3-6.

Ward, D.A. 1998. Clinical ophthalmic pharmacology and therapeutics. In Veterinary Ophthalmology, Eds., Gelatt, K.N., 3rd ed. Lippincott/Williams&Wilkins, Philadelphia, pp: 291-354.

Wu, S.C., Lee, Y.S., Wu, W.C. and Chang, S.H. 2015. Acute angle-closure glaucoma in retinopathy of prematurity following pupil dilation. BMC Ophthalmol. 15, 96. doi: 10.1186/s12886-015-0099-7.

Glucosamine and chondroitin use in canines for osteoarthritis

Angel Bhathal[1], Meredith Spryszak[2], Christopher Louizos[2] and Grace Frankel[2,*]

[1]*Faculty of Pharmacy and Pharmaceutical Sciences, University of Alberta, Edmonton, Alberta T6G 2H7, Canada*
[2]*College of Pharmacy, Faculty of Health Sciences, University of Manitoba, Winnipeg, Manitoba R3E 0T5, Canada*

Abstract

Osteoarthritis is a slowly progressive and debilitating disease that affects canines of all breeds. Pain and decreased mobility resulting from osteoarthritis often have a negative impact on the affected canine's quality of life, level of comfort, daily functioning, activity, behaviour, and client-pet companionship. Despite limited and conflicting evidence, the natural products glucosamine hydrochloride (HCl) and chondroitin sulfate are commonly recommended by veterinarians for treating osteoarthritis in dogs. There is a paucity of well-designed clinical veterinary studies investigating the true treatment effect of glucosamine and chondroitin. The purposes of this review article are to provide a brief background on glucosamine and chondroitin use in canine osteoarthritis and to critically review the available literature on the role of these products for improving clinical outcomes. Based on critical review, recommendations for practice are suggested and a future study design is proposed.

Keywords: Canine, Chondroitin, Glucosamine, Osteoarthritis, Veterinary.

Introduction

Osteoarthritis is a slowly progressive, degenerative, and debilitating disease affecting 20% of the canine population over the age of one (Johnston, 1997; Johnson *et al.*, 2001; Roush *et al.*, 2002; Aragon *et al.*, 2007). Large-breed dogs may develop more severe clinical signs and initial symptoms of osteoarthritis; however, dogs of all sizes and breeds are affected by the disease as they age (Rychel, 2010).

The etiology of osteoarthritis' pathology may include defective articular cartilage structure, inadequate cartilage biosynthesis, joint trauma, instability, and inflammatory mechanisms. The disease presents with symptoms such as pain, stiffness, lameness, and disability (D'Altilio *et al.*, 2007).

Pain and decreased mobility resulting from osteoarthritis often have a negative impact on the affected canine's quality of life, level of comfort, daily functioning (i.e. standing, walking), exercise tolerance, activity (i.e. playing, climbing stairs), behaviour, urinary and fecal habits, and client-pet companionship. Owners of severely affected dogs may decide to euthanize their pet (Rychel, 2010; Epstein *et al.*, 2015). Once a canine develops osteoarthritis, exploring treatment options becomes essential for minimizing the negative consequences of the disease. Non-pharmaceutical treatment options may include surgery, weight loss, exercise modification, and physical therapy (Beale, 2004).

Non-steroidal anti-inflammatory drugs (NSAIDs) are the current gold-standard pharmaceutical therapy for dogs with osteoarthritis; however, NSAIDs may cause gastrointestinal ulceration as an adverse effect and are contraindicated in the presence of renal insufficiency or dehydration. Other pharmaceutical options include diacerhein, corticosteroids, and hyaluronic acid (Henrotin *et al.*, 2005). Select nutraceuticals such as glucosamine, chondroitin, pentosane polysulphate, avocado/soybean unsaponifiables, green-lipped mussel, and milk protein have also been used (Henrotin *et al.*, 2005).

Glucosamine hydrochloride (HCl) and chondroitin sulfate (CS) are commonly recommended natural health products for treating osteoarthritis in dogs (Rychel, 2010). Glucosamine regulates the synthesis of collagen in cartilage and may provide mild anti-inflammatory effects while chondroitin sulfate inhibits destructive enzymes in joint fluid and cartilage. The two nutraceuticals also contribute to the synthesis of glycoaminoglycans and proteoglycans, which are building blocks for the formation of cartilage (Beale, 2004).

In humans, glucosamine is available in several dosage forms; glucosamine hydrochloride (HCl), glucosamine sulfate (stabilized with different salts, usually potassium chloride) and crystalline glucosamine sulfate. N-acetyl glucosamine is another available salt form, but it appears to have no clinical activity as compared to the other salt forms (Beale, 2004).

In terms of efficacy, crystalline glucosamine sulfate has shown the greatest efficacy for osteoarthritis of the knee which is likely due to an improved oral bioavailability (25%-44%) as compared to other glucosamine salts (Setnikar and Rovati, 2001; Persiani

*Corresponding Author: Grace Frankel. College of Pharmacy, Faculty of Health Sciences, University of Manitoba, Apotex Centre 750 McDermot Ave, Winnipeg, Manitoba, R3E 0T5, Canada. Email: *Grace.Frankel@umanitoba.ca*

et al., 2005; Altman, 2009). Crystalline glucosamine sulfate is a pharmaceutical-grade prescription product in Europe (but not in the United States or Canada) that consists of glucosamine, sulfate, sodium and chloride ions in a specific stoichiometric ratio (Altman, 2009). The other glucosamine salt forms (HCl, sulfate salts) have demonstrated variable efficacy in humans (Sawitzke et al., 2010; Rovati et al., 2012). This is primarily due to inconsistency in glucosamine content amongst nutraceutical products and poor oral bioavailability, especially in combination with other nutraceutical additives (Altman, 2009; Sawitzke et al., 2010; Wandel et al., 2010).

Similar to human products, there are various manufactured glucosamine and chondroitin products marketed for canines that differ in terms of strength, formulation, and additional active ingredients. Table 1 provides reference to various examples of glucosamine and chondroitin products marketed for canines. It should be noted that the majority of veterinary supplements contain glucosamine HCl, which is already known to have poorer bioavailability and poor clinical effect in humans.

There are several hypothesized reasons for this salt choice in veterinary products. First, the hydrochloride salt from a chemical perspective provides a greater amount of glucosamine per gram than does the sulfate salt despite the fact previous studies report overall lower oral bioavailability (Beale, 2004). The sulfate salt is often stabilized with sodium chloride (NaCl) or potassium chloride (KCl), which may be undesirable in aging canines with potential co-morbid medical conditions such as heart failure, hypertension or renal decline. Although this is a theoretical concern, human clinical trials have not demonstrated increases in blood pressure with NaCl content of crystallized glucosamine sulfate (Herrero-Beaumont et al., 2007; Rovati et al., 2012).

Last, the hydrochloride salt is much cheaper to produce; keeping in mind that crystalline glucosamine sulfate is manufactured as pharmaceutical-grade with strict quality control standards (Altman, 2009).

There is currently a lack of evidence to confirm a specific therapeutic dose of glucosamine in canines, yet, an adjunctive chondroitin dose of 15-30mg/kg has been suggested (Plumb, 2015). Few in vitro studies have provided bioavailability and pharmacokinetic data differentiating the most optimally absorbed glucosamine formulation in canines.

In horses, crystalline glucosamine sulfate achieves higher concentrations than glucosamine HCl (Meulyzer et al., 2008). One study in dogs demonstrated oral bioavailability of 12% and 5% for glucosamine hydrochloride and chondroitin sulfate respectively. (Adebowale et al., 2002).

Table 1. Examples of Nutraceutical Products Marketed for Canines with Osteoarthritis (Henrotin et al., 2005) and their Various Ingredients.

Propriety Name	Containing Ingredients/Tablet
ProMotion for Medium Large Dogs (PetMed Express Inc., 2016).	Glucosamine HCl 700 mg, Manganese 10 mg, Zinc 2 mg, Ascorbic Acid 25 mg, Cysteine 25 mg.
Dasuquin with MSM (Nutramax Laboratories Veterinary Sciences Inc., 2016b).	Large Dogs: Glucosamine HCl 900 mg, 350 mg CS, 90 mg Avocado/Soybean Unsaponifiables, 800 mg MSM. Small Dogs: Glucosamine HCl 600 mg, 250 mg CS, 45 mg Avocado/Soybean Unsaponifiables, 400 mg MSM.
Glyco-Flex III Soft Chews (Vetri-Science Laboratories, 2016).	Glucosamine HCl 1000 mg, MSM 1000 mg, Green Lipped Mussel 600 mg, DMG 100 mg, dl-alpha Tocopheryl Acetate 50 IU, Calcium Ascorbate 30 mg, Ascorbic Acid 24 mg, Mg 10 mg, Grape Seed Extract 5 mg, L-Glutathione 2 mg.
TerraMax Pro Hip & Joint Supplement (TerraMax Pro, 2016).	1600 mg Glucosamine HCl, 1200 mg Chondroitin Sulfate, 1000 mg Opti-MSM.
Extend K9 Health Formula Joint Care (Extend Joint Care, 2016).	Glucosamine HCl 300 mg, MSM, Type II Collagen, and Ascorbic Acid 400 mg, other quantities not specified.
Pet Naturals Hip & Joint Tablets (Pet Naturals of Vermont, 2016).	750 mg Glucosamine HCl, 400 mg Chondroitin Sulfate, MSM 400 mg, Ascorbic Acid 100 mg, Magnesium Proteinate 5 mg.
Cosequin DS (Nutramax Laboratories Veterinary Sciences Inc., 2016a).	Glucosamine HCl 500 mg, Chondroitin Sulfate 500 mg, Manganese 3 mg.
Liquid Health K9 Glucosamine (Liquid Health Inc., 2016).	Glucosamine HCl 1600 mg, CS 1200 mg, MSM 1000 mg, Manganese Chelate 7 mg, Hyaluronic Acid 10 mg.

(CS): Chondroitin sulfate; (DMG): Dimethylglycine; (HCL): Hydrochloride; (IU): International units; (MSM): Methyl-sulfonyl-methane.

Some studies have indicated that when administered to dogs as a combination, glucosamine and chondroitin are absorbed in as little as two hours (Beale, 2004). One commentary notes that glucosamine HCl and chondroitin sulfate require 10 to 20 times the quantity used in in vitro studies to reach a plasma concentration that will result in biological activity (Comblain et al., 2016).

It has been suggested that 2-6 weeks of treatment with glucosamine and chondroitin may be necessary for any therapeutic effect to become apparent (Plumb, 2015), but there is a lack of clinical evidence to support this statement. Potential adverse effects include hypersensitivity and minor gastrointestinal effects such as flatulence and stool softening (Plumb, 2015).

Veterinarians commonly recommend glucosamine and chondroitin for treating osteoarthritis in canines despite the lack of compelling scientific evidence demonstrating clinical benefit.

Clinical trials to date have used different products, salt forms, doses, and dosing regimens such that comparing the results to draw meaningful conclusions about therapeutic efficacy is difficult (Addleman, 2010). In addition, pharmacists are often approached by pet owners with questions about the use of over-the-counter natural products in pets due to the availability of these products in pharmacies.

Unfortunately, the lack of high-quality research on natural product use in pets makes it difficult to offer informed recommendations to pet owners with regard to glucosamine and chondroitin.

The purpose of this review is to critically appraise the available literature on the role of glucosamine and chondroitin in improving clinical outcomes in canines with osteoarthritis. We will propose evidence-based recommendations for practice and provide suggestions regarding the design of future clinical studies.

Evidence summary

Clinical trial: Glucosamine and chondroitin versus NSAID or placebo

Moreau *et al.* (2003) conducted a prospective, randomized, double-blinded study including 71 client-owned dogs >12 months old and >20 kg with owner-reported lameness and radiographic signs of osteoarthritis.

The trial consisted of four arms in which the subjects received either: 1) glucosamine HCl, chondroitin sulfate, and magnesium ascorbate (GSCM), 2) carprofen, 3) meloxicam, or 4) placebo. For complete dosing and titration schedules, please see Table 2.

Primary outcomes included treatment efficacy, tolerability and ease of administration. Efficacy was measured objectively through ground reaction force (GRF) values and subjectively through owner and orthopaedic surgeon assessments at 0, 30 and 60 days of treatment. Blood and faecal analyses were conducted on the same schedule to determine treatment safety. The placebo and GCSM arms did not experience statistically significant improvements in any of the outcome measures by trial end.

In contrast, both NSAID arms experienced significant improvements in GRF values and orthopaedic surgeon assessment scores; however, only the meloxicam arm experienced a significant improvement according to owner assessment.

The Moreau *et al.* (2003) trial had several strengths. The study was double-blinded, prospective and subjects were randomized to treatment groups. Additionally, the authors claimed that mean age, weight, affected limb GRF values, radiographic scores, and subjective scores of the dogs in the four study arms were all similar at baseline, although data to support this claim was not provided. Weaknesses of the trial included that glucosamine and chondroitin doses are much lower in comparison to other clinical trials and the treatment regimens differed between study arms.

The meloxicam arm received a loading dose, the GCSM dose was decreased over the course of the trial, and the placebo arm was discontinued after 30 days while all other interventions continued for 60 days. While the GCSM arm did not experience any significant outcome improvements by trial end, it is possible that the intervention was ineffective due to the absence of a GCSM loading dose, the use of sub-therapeutic GCSM doses throughout the trial, and/or an insufficient trial length. The fact that the improvement in GRF values experienced by the carprofen arm was not accompanied by an improvement in subjective owner assessment scores questions the clinical significance of GRF values. Eight of the 71 subjects (11.3%) were lost to follow-up and the authors did not disclose which study arms were affected by dropout.

Mean assessment scores with confidence intervals for GRF, orthopaedic surgeon assessment and owner assessment were not provided. The primary outcome stated by investigators was to identify the "best" treatment for dogs with osteoarthritis which requires appropriately designed statistical methods to compare treatment arms. However, statistical comparisons and treatment rankings were not provided and the magnitudes of the treatment effects were not reported.

Clinical trial: glucosamine and chondroitin versus placebo or NSAID

Investigators in the McCarthy *et al.* (2007) group conducted a prospective, randomized, double-blinded study that included 42 client-owned dogs, with 35 completing the trial. The dogs could be of any breed or sex, presenting with clinical signs of chronic lameness, stiffness, joint pain, and radiological evidence of osteoarthritis of the hips and/or elbows. The trial consisted of two arms in which the subjects received either: 1) glucosamine HCl, chondroitin sulfate, N-acetyl-D-glucosamine, ascorbic acid, and zinc sulfate or 2) carprofen. For complete dosing and titration schedules, please see Table 2. The primary outcome of efficacy in the treatment of osteoarthritis was determined through subjective veterinarian assessment at 0, 14, 42, 70 and 98 days of treatment.

Table 2. Literature Overview on Glucosamine and Chondroitin Use in Canines for Osteoarthritis.

Reference	Design, Subjects, & Duration	Intervention(s)	Findings/Results
Systematic Reviews			
Aragon *et al.* (2007)	Included 1 trial: - Moreau trial.	See Moreau trial summary below.	No subjective or objective improvements in comparison to placebo. Insufficient design quality for generalizability.
Vandeweerd *et al.* (2012)	Included 2 trials: - McCarthy trial. - Moreau trial.	See McCarthy & Moreau trial summaries below.	Trials used different compounds and had conflicting results. The McCarthy trial showed beneficial effects while the Moreau trial showed no effect; however, the Moreau trial used a combination of GHCl + CS + MA. Efficacy evidence is of low quality and MA may have contributed to the results.
Clinical Trials			
Moreau *et al.* (2003)	***Design:*** Prospective, randomized (via computer-generated list), double-blinded trial ***Subjects:*** 71 client-owned dogs with OA who were >12 months old and >20 kg with chronic and stable lameness reported by the owner plus radiographic signs of OA in one or two elbows, stifles, or hips; compared to pure-breed dogs with normal GRF measurements ***Exclusion criteria:*** Pregnancy; hypersensitivity to NSAIDs; neurological or musculoskeletal pathology; orthopaedic surgery within the same year; gait abnormalities involving both hind and fore limbs; concurrent osteoarthritis treatment ***Outcomes:*** Efficacy, tolerance, and ease of administration, measured at days 30 and 60 ***Objective outcome measures:*** GRF measurements (provided data about the level of pain-related functional impairment present) ***Subjective outcome measures:*** Gait, articular mobility, articular pain and discomfort (indicated by vocalization), lameness, and activity ***Duration:*** 30 or 60 days	***Number of study arms:*** Four ***Intervention:*** GHCl 500 mg + CS 400 mg + MA 75 mg dosed as either 2 caps AM and 1 cap in the afternoon for 30 days followed by 1 cap q12h for 30 days if <45 kg or 2 caps BID for 30 days followed by 2 caps AM and 1 cap at noon for 30 days if >45 kg ***Comparator arms:*** 1) Carprofen 2.2 mg/kg q12h for 60 days 2) Meloxicam 0.2 mg/kg for the first day followed by 0.1 mg/kg for 59 days 3) Placebo for 30 days	***Efficacy:*** The GHCl + CS + MA and placebo arms did not experience statistically significant improvements in any of the outcome measures by trial end. The carprofen arm experienced statistically significant improvements in GRF values and orthopaedic surgeon assessment scores, but not in subjective owner assessment scores. The meloxicam arm experienced statistically significant improvements in GRF values, orthopaedic surgeon assessment scores, and owner assessment scores ***Safety:*** One dog in the meloxicam arm experienced vomiting. One dog in the carprofen arm experienced anorexia, lethargy, jaundice, and vomiting and was diagnosed with toxic idiosyncratic hepatitis to carprofen. Both dogs were withdrawn from the trial.

Table 2: Literature Overview on Glucosamine and Chondroitin Use in Canines for Osteoarthritis (*Cont.*).

McCarthy *et al.* (2007)	*Design:* Multi-centered, prospective, randomized (alternating order of enrollment), double-blinded trial. *Subjects:* 42 client-owned dogs of any breed or sex presenting with clinical signs of chronic lameness (present for at least 1 month), stiffness, joint pain, and radiological evidence of OA of the hips and/or elbows; 35 completed the trial. *Exclusion criteria:* Pregnancy; current use of other medications; hepatic, renal, and/or CV disease; gastrointestinal ulceration; bleeding disorder; lameness due to infectious, immune-mediated, neurological, or neoplastic disease; previous use of drugs and/or dietary supplements for the treatment of OA. *Outcomes:* Efficacy in the treatment of confirmed OA, measured at days 14, 42, and 70; additionally, compliance was assessed by counting the number of capsules remaining at each visit. *Subjective outcome measures:* Scores for lameness, joint mobility, pain on palpation, weight-bearing, and an overall score for clinical condition; severity of condition, subjective veterinarian evaluation, and withdrawal symptoms were also measured. *Duration:* 70 days.	*Number of study arms:* Two *Intervention:* GHCl 475 mg/g, CS 350 mg/g, NADG 50 mg/g, AA 50 mg/g, and ZS 30 mg/g with total doses of 1 g, 1.5 g, or 2 g of active ingredient BID for 42 days for dogs weighing 5-19.9 kg, 20-40 kg, or >40 kg respectively, followed by a dose decrease by one-third of the original dose for the subsequent 28 days; administered with food. *Comparator arm:* Carprofen 2 mg/kg BID for 7 days followed by 2 mg/kg SID for the subsequent 63 days; administered with food.	*Efficacy:* The GHCl + CS + NADG + AA + ZS arm showed statistically significant improvements from baseline with regard to pain, weight-bearing, and overall condition scores at 70 days. Lameness and joint mobility scores did not improve significantly by trial end. The carprofen arm showed significant improvements from baseline with regard to all five parameters at or before 70 days. *Safety:* Two dogs in the GHCl + CS + NADG + AA + ZS arm experienced unspecified adverse drug reactions and were withdrawn from the trial.
Gupta *et al.* (2012)	*Design:* Prospective, randomized, controlled, double-blinded trial. *Subjects:* 31-37 client-owned dogs (each of the four trial arms consisted of 7-10 dogs) weighing >40 lbs with moderate OA. *Exclusion criteria:* Serious concomitant diseases or complications. *Outcomes:* Therapeutic efficacy, tolerability, and safety, measured on a monthly basis. *Objective outcome measures:* Peak vertical force and impulse area measurements obtained with a piezoelectric sensor-based ground force plate (indicators of lameness due to pain); physical, hepatic, and renal functions were monitored via body weight, temperature, pulse, ALP, ALT, bilirubin, BUN, and Cr measurements. *Subjective outcome measures:* Overall pain, pain upon limb manipulation (vocalization), pain after physical exertion (limping and limb rigidity), signs of pain, signs of lameness, severity of pain during various activities (i.e. playing), and overall performance assessments (running, participation in activities, movement, change between sitting and standing). *Duration:* 150 days.	*Number of study arms:* Four *Interventions:* 1) GHCl 2000 mg + CS 1600 mg + UCII 10 mg given daily 2) GHCl 2000 mg + CS 1600 mg given daily 3) UCII 10 mg given daily *Comparison arm:* Placebo given daily.	*Efficacy:* The placebo arm did not experience statistically significant changes in any of the outcome measures by trial end. The GHCl + CS arm exhibited a significant reduction in pain by day 90 with maximal effects observed on day 150. Specifically, overall pain had decreased by 51%, pain after limb manipulation had decreased by 48%, and pain after physical exertion had decreased by 43% from baseline at 150 days. Ground force plate-based parameters remained significantly unchanged by trial end. Supplementing GHCl + CS with UCII did not provide any additional benefit. *Safety:* None of the dogs receiving dietary supplements showed any signs of adverse effects.

Table 2. Literature Overview on Glucosamine and Chondroitin Use in Canines for Osteoarthritis (*Cont.*).

D'Altilio *et al.* (2007)	*Design:* Prospective, randomized, controlled, double-blinded trial. *Subjects:* 20 client-owned dogs presenting with joint stiffness, lameness, moderate pain, swollen joints, difficulty getting up/down, and difficulty walking in horizontal areas or stairs due to OA. *Outcomes:* Therapeutic efficacy and safety, measured on a monthly basis. *Objective outcome measures:* Body weight, hepatic function (ALT, bilirubin), and renal function (BUN, Cr) were measured to monitor for adverse effects. *Subjective outcome measures:* Overall pain (trouble changing between sitting and standing, vocalization, crying), pain upon limb manipulation (vocalization), and exercise-associated lameness (limping, holding limb up, limb rigidity). *Duration:* 120 days of intervention exposure followed by a 30-day withdrawal period.	*Number of study arms:* Four *Interventions:* 1) GHCl 2000 mg + CS 1600 mg + UCII 10 mg given daily 2) GHCl 2000 mg + CS 1600 mg given daily 3) UCII 10 mg given daily *Comparison arm:* Placebo given daily	*Efficacy:* The placebo arm did not experience statistically significant changes in any of the outcome measures by trial end. The GHCl + CS arm experienced a reduction in pain that was not significant and showed relapse following the 30-day treatment withdrawal period. Supplementing GHCl + CS with UCII did reduce overall pain, pain upon limb manipulation, and exercise induced lameness to a significant extent, although this benefit was also lost following the 30-day treatment withdrawal period. *Safety:* None of the dogs receiving dietary supplements showed any signs of adverse effects.
In Vitro Studies Anderson *et al.* (1999)	N=2 adult female dogs recently euthanized for reasons unrelated to orthopedic abnormalities. Measured chondrocytes for viable cells, PGE2 and GAG concentrations at days 3, 6, and 12.	*Number of study arms:* Three *Interventions:* 1) Chondrocytes cultured in glucosamine 100 mcg/mL. 2) Chondrocytes cultured in acetylsalicylate 18 mcg/mL. 3) Chondrocytes cultured in a control medium.	Chondrocytes in all three mediums had characteristics indicative of viability and differentiation.
Adebowale *et al.* (2002)	Randomized three-way single dose cross-over study and multiple dose open study. N=8 male beagle dogs of age >6 months weighing approximately 9 kg. Bioavailability and pharmacokinetics of single and multiple doses were measured through blood and plasma samples. A typical blood sampling scheme was measured pre-dose and at 0.5, 1, 2, 4, 6, 8, 10, 12, 14, and 24 hours following drug administration.	*Number of study arms:* Four *Interventions:* 1) IV GHCl 500 mg + LMWCS 400 mg for 14 days. 2) PO GHCl 1500 mg + LMWCS 1200 mg for 14 days. 3) PO GHCl 2000 mg + LMWCS 1600 mg for 14 days. 4) PO GHCl 1500 mg + LMWCS 1200 mg on days 1-7 followed by PO GHCl 3000 mg + LMWCS 2400 mg on days 8-14.	GHCl and LMWCS are bioavailable after oral dosing. LMWCS results in significant accumulation upon multiple dosing. GHCl and LMWCS BA were 12% and 5%, respectively. Cmax=8.95 mcg/mL and Tmax=1.5 hours following 1500 mg dose of GHCl. Cmax=21.5 mcg/mL following 1600 mg dose of CS.

Table 2. Literature Overview on Glucosamine and Chondroitin Use in Canines for Osteoarthritis (*Cont.*).

Surrogate Outcome Trials			
Johnson *et al.* (2001)	N=16 pure-bred dogs weighing 23-32 kg with surgically-induced OA; not client-owned. Measured concentrations of synovial fluid markers at 0, 1, 3, & 5 months.	***Number of study arms:*** Four ***Interventions:*** 1) GHCl 250 mg + CS 200 mg + MA 5 mg + CCL reconstruction. 2) GHCl 250 mg + CS 200 mg + MA 5 mg + sham CCL reconstruction. 3) Sham CCL reconstruction 4) CCL reconstruction.	Heterogeneity of results from synovial fluid analyses reported. GHCl + CS + MA arms had significantly higher levels of beneficial synovial fluid markers; however, concentrations were not localized to joints.
Canapp *et al.* (1999)	N=32 skeletally mature mixed-breed dogs of age 1-5 years weighing 4.5-11 kg with chemically-induced synovitis. Measured SA at days 13, 20, 27, 34, 41, and 48 post-SI; measured lameness at days 1-48 post-SI.	***Number of study arms:*** Four ***Interventions:*** 1) GHCl 500 mg + CS 400 mg + manganese 10 mg + ascorbate 66 mg (GlAm-CS) q8h for 21 days pre-SI, then GlAm-CS for 48 days post-SI. 2) Placebo for 21 days pre-SI, then GlAm-CS for 48 days post-SI. 3) Placebo for 21 days pre-SI, then GlAm-CS + SAMe 200 mg for 48 days post-SI 4) Placebo for 21 days pre-SI, then placebo for 48 days post-SI.	Dogs given pre-SI GlAm-CS showed significantly less soft-tissue SA at day 48 and significantly less bone SA at days 41 and 48 compared to the other study arms, with less SA being suggestive of a protective effect against synovitis. Dogs given pre-SI GlAm-CS showed a significant decrease in lameness on days 12, 19, 23, and 24 compared to the other study arms. Significant differences in SA and lameness were not found at any time among the study arms that did not receive pre-SI therapy.
Review Articles			
Pascoe (2002)	Not applicable.	Glucosamine & chondroitin.	Article reviews studies in humans, horses, and dogs.
Henrotin *et al.* (2005)	Not applicable.	Glucosamine sulfate & CS.	*In vitro* studies show increased production of proteoglycans by chondrocytes; however, results cannot be extrapolated to different preparations. No scientifically conducted trials demonstrate disease-modifying properties.
Johnston *et al.* (2008)	Not applicable.	GHCl & CS.	Refers to Moreau and McCarthy trials. Concludes that based on the quality of the trials, one can be moderately comfortable with the results despite their lack of consistency.
Addleman (2010)	Not applicable.	Glucosamine & chondroitin.	Purity, quality, efficacy, dosing, and absorption of glucosamine and chondroitin vary and evidence is limited. There is a need for validated owner questionnaires, long-term studies with objective measures, and a better understanding of their mode of action.
McKenzie (2010)	Not applicable	Glucosamine & chondroitin	The evidence is limited in terms of quantity and quality and the results are mixed.

Table 2. Literature Overview on Glucosamine and Chondroitin Use in Canines for Osteoarthritis (*Cont.*).

KuKanich (2013)	Not applicable.	Glucosamine & chondroitin dosed q24h.	Current literature does not support the use of glucosamine and chondroitin for the control of osteoarthritis pain in dogs.
Comblain *et al.* (2016)	Not applicable.	Glucosamine & chondroitin.	Studies have contrasting results.
Neil *et al.* (2005)	Not applicable.	Glucosamine & chondroitin.	*In vitro* studies indicate rapid absorption, a good safety profile, and chondroprotective effects in dogs. Minimal effective concentrations of these compounds and beneficial effects in dogs require further investigation.

(AA): Ascorbic acid; (ALP): Alkaline phosphatase; (ALT): Alanine transaminase; (AM): Morning, (BA): Bioavailability; (BID): Twice daily; (BUN): Blood urea nitrogen; (CCL): Cranial cruciate ligament; (Cmax): Maximum or peak serum concentration; (Cr): Creatinine; (CS): Chondroitin sulfate; (CV): Cardiovascular; (GAG): Glycosaminoglycan; (GHCl): Glucosamine hydrochloride; (GlAm-CS): Glucosamine and chondroitin sulfate; (GRF): Ground reaction force; (IV): Intravenous; (LMWCS): Low molecular weight chondroitin sulfate; (MA): Manganese ascorbate; (MSM): Methyl-sulfonyl-methane; (N): Number of study subjects; (NADG): N-acetyl-D-glucosamine; (OA): Osteoarthritis; (PGE2): Prostaglandin E2; (PO): By mouth; (q12H): Every 12 hours; (SAMe): S-adenosyl-L-methionine; (SA): Scintigraphic activity; (SI): Synovitis induction; (SID): Once daily; (Tmax): Time to reach maximum concentration; (UCII): Undenatured collagen type II; (ZS): Zinc sulfate.

The outcome measures included scores for joint mobility, lameness, pain on palpation, weight-bearing, and an overall score for clinical condition. In the carprofen arm, statistically significant improvements were found between the pre-treatment and change scores for all five efficacy parameters at or before 70 days. In contrast, the glucosamine and chondroitin arm showed statistically significant improvements in pain, weight-bearing, and overall condition for the first time at 70 days, while lameness and joint mobility did not improve to a significant extent by trial end. The authors also concluded that glucosamine and chondroitin therapy was non-inferior to carprofen therapy at day 70 in the treatment of osteoarthritis in dogs.

The McCarthy *et al.* (2007) trial was multi-centered, randomized, double-blinded, and prospective which is an ideal study design. However, the method of randomization was determined by order of presentation (alternating), which introduces the risk of selection bias since the ability to anticipate treatment allocation may potentially influence the order of enrollment. Baseline characteristics of the two groups of canines had some variation in terms of mean weight, age, and affected joints.

Therapeutic efficacy scores were based on subjective assessments conducted by veterinarians, which could be highly variable between clinicians. Six dogs from the glucosamine and chondroitin arm failed to complete the study, two of which were withdrawn due to experiencing unspecified adverse drug reactions. One dog from the carprofen arm failed to complete the study. With seven dropouts, the loss to follow-up was high (16.7%). The collected data underwent a per-protocol analysis (versus intention-to-treat) therefore we cannot comment on the robustness of the results.

The reported result of therapeutic efficacy in the carprofen arm did support the validity of the results for the glucosamine and chondroitin arm. However, the absence of a comparator placebo arm in the study design calls into question whether the glucosamine and chondroitin arm was more or less effective as compared to placebo.

The authors claimed that glucosamine and chondroitin therapy was *non-inferior* to carprofen therapy at day 70. Non-inferiority studies often require large sample sizes and rigorous statistical methods to demonstrate non-inferiority between two treatments. The decision to use a sample size that provided 78% power to detect a difference in the median subjective veterinarian assessment score of one point was questionable and lacking in transparency of statistical method design. A median reduction of one point in the subjective veterinarian assessment score represented a clinically significant improvement in the canines' condition, but justification for selection of this score was absent.

Clinical trials: Glucosamine/chondroitin versus undenatured collagen type II, placebo, or glucosamine/chondroitin/undenatured collagen type II

Gupta *et al.* (2012) conducted a prospective, randomized, double-blinded study that included approximately 31-37 client-owned dogs weighing >40 lbs with moderate osteoarthritis. The trial consisted of four arms in which the subjects received either 1) glucosamine HCl, chondroitin sulfate, and undenatured collagen type II (UCII), 2) glucosamine HCl and chondroitin sulfate, 3) UCII, or 4) placebo. For complete dosing schedules, please see Table 2. Outcomes included therapeutic efficacy, tolerability, and safety. Efficacy was measured objectively through peak vertical force and impulse area measurements obtained with a piezoelectric sensor-based ground force plate (GFP) and subjectively through observational pain assessments on a monthly basis for 150 days. Additionally, the physical, hepatic, and renal functions of the dogs were monitored each month via body weight, temperature, pulse, alkaline phosphatase (ALP), alanine transaminase (ALT), bilirubin, blood urea nitrogen (BUN), and creatinine (Cr) measurements. The placebo arm showed no statistically significant changes in any of the outcome measures by trial end. The glucosamine and chondroitin arm exhibited a significant reduction in subjectively-assessed pain at 90 days with maximal effects observed at 150 days. The GFP-based parameters remained significantly unchanged by trial end. Supplementing glucosamine and chondroitin with UCII did not provide any additional benefit. None of the dogs receiving dietary supplements showed any signs of adverse effects.

Strengths of the Gupta *et al.* (2012) trial were that it was prospective, randomized, controlled, and double-blinded. Weaknesses of the trial were that baseline patient characteristic information was not provided and the analysis protocol was vague.

Investigators in the D'Altilio *et al.* (2007) group conducted a prospective, randomized, double-blinded study that included 20 client-owned dogs with joint stiffness, lameness, moderate pain, swollen joints, difficulty getting up/down, and difficulty walking in horizontal areas or stairs due to osteoarthritis. The trial consisted of four arms in which the interventions were identical to those in the Gupta *et al.* (2012) trial. However, in contrast, intervention exposure lasted only 120 days followed by a 30-day withdrawal period. Outcomes included therapeutic efficacy and safety. Efficacy was measured subjectively through observational pain assessments on a monthly basis for 150 days. Additionally, body weight, hepatic function (ALT, bilirubin), and renal function (BUN, Cr) were measured each month to monitor for adverse effects. While the placebo arm exhibited no statistically significant changes in any of the outcome measures by trial end, the other results of the D'Altilio *et al.* (2007) trial differed from those of the Gupta *et al.* (2012) trial. The glucosamine and chondroitin arm showed a reduction in pain that was not significant and relapsed following the withdrawal of treatment for 30 days. As well, supplementing glucosamine and chondroitin with UCII did provide additional benefit to the point of reducing pain to a significant extent, although this benefit was also lost following the withdrawal of treatment for 30 days. None of the dogs receiving dietary supplements showed any signs of adverse effects. Strengths of the D'Altilio *et al.* (2007) trial were that it was prospective, randomized, controlled, and double-blinded. Weaknesses of the trial were that the baseline patient characteristics were unspecified and the follow-up and analysis protocol were unclear.

Surrogate endpoint/in vitro studies

In vitro studies investigating surrogate outcomes related to osteoarthritis treatment in dogs suggest that the use of glucosamine and chondroitin produces chondroprotective effects (Anderson *et al.*, 1999). Currently, good-quality evidence does not exist to suggest that *in vitro* studies using surrogate endpoints translate into clinically meaningful improvements in canine osteoarthritis symptoms. Table 2 provides a brief summary of surrogate endpoint/*in vitro* trials for reader interest.

Review articles

Eight commentaries reviewing the evidence around glucosamine and chondroitin use in canines with osteoarthritis were available in the literature. These commentaries are presented below in chronological order from the time of publication.

The Pascoe (2002), Henrotin *et al.* (2005), and Neil *et al.* (2005) commentaries pre-date or opt not to discuss clinical trials investigating the use of glucosamine and chondroitin for pain reduction and improved mobility in canines. However, Pascoe (2002) notes that despite the lack of clinical evidence, 62% of surveyed veterinary practitioners reported recommending products containing glucosamine and chondroitin for canines because they believed that they were seeing beneficial effects with their use. Similarly, Henrotin *et al.* (2005) appear to give precedence to anecdote over scientific evidence by concluding that glucosamine and chondroitin have clearly demonstrated symptomatic action. Neil *et al.* (2005) concludes that the determination of the minimal effective concentrations of glucosamine and chondroitin and their beneficial effects in canines require further investigation.

The Johnston *et al.* (2008) commentary refers to the Aragon *et al.* (2007) systematic review, the Moreau *et al.* (2003) trial, and the McCarthy *et al.* (2007) trial. The authors conclude that despite having conflicting results, the two studies shared similar strengths such that one can have a moderate level of comfort with the results from both studies. In contrast, the Addleman commentary (Addleman, 2010) identifies the lack of high-quality clinical trials and objective measures of efficacy as well as the unknown absorption and duration of effect of nutraceuticals as limitations in the current evidence around glucosamine and chondroitin use in canines with osteoarthritis.

The author concludes that objective methods for measuring joint disease symptoms, mobility, and pain using force plate gait analysis, accelerometers, and validated pain scales need to be established and that effective glucosamine and chondroitin dosing needs to be determined using dogs as the study subjects, as canine dosing is currently extrapolated from studies conducted in other species and therefore suboptimal. Similarly, the McKenzie (2010) commentary concludes that clinical trial evidence is severely limited. The author calls for veterinarians to translate the uncertainty around the usefulness of glucosamine and chondroitin therapy when discussing this treatment option with dog owners. McKenzie (2010) points out that there is a lack of literature addressing the use of glucosamine and chondroitin as an adjunct to NSAID therapy.

KuKanich (2013) commentary concludes that current literature does not support the use of glucosamine and chondroitin for the control of osteoarthritis in dogs, although this conclusion appears to be based solely on the Moreau et al. (2003) trial. Finally, the Comblain et al. (2016) commentary objectively presents the negative results of the Moreau et al. (2003) trial in contrast to the relatively positive results of the McCarthy et al. (2007), D'Altilio et al. (2007), and Gupta et al. (2012) trials without offering any conclusions or recommendations.

Discussion

Nutraceuticals are not considered medicinal products and are consequently not regulated by the United States Food and Drug Administration (FDA); therefore manufacturers are not required to provide scientific information to legal authorities for approval (Vandeweerd et al., 2012).

Health Canada, through the Veterinary Drugs Directorate (VDD) has the mandate to set standards for, evaluate and monitor the safety, quality, and effectiveness of, and promote the prudent use of veterinary drugs including veterinary natural health products (Health Canada, 2013). Despite the trend towards more stringent criteria for veterinary nutraceutical products, the research community continues to conduct and publish novel, low-quality studies without consistent evaluation methods and varying products/doses.

The lack of high-quality, peer-reviewed literature makes it difficult to draw conclusions about therapies. Nutraceutical studies commonly have limitations related to methods of participant recruitment and randomization, baseline characteristic data reporting, intervention standardization and concealment, blinding, participant retention, follow-up procedures, and overall protocol. In contrast, background, objectives, interventions, and statistical results tend to be well-reported (Vandeweerd et al., 2012).

Based on the available literature, the potential benefits of glucosamine and chondroitin use in osteoarthritic canines can neither be confirmed nor denied. Glucosamine and chondroitin use in canines requires further clinical study using improved methodology. Clinical trials conducted to date have yielded mixed results.

These results are of questionable validity due to several trial shortcomings. First is the absence of therapeutic standardization. The sources of active ingredients, manufacturers of products, formulations, combinations of active ingredients, treatment doses, regimens, and durations of therapy differed significantly between trials. Second, multiple potential sources of bias were present in the trials, including the lack of a standardized follow-up timeframe, unexplained loss to follow-up, flawed study protocols, and incomplete data sets. Moreover, all of the clinical trials relied on subjective outcome measures to some extent, and the absence of standardized owner and veterinarian assessments increased the risk of bias in the reported results and diminished internal study validity.

The trials generally lacked peer review and were at risk of funding bias due to company sponsorship. Finally, there was an overall lack of generalizability of trial results. The trials were small in terms of the number of subjects used and subject baseline characteristics were not always disclosed. We cannot confidently extrapolate results from in-vitro studies using dogs with surgically/chemically-induced osteoarthritis to the client-owned dogs with naturally occurring osteoarthritis seen in practice.

Future study design proposal

From the above discussion, there is a clear need for a high-quality clinical study to evaluate the effect of glucosamine and chondroitin in canines with osteoarthritis. Table 3 proposes an ideal study design for a randomized clinical trial.

Our rationale for the study design aims to rectify common criticisms of previous study designs. We recommend conducting a multi-centered trial facilitated within veterinary orthopaedic surgery institutions and/or veterinary college institutions to eliminate funding bias. Client-owned dogs with naturally occurring osteoarthritis would be recruited and stratified according to disease severity (mild, moderate, or severe) using objective guideline measurements (i.e. radiographic imaging and semi-objective veterinary guideline assessment measurements).

Radiographic imaging to evaluate efficacy would include joint capsular distention, soft tissue thickening, and narrowed joint spaces. However, it is important to note that radiographic severity often does not correlate with clinical severity of disease. Thus, a standardized, semi-objective veterinary assessment would also be necessary for assessing disease severity and progression (Tilley and Smith, 2015). Once stratified, the dogs would be randomized into study arms using a central computerized system. All data collectors, analyzers, investigators, pet owners, subjects, and clinicians involved in the study would be blinded to the allocation of treatment.

Table 3. Future Study Design Proposal.

Patients	Client-owned dogs with naturally occurring osteoarthritis.
Inclusion	All breeds Age >1 year Weight >20 kg
Exclusion	Pregnancy; use of medications; hepatic, renal, or CV disease; gastrointestinal ulceration; bleeding disorder; lameness due to infectious, immune-mediated, neurological, or neoplastic disease.

Intervention	Dosages and regimen: 4 treatment arms
	   1) GHCl monotherapy
	       GHCl 475mg BID for dogs 5-19.9 kg
	       GHCl 712.5mg BID for dogs 20-40 kg
	       GHCl 950mg for dogs >40 kg
	   2) GHCl and CS combination
	       GHCl 475mg/CS 350mg BID for dogs 5-19.9 kg
	       GHCl 712.5mg/ CS 525mg BID for dogs 20-40 kg
	       GHCl 950mg/CS 700mg BID for dogs >40 kg
	   3) Crystalline glucosamine sulfate (unknown dose)
	   4) Placebo (control)
	Formulation: Liquid (appears to produce higher peak concentrations in comparison to tablets) (Maxwell et al., 2016).
	Administration: With food (typical home environments would have intervention administered in conjunction with food) (Maxwell et al., 2016).

Control	Placebo (liquid).
Open Label NSAID	Carprofen 2.2 mg/kg q12h.
Randomization	Stratified randomization based on disease severity.
Allocation Concealment	Central computerized random allocation, with all assessors, investigators, analyzers, owners, clinicians, and subjects blinded to treatment allocation.
Outcome	Primary outcomes: 1. Subjective: The owner's assessment of the pet's clinical presentation and quality of life using a standardized OA pain questionnaire (i.e. LOAD) 2. Semi-objective: A standardized clinical pain and OA assessment by a veterinarian 3. Objective: Radiographic changes, force plate gait analysis, static load bearing (to quantify reduced limb loading (Tilley and Smith, 2015)), and kinematics Secondary outcomes: Pharmacokintic characteristics of each dosage form, use of open-label NSAID, safety outcomes (adverse effects) and client/patient adherence.
Size	Calculated using the clinically significant difference in primary outcome score, expected standard deviation, and desired levels of confidence and power.
Baseline Characteristics Reported	Disease severity, number and location(s) of affected joints, weight, age, breed, athletic history, disorders that affect collagen or cartilage synthesis (Cushing's disease, diabetes mellitus, hypothyroidism) (Tilley and Smith, 2015).
Centre	Multi-centred, using veterinary or orthopaedic college institution(s).
Duration	≥90 days (potentially 1 year of follow-up if funding permits).

(CS): Chondroitin sulfate; (GHCl): Glucosamine hydrochloride; (LOAD): Liverpool Osteoarthritis in Dogs; (OA): osteoarthritis.

Baseline characteristics including age, number of affected joints, location of affected joints, breed, weight, comorbidities, and other medications used would be included in the study. Appropriate inclusion and exclusion criteria would be pre-specified. The study size would need to be sufficiently large to ensure internal validity through statistical adjudication.

The intervention in our proposed study would ideally be a multi-arm trial. A prospective superiority trial would consist of 4 treatment arms: 1) glucosamine HCl monotherapy, 2) glucosamine HCl and chondroitin sulfate in combination, 3) crystalline glucosamine sulfate and 4) placebo. Glucosamine and chondroitin are slow-acting agents; therefore, a study examining their long-term use would be appropriate. Serial blood samples would be helpful to determine pharmacokinetic characteristics of the different dosage forms. We would recommend a trial of at least 90 days in duration, with possible extension to 1 year of follow-up. However, longer treatment duration is often limited by cost and client/patient adherence to medication regimen. Conditions of treatment administration could be further defined once efficacy has been established. A method of measuring compliance such as a client-completed dosing journal would be superior to reviewing the product returned by the owner, as dose absence does not necessarily equate to the successful administration of the dose. Additionally, analysing the data using both intention-to-treat and per-protocol analyses would establish the robustness of the results and reduce bias. For ethical reasons, allowing the open-label use of a standardized NSAID regimen (carprofen or meloxicam) for all subjects as needed would be ethically appropriate. NSAID use would be documented for both study arms and could be reported as a secondary outcome. The risks of all the interventions would be presented and explained to each dog owner using informed consent.

It is important to note that when drawing conclusions from a study, statistically significant results are not always indicative of clinical importance (Addleman, 2010). Pre-defining clinically meaningful results prior to the trial would help to establish whether or not the glucosamine and chondroitin intervention would be advantageous for use. Minimizing the risk of type 1 or type 2 errors by conducting a proper sample size calculation is also essential for producing trustworthy study results.

Objective guidelines and measures would be used to assess the baseline severity of osteoarthritis, clinical disease progression, and benefits of therapy. Primary outcomes would also be measured with a semi-objective standardized clinical assessment conducted by veterinarians or orthopedic surgeons. A thorough history, physical examination, and standardized pain-rating scale as well as objective measures such as radiograph, force plate gait analysis, and kinematic results would all be essential for generating a complete picture of the canines in the trial.

Additionally, standardized pain and activity scoring tools completed by the dog owners would provide subjective data as an adjunct to the objective and semi-objective data. The Liverpool Osteoarthritis in Dogs' Clinical Metrology Instrument (LOAD) is a good option for gathering subjective data from the dog owners as it is easy to use, validated, and has demonstrated a correlation with force-platform data (Walton et al., 2013).

The LOAD tool considers the pet's background, lifestyle, and mobility; specifically, it assesses the pet's level of exercise, activity, lameness, and stiffness, as well as the effects of the weather. As mentioned earlier, secondary outcomes to measure may include the frequency of open-label NSAID use.

Future studies require greater transparency to promote educated recommendations by veterinarians and pharmacists to dog owners. Studies should always disclose complete information with regard to the ingredients present in an intervention, subject baseline data, dates of recruitment and follow up, references of publications used, data for every item measured, and data analysis methods used such that readers can interpret the results independently.

Studies should also report the flux of participants using a flow chart that specifies the number of patients that were eligible, excluded, included, stratified, randomized, treated as intended, analyzed for the primary outcome(s), and lost to follow-up (Vandeweerd et al., 2012). Reporting the number of patients lost to follow-up and documented reasons for drop-out is standard safety reporting for clinical trials. Authors should determine the risk versus benefit ratios objectively. Lastly, the authors' conclusions and interpretations should be consistent with the study results.

Once higher-quality randomized controlled trials have been conducted, the quality of systematic reviews would also increase. Additionally, well-structured observational studies would help limit the heterogeneity of the results and ensure that fair comparisons between studies are made (Addleman, 2010). Literature should also be peer-reviewed to make the interpretation of study results and their application to practice easier.

Conclusion

Glucosamine and chondroitin are commonly recommended by veterinarians as an alternative for treating osteoarthritis in canines unable to tolerate the adverse effects of NSAIDs, or as add-on therapy. Although glucosamine and chondroitin have benign adverse effect profiles, the clinical benefit of using these agents remains questionable. The available evidence is difficult to interpret due to the use of different manufacturers, salt forms, compositions, sources, strengths, regimens, therapy durations, and combinations of active ingredients. Further study is required in order to clarify the uncertainty around the clinical benefit of using these agents and quantify any treatment effect that exists.

Conflict of interest statement

The authors declare that there are no conflicts of interest regarding the writing of this paper.

References

Addleman, A. 2010. Evaluation of glucosamine hydrochloride/chondroitin sulfate nutraceuticals as a treatment to improve symptoms associated with canine and feline joint disease. Retrieved from https://www.banfield.com/Banfield/media/PDF/Downloads/CriticallyAppraisedTopics/2010_Winter_CAT_Evaluation-of-Nutraceuticals.pdf

Adebowale, A., Du, J., Liang, Z., Leslie, J.L. and Eddington, N.D. 2002. The bioavailability and pharmacokinetics of glucosamine hydrochloride and low molecular weight chondroitin sulfate after single and multiple doses to beagle dogs. Biopharm. Drug Dispos. 23(6), 217-225.

Altman, R.D. 2009. Glucosamine therapy for knee osteoarthritis: pharmacokinetic considerations. Expert Rev. Clin. Pharmacol. 2(4), 359-371.

Anderson, C.C., Cook, J.L., Kreeger, J.M., Tomlinson, J.L. and Wagner-Mann, C.C. 1999. In vitro effects of glucosamine and acetylsalicylate on canine chondrocytes in three-dimensional culture. Am. J. Vet. Res. 60(12), 1546-1551.

Aragon, C.L., Hofmeister, E.H. and Budsberg, S.C. 2007. Systematic review of clinical trials of treatments for osteoarthritis in dogs. J. Am. Vet. Med. Assoc. 230(4), 514-521.

Beale, B.S. 2004. Use of nutraceuticals and chondroprotectants in osteoarthritic dogs and cats. Vet. Clin. North Am. Small Anim. Pract. 34(1), 271-289.

Canapp, S.O.Jr., McLaughlin, R.M.Jr., Hoskinson, J.J., Roush, J.K. and Butine, M.D. 1999. Scintigraphic evaluation of dogs with acute synovitis after treatment with glucosamine hydrochloride and chondroitin sulfate. Am. J. Vet. Res. 60(12), 1552-1557.

Comblain, F., Serisier, S., Barthelemy, N., Balligand, M. and Henrotin, Y. 2016. Review of dietary supplements for the management of osteoarthritis in dogs in studies from 2004 to 2014. J. Vet. Pharmacol. Ther. 39(1), 1-15.

D'Altilio, M., Peal, A., Alvey, M., Simms, C., Curtsinger, A., Gupta, R.C., Canerdy, T.D., Goad, J.T., Bagchi, M. and Bagchi, D. 2007. Therapeutic Efficacy and Safety of Undenatured Type II Collagen Singly or in Combination with Glucosamine and Chondroitin in Arthritic Dogs. Toxicol. Mech. Methods 17(4), 189-196.

Epstein, M., Rodan, I., Griffenhagen, G., Kadrlik, J., Petty, M., Robertson, S. and Simpson, W. 2015. 2015 AAHA/AAFP Pain Management Guidelines for Dogs and Cats. Retrieved from https://www.aaha.org/public_documents/professional/guidelines/2015_aaha_aafp_pain_management_guidelines_for_dogs_and_cats.pdf

Extend Joint Care. 2016. Extend For a Longer, Better Life. Retrieved from https://www.extendpetcare.com/

Gupta, R.C., Canerdy, T.D., Lindley, J., Konemann, M., Minniear, J., Carroll, B.A., Hendrick, C., Goad, J.T., Rohde, K., Doss, R., Bagchi, M. and Bagchi, D. 2012. Comparative therapeutic efficacy and safety of type-II collagen (UC-II), glucosamine and chondroitin in arthritic dogs: pain evaluation by ground force plate. J. Anim. Physiol. Anim. Nutr. (Berl) 96(5), 770-777.

Health Canada. 2013. Drugs and Health Products: Veterinary Drugs. Retrieved from http://www.hc-sc.gc.ca/dhp-mps/vet/index-eng.php.

Henrotin, Y., Sanchez, C. and Balligand, M. 2005. Pharmaceutical and nutraceutical management of canine osteoarthritis: present and future perspectives. Vet. J. 170(1), 113-123.

Herrero-Beaumont, G., Ivorra, J.A., Del Carmen Trabado, M., Blanco, F.J., Benito, P., Martin-Mola, E., Paulino, J., Marenco, J.L., Porto, A., Laffon, A., Araujo, D., Figueroa, M. and Branco, J. 2007. Glucosamine sulfate in the treatment of knee osteoarthritis symptoms: a randomized, double-blind, placebo-controlled study using acetaminophen as a side comparator. Arthritis Rheum. 56(2), 555-567.

Johnson, K.A., Hulse, D.A., Hart, R.C., Kochevar, D. and Chu, Q. 2001. Effects of an orally administered mixture of chondroitin sulfate, glucosamine hydrochloride and manganese ascorbate on synovial fluid chondroitin sulfate 3B3 and 7D4 epitope in a canine cruciate ligament transection model of osteoarthritis. Osteoarthritis Cartilage 9(1), 14-21.

Johnston, S.A. 1997. Osteoarthritis. Joint anatomy, physiology, and pathobiology. Vet. Clin. North Am. Small Anim. Pract. 27(4), 699-723.

Johnston, S.A., McLaughlin, R.M. and Budsberg, S.C. 2008. Nonsurgical management of osteoarthritis in dogs. Vet. Clin. North Am. Small Anim. Pract. 38(6), 1449-1470.

KuKanich, B. 2013. Outpatient oral analgesics in dogs and cats beyond nonsteroidal antiinflammatory drugs: an evidence-based approach. Vet. Clin. North Am. Small Anim. Pract. 43(5), 1109-1125.

Liquid Health Inc. 2016. K9 Glucosamine for Dogs Joint Supplement. Retrieved from http://liquidhealthpets.com/products/k9-glucosamine-for-dogs.

Maxwell, L.K., Regier, P. and Achanta, S. 2016. Comparison of Glucosamine Absorption After Administration of Oral Liquid, Chewable, and Tablet Formulations to Dogs. J. Am. Anim. Hosp. Assoc. 52(2), 90-94.

McCarthy, G., O'Donovan, J., Jones, B., McAllister, H., Seed, M. and Mooney, C. 2007. Randomised double-blind, positive-controlled trial to assess the efficacy of glucosamine/chondroitin sulfate for the treatment of dogs with osteoarthritis. Vet. J. 174(1), 54-61.

McKenzie, B.A. 2010. What is the evidence? There is only very weak clinical trial evidence to support the use of glucosamine and chondroitin supplements for osteoarthritis in dogs. J Am Vet Med Assoc, 237(12), 1382-1383.

Meulyzer, M., Vachon, P., Beaudry, F., Vinardell, T., Richard, H., Beauchamp, G. and Laverty, S. 2008. Comparison of pharmacokinetics of glucosamine and synovial fluid levels following administration of glucosamine sulphate or glucosamine hydrochloride. Osteoarthritis Cartilage, 16(9), 973-979.

Moreau, M., Dupuis, J., Bonneau, N.H. and Desnoyers, M. 2003. Clinical evaluation of a nutraceutical, carprofen and meloxicam for the treatment of dogs with osteoarthritis. Vet. Rec. 152(11), 323-329.

Neil, K.M., Caron, J.P. and Orth, M.W. 2005. The role of glucosamine and chondroitin sulfate in treatment for and prevention of osteoarthritis in animals. J. Am. Vet. Med. Assoc. 226(7), 1079-1088.

Nutramax Laboratories Veterinary Sciences Inc. 2016a. Cosequin Joint Health Supplement. Retrieved from http://www.cosequin.com/dogs/joint-and-bone/cosequin-professional-line/cosequin-ds-maximum-strength

Nutramax Laboratories Veterinary Sciences Inc. 2016b. Dasuquin with MSM. Retrieved from http://www.nutramaxlabs.com/dog/dog-joint-bone-health/dasuquin-for-dogs

Pascoe, P.J. (2002). Alternative methods for the control of pain. J. Am. Vet. Med. Assoc. 221(2), 222-229.

Persiani, S., Roda, E., Rovati, L.C., Locatelli, M., Giacovelli, G. and Roda, A. 2005. Glucosamine oral bioavailability and plasma pharmacokinetics after increasing doses of crystalline glucosamine sulfate in man. Osteoarthritis Cartilage, 13(12), 1041-1049.

Pet Naturals of Vermont. 2016. Animal Health Products: Hip + Joint Extra Strength. Retrieved from http://www.petnaturals.com/index.php?l=product_detail&p=700523120

PetMed Express Inc. 2016. ProMotion for Medium Large Dogs. Retrieved from http://www.1800petmeds.com/ProMotion+For+Medium+Large+Dogs-prod10490.html

Plumb, D.C. 2015. Glucosamine/Chondroitin Sulfate. In: Plumb's Veterinary Drug Handbook (Eighth ed.). Stockholm, Wiscoconsin, USA: Pharma Vet Inc.

Roush, J.K., McLaughlin, R.M. and Radlinsky, M.G. 2002. Understanding the pathophysiology of osteoarthritis. Vet Med. 97, 108-117.

Rovati, L.C., Girolami, F. and Persiani, S. 2012.

Crystalline glucosamine sulfate in the management of knee osteoarthritis: efficacy, safety, and pharmacokinetic properties. Ther. Adv. Musculoskelet. Dis. 4(3), 167-180.

Rychel, J.K. 2010. Diagnosis and treatment of osteoarthritis. Top Companion Anim. Med. 25(1), 20-25.

Sawitzke, A.D., Shi, H., Finco, M.F., Dunlop, D.D., Harris, C.L., Singer, N.G., Bradley, J.D., Silver, D., Jackson, C.G., Lane, N.E., Oddis, C.V., Wolfe, F., Lisse, J., Furst, D.E., Bingham, C.O., Reda, D.J., Moskowitz, R.W., Williams, H.J. and Clegg, D.O. 2010. Clinical efficacy and safety of glucosamine, chondroitin sulphate, their combination, celecoxib or placebo taken to treat osteoarthritis of the knee: 2-year results from GAIT. Ann. Rheum. Dis. 69(8), 1459-1464.

Setnikar, I. and Rovati, L.C. 2001. Absorption, distribution, metabolism and excretion of glucosamine sulfate. A review. Arzneimittelforschung 51(9), 699-725.

TerraMax Pro. 2016. Hip & Joint Supplement for Dogs. Retrieved from http://terramaxpro.com/product/hipjoint/

Tilley, L.P. and Smith, F.W.K.Jr. 2015. Arthritis (Osteoarthritis). In: Blackwell's Five-Minute Veterinary Consult: Canine and Feline (Sixth ed.): Wiley Blackwell.

Vandeweerd, J.M., Coisnon, C., Clegg, P., Cambier, C., Pierson, A., Hontoir, F., Saegerman, C., Gustin, P. and Buczinski, S. 2012. Systematic review of efficacy of nutraceuticals to alleviate clinical signs of osteoarthritis. J. Vet. Intern. Med. 26(3), 448-456.

Vetri-Science Laboratories. 2016. Glyco-Flex III Soft Chews. Retrieved from http://www.glycoflex3.com/info.html

Walton, M.B., Cowderoy, E., Lascelles, D. and Innes, J.F. 2013. Evaluation of construct and criterion validity for the 'Liverpool Osteoarthritis in Dogs' (LOAD) clinical metrology instrument and comparison to two other instruments. PLoS One 8(3), e58125. doi:10.1371/journal.pone.0058125.

Wandel, S., Juni, P., Tendal, B., Nuesch, E., Villiger, P.M., Welton, N.J., Reichenbach, S. and Trelle, S. 2010. Effects of glucosamine, chondroitin, or placebo in patients with osteoarthritis of hip or knee: network meta-analysis. BMJ. 341, c4675. doi:10.1136/bmj.c4675

7

Proliferation, angiogenesis and differentiation related markers in compact and follicular-compact thyroid carcinomas in dogs

P. Pessina[1,*], V.A. Castillo[2], D. César[3], I. Sartore[1] and A. Meikle[1]

[1]*Laboratorio de Técnicas Nucleares, Facultad de Veterinaria, Universidad de la República, Lasplaces 1550, Montevideo, Uruguay*
[2]*Cat. Clin. Méd. Peq. An. and U. Endocrinología, Escuela Medicina Veterinaria, Facultad de Ciencias Veterinarias, Universidad de Buenos Aires. Av. Chorroarín 280, C. Autónoma de Buenos Aires, Argentina*
[3]*Instituto Plan Agropecuario, Br. Artigas 3802, Montevideo, Uruguay*

Abstract

Immunohistochemical markers (IGF-1, IGF-1R, VEGF, FGF-2, RARα and RXR) were evaluated in healthy canine thyroid glands (n=8) and in follicular-compact (n=8) and compact thyroid carcinomas (n=8). IGF-1, IGF-1R and VEGF expression was higher in fibroblasts and endothelial cells of compact carcinoma than in healthy glands ($P < 0.05$). Compared to follicular-compact carcinoma, compact carcinoma had higher IGF-1R expression in fibroblasts, and higher FGF-2 expression in endothelial cells ($P < 0.05$). RARα expression was higher in endothelial cells of compact carcinoma than in those of other groups ($P < 0.05$). The upregulation of these proliferation- and angiogenesis-related factors in endothelial cells and/or fibroblasts and not in follicular cells of compact carcinoma compared to healthy glands supports the relevance of stromal cells in cancer progression.

Keywords: Canine, Histology, Immunohistochemistry, Thyroid carcinoma.

Introduction

Similar to humans, thyroid cancer is the most common endocrine malignancy in dogs and the leading cause of death among endocrine cancers (Barber, 2007). Ninety percent of canine thyroid tumours are carcinomas, and 16–38%, and even up to 60%, of patients show evidence of metastasis at the time of diagnosis (Wucherer and Wilke, 2010; Campos et al., 2012). In dogs, the most frequent thyroid tumour types are derived from follicular epithelial cells, and the most common histological patterns are follicular, follicular-compact and compact (Ramos-Vara et al., 2002; Nadeau and Kitchell, 2011). Most canine thyroid tumours are well to moderately differentiated (Klein et al., 1995). Although surgery is often successful in the early stages of the disease, unsatisfactory results are obtained in advanced tumours. Therefore, a better understanding of the molecular mechanisms and intracellular networks associated with oncogenesis may help discover new therapeutic options for these malignancies (Malaguarnera et al., 2012).

Alterations in the expression of growth factors such as insulin-like growth factor (IGF)-1, vascular endothelial growth factor (VEGF) and fibroblast growth factor (FGF)-2, and their receptors, play a role in the progression of thyroid cancer in humans and dogs (de Araujo-Filho et al., 2009; Redler et al., 2013; Campos et al., 2014). The activation of the IGF system is associated with the pathogenesis of a variety of human neoplasias because of the mitogenic and anti-apoptotic properties of its cognate receptor (Vella et al., 2001; Ciampolillo et al., 2007). IGF-1, a potent mitogen in many cell types, promotes the progression of mitosis via the induction of DNA synthesis and has long-term effects on cell proliferation, differentiation and apoptosis (Jones and Clemmons, 1995). Experimental evidence suggests that IGF-1 plays a significant role in the transformation, infiltrative growth and metastasis of tumour cells (LeRoith and Roberts, 2003; Liu and Brown, 2011). Moreover, IGF-1/IGF-1R are overexpressed in some types of thyroid carcinomas in humans, and it is correlated with poor prognosis (Liu et al., 2013).

In the absence of vascular support, tumours may become necrotic or even apoptotic (Holmgren et al., 1995). New growth in the vascular network is important because the proliferation, as well as metastatic spread, of cancer cells depends on an adequate supply of oxygen and nutrients, and the removal of waste products (Nishida et al., 2006). In addition, tumour angiogenesis is controlled by positive and negative modulators produced by neoplastic, stromal and tumour-infiltrating cells (Carmeliet and Jain, 2000). Studies showed that vascular tumour markers, such as VEGF expression, are increased in association with poor outcome in some canine compact tumours (Restucci et al., 2003). VEGF is essential for the growth of new vessels under normal physiological

*Corresponding Author: Dr. Paula Pessina. Laboratorio de Técnicas Nucleares, Facultad de Veterinaria, UDELAR, Montevideo, Uruguay. Email: *paulapessina@gmail.com*

conditions as well as in tumour cells, and it plays an important role in the development of distant metastases (Lin and Chao, 2005). In dogs, VEGF is expressed at higher levels in endothelial cells of canine thyroid glands with carcinoma than in those of healthy glands, which is consistent with the higher number of blood vessels and cell density (Campos *et al.*, 2014; Pessina *et al.*, 2014). FGF-2 is also implicated in abnormal human thyroid growth, both as a potential follicular cell mitogen and as a stimulator of thyroid endothelial cell growth. Reports on FGF-2 levels in thyroid carcinoma are contradictory (Kondo *et al.*, 2007), and its expression may depend on the degree of differentiation (Boelaert *et al.*, 2003).

Differentiating factors redirect cells toward their normal phenotype and may reverse or suppress carcinogenesis (Miller, 1998). Retinoids are natural or synthetic derivatives of vitamin A that modulate cell growth, differentiation and apoptosis (de Mello Souza *et al.*, 2014). In dogs, retinoids are used to treat various types of cancer such as cutaneous lymphoma, mast cell tumours and corticotroph adenoma of the pituitary (White *et al.*, 1993; Miyajima *et al.*, 2006; Ohashi *et al.*, 2006; Castillo *et al.*, 2006; Castillo and Gallelli, 2010), and recently in thyroid carcinoma (Castillo *et al.*, 2016). The action of retinoic acid is mediated by retinoic acid receptors (RARs) and the retinoid X receptors (RXRs) (Kasimanickam *et al.*, 2013). Both receptors are expressed in cutaneous lymphoma in dogs (de Mello Souza *et al.*, 2010); however, their expression in the thyroid gland has not been described to date.

Based on evidence showing that primary tumours are composed of a multitude of stromal cell types in addition to cancerous cells (Tlsty and Coussens, 2006), we investigated different markers (VEGF, FGF-2, IGF-1, IGF-1R, RARα and RXR) in compact and follicular-compact canine thyroid carcinomas.

Materials and Methods

Experimental design

All experiments were performed in accordance with the regulations of the Animal Experimentation Committees of the Faculty of Veterinary Medicine, Universidad de la República, Uruguay, and the Faculty of Veterinary Sciences, University of Buenos Aires, Argentina.

Tissue samples

Tissue samples were collected from the Endocrinology Unit, Faculty of Veterinary Medicine, University of Buenos Aires, Argentina, and the Veterinary Hospital, Faculty of Veterinary Medicine, University of Uruguay. Canine tissue samples were selected as follows: normal thyroid tissues were obtained from dogs that had been euthanised for reasons unrelated to thyroid disease (traumatized or aggressive patients) and had histopathologically normal thyroid glands (healthy group, n = 8); thyroid follicular carcinomas were

obtained postsurgically (carcinoma group, n = 16). Tumours were classified according to the World Health Organization (WHO).

Haematoxylin and eosin stained specimens were classified into two categories, namely, follicular-compact carcinoma (n = 8) and compact carcinoma (n = 8), according to the predominant histological pattern and following established criteria for thyroid neoplasms. Classification of thyroid tumours according to thyroglobulin and calcitonin immunohistochemistry was performed as previously described (Patnaik and Lieberman, 1991); all tumours included in this study were positive for the former and negative for the latter. All samples were processed in the Laboratory of Nuclear Techniques, Faculty of Veterinary Medicine, University of Uruguay.

Immunohistochemistry

Samples were fixed in 4% paraformaldehyde in phosphate-buffered saline (PBS) and embedded in paraffin for immunohistochemistry. Immunoreactivity against VEGF, FGF-2, IGF-1, IGF-1R, RARα, RXR, thyroglobulin and calcitonin was assessed in transverse 5 μm sections of healthy thyroid gland and thyroid carcinoma specimens using the avidin-biotin peroxidase immunohistochemical technique, as previously described (Pessina *et al.*, 2014). Paraffin embedded tissue sections were de-waxed and re-hydrated, and antigen retrieval was performed. Sections were pretreated in a microwave oven at 900 W in 0.01 M sodium citrate buffer (pH 6.0) for 9 min, and then allowed to cool for 20 min. After washing in buffer (0.01 M PBS, pH 7.4), non-specific endogenous peroxidase activity was blocked by exposure to 3% hydrogen peroxide in methanol for 10 min at room temperature. After another wash in buffer (10 min), sections were blocked in normal horse or goat serum diluted in PBS (Vectastain, Vector Laboratories, Burlingame, CA) for 30 min at room temperature in a humidified chamber. Sections were incubated with the primary antibodies for one hour a humidity chamber at room temperature (Table 1).

Negative control immunolabeling was performed for each receptor by replacing the primary antibody with non-immune IgG (Santa Cruz Biotechnology), diluted 1:100 in PBS. After primary antibody binding, sections were incubated with a biotinylated secondary antibody (horse anti-mouse or goat anti-rabbit IgG; Vector Laboratories), diluted 1:200 in normal horse (thyroglobulin and IGF-1) or goat serum (the remaining antibodies). A Vectastain ABC kit (Vector Laboratories) was used for the detection of all proteins. The site of the bound enzyme was visualised by 3, 3'-diaminobenzidine (DAB), a chromogen that produces a brown insoluble precipitate when incubated with the enzyme, in H_2O_2 using a DAB kit (Vector Laboratories).

Table 1. Primary antibodies used for immunohistochemistry.

Antibody	Antibody Name	Antibody Type	Dilution
Calcitonin	A 0576[a]	Rabbit polyclonal	1:1000
Thyroglobulin	sc-365997[b]	Mouse monoclonal	1:75
VEGF	sc-152[b]	Rabbit polyclonal	1:200
FGF-2	sc-79[b]	Rabbit polyclonal	1:200
IGF-1	sc-1422[b]	Goat polyclonal	1:50
IGF-1R	ab 5497[c]	Rabbit polyclonal	1:50
RARα	sc-551[b]	Rabbit polyclonal	1:100
RXR	sc-831[b]	Rabbit polyclonal	1:100

[a]Dako, Glostrup, Denmark. [b]Santa Cruz Biotechnology, Inc, Dallas, TX. [c]Abcam, Cambridge, USA.

Sections were counterstained with haematoxylin and dehydrated before mounting with Entellan® (Merck, Darmstadt, Germany). For each protein, all samples were analysed using same immunohistochemical assay.

Image analysis

Cell density (number of cells/field) and number of blood vessels were counted in 15 images captured from each histological section at 40× magnification. Three cell types, namely, follicular cells, endothelial cells and fibroblasts, were evaluated in the same images. Immunolabeling of the nucleus or cytoplasm was scored as negative (-), faint (+), moderate (++) or intense (+++) by two independent observers who were blinded to the treatment groups (Pessina *et al.*, 2014). The average labeling intensity was calculated as $(1 \times n1) + (2 \times n2) + (3 \times n3)$, where n is the number of cells in each field exhibiting faint (n1), moderate (n2) and intense (n3) labeling (Boos *et al.*, 1996). The average of the abovementioned variables in the 15 images captured from each histological section was used for statistical analysis.

Statistical analysis

Univariate analyses were performed on all variables to identify outliers and to verify the normality of residuals. Antigen immunolabeling intensity was evaluated by analysis of variance using a mixed model (Statistical Analysis System, SAS Institute, Cary, NC). The statistical model used to assess labeling intensity included observer effects, animal group (healthy thyroid gland, follicular-compact carcinoma and compact carcinoma), and cell type (follicular cells, fibroblasts and endothelial cells) and their interactions. Cell density was analysed by PROC MIXED (SAS, V9.0) with the animal group included in the model. Since blood vessels were not detected in the images of most healthy animals (7/8), the number of blood vessels was analysed by PROC GENMOD using a binomial distribution (presence or not of vessels) including the animal group in the model. Data are presented as the least square mean ± pooled S.E.M. The level of significance was set at P < 0.05.

Results

Number of blood vessels and cell density

Cell density was higher in compact carcinomas and follicular-compact carcinomas than in healthy glands (cells per field: 288 ± 24, 221 ± 24 and 142 ± 24, respectively, $P < 0.03$). Moreover, the number of cells per field tended to be higher in compact carcinomas than in follicular-compact carcinomas ($P = 0.06$). A significant group effect was observed regarding the number of blood vessels ($P = 0.007$), with a greater number of blood vessels observed in thyroid follicular-compact carcinomas than in healthy thyroid tissue ($P = 0.01$), and in compact carcinomas than in the healthy group ($P < 0.1$), although the latter did not reach statistical significance.

Protein localisation

Positive immunolabeling for IGF-1, IGF-1R, VEGF, FGF-2, RARα and RXR was observed in the cytoplasm in all cell types analysed (Figs. 1, 2 and 3). Five carcinoma samples (two compact and three follicular-compact) had positive labeling for nuclear IGF-1R, although the percentage of positive cells was too low for statistical analysis. Nuclear RARα and RXR labeling was also detected in follicular cells in eight (three compact and five follicular-compact) and two (one compact and one follicular-compact) carcinoma samples. For all assays, no immunolabeling was observed when the primary antibody was replaced by non-specific IgG.

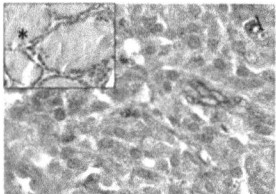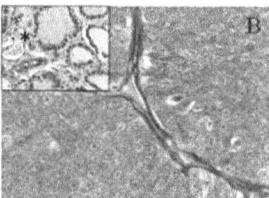

Fig. 1. Immunoreactivity of insulin-like growth factor-1 (IGF-1, A) and insulin-like growth factor-1 receptor (IGF-1R, B) in thyroid compact carcinoma. Cytoplasmic labeling in follicular cells is shown. The asterisk (*) shows expression in healthy thyroid tissue. All images were captured at a magnification of 400×.

Overall, IGF-1 and IGF-1R labeling intensities were higher in compact carcinoma than in healthy thyroid tissues, although the differences did not reach statistical significance ($P = 0.09$ and $P = 0.07$, respectively). IGF-1 and IGF-1R expression was higher in fibroblasts and endothelial cells of compact carcinomas than in those of healthy thyroid tissues ($P < 0.05$), whereas no differences were observed for follicular cells (Fig. 4A and B).

No differences were observed between compact and follicular-compact carcinomas, except in fibroblasts, where compact carcinomas showed higher IGF-1R labeling intensity ($P < 0.05$).

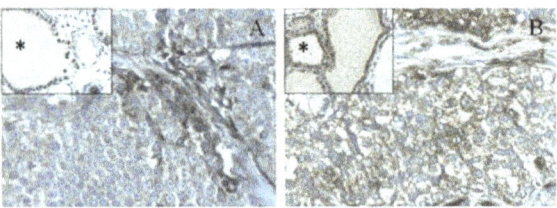

Fig. 2. Vascular endothelial growth factor (VEGF, A) and fibroblast growth factor-2 (FGF-2, B) cytoplasmic labeling in thyroid compact carcinoma. The asterisk (*) shows expression in healthy thyroid tissues. All images were captured at a magnification of 400×.

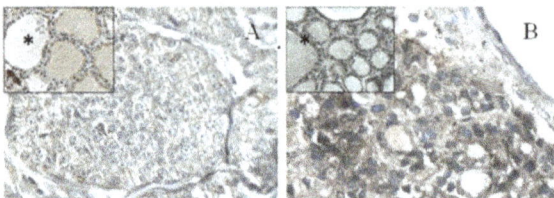

Fig. 3. Cytoplasmic immunolabeling of retinoic acid receptor alpha (RARα, A) and retinoid X receptor (RXR, B) in thyroid compact carcinoma. All images were captured at a magnification of 400×.

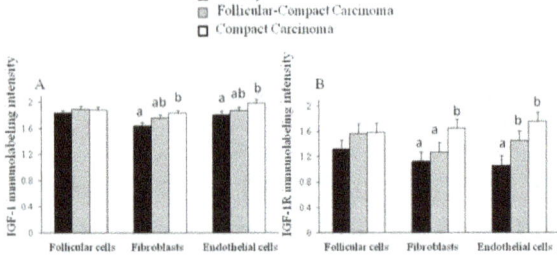

Fig. 4. Immunolabeling intensity of insulin-like growth factor-1 (IGF-1, A) and insulin-like growth factor-1 receptor (IGF-1R, B). Data are expressed as the least square mean ± pooled S.E.M. Different letters within the same cell type indicate differences, P < 0.05.

Overall, VEGF expression was higher in compact carcinomas than in healthy thyroid tissues (P < 0.05) and follicular-compact carcinomas (P < 0.1). Stronger labeling for VEGF was detected in fibroblasts and endothelial cells of compact carcinomas than in those of normal thyroid tissues (P < 0.05) (Fig. 5A). No differences in FGF-2 labeling intensity were detected in follicular cells and fibroblasts, whereas endothelial cells of compact carcinomas showed higher FGF-2 immunolabeling than the other two groups (P < 0.05) (Fig. 5B).

In endothelial cells, RARα immunolabeling was higher in compact carcinomas than in the other two groups (P < 0.01). An altered pattern of RARα expression in different cells types according to group was observed; a stronger labeling in follicular cells than fibroblasts and endothelial cells of healthy glands was found (P <

0.05), whereas no differences according to cells types in follicular compact carcinoma were observed, and endothelial cells presented greater RARα labeling than fibroblasts in compact carcinoma (P < 0.05) (Fig. 6A). Similar profile of RXR expression was observed, with stronger labeling in follicular cells than fibroblasts and endothelial cells of healthy glands (P < 0.05), whereas RXR expression in both types of carcinomas did not differ according to cell type (Fig. 6B).

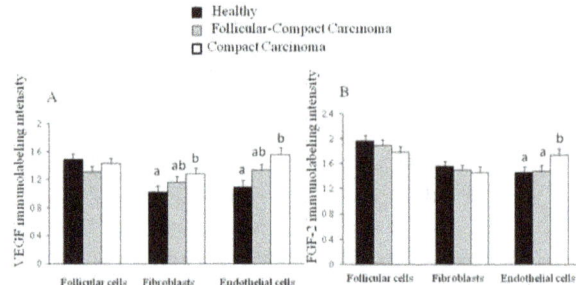

Fig. 5. Immunolabeling intensity of vascular endothelial growth factor (VEGF, A) and fibroblast growth factor-2 (FGF-2, B). Data are expressed as the least square mean ± pooled S.E.M. Different letters within the same cell type indicate differences, P < 0.05.

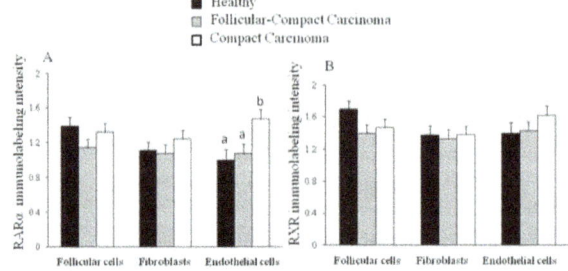

Fig. 6. Immunolabeling intensity of retinoic acid receptor alpha (RARα, A) and retinoid X receptor (RXR, B). Data are expressed as the least square mean ± pooled S.E.M. Different letters within the same cell type indicate differences, P < 0.05.

Discussion

Most canine thyroid tumours arise from the follicular epithelium and are classified as follicular, compact or a mixture of the two patterns (follicular-compact) (Barber, 2007). As reported previously (Pessina *et al.*, 2014), cell density and the number of blood vessels were higher in thyroid carcinoma tissues than in healthy glands. Cell density was increased in compact carcinomas when compared to follicular-compact carcinomas, which is consistent with their corresponding histological classification.

To the best of our knowledge, this is the first report showing simultaneous detection of immunoreactive IGF-1/IGF-1R in healthy and carcinomatous thyroid glands in dogs. Cytoplasmic immunoreactivity of both factors was observed in follicular cells, fibroblasts and endothelial cells, as reported previously for other cancers in dogs (Buishand et al., 2012; Maniscalco et al., 2014). In carcinomas, a portion of thyroid follicular cells had positive immunolabeling for nuclear IGF-1R, which is consistent with the findings of Sarfstein et al. (2012), who described the translocation of IGF-1R to the nucleus in breast cancer cells and identified a novel mechanism of IGF-1R gene autoregulation. In the present study, IGF-1 and IGF-1R labelling intensity was higher in fibroblasts and endothelial cells of compact carcinoma than in those of healthy thyroid tissues, while follicular-compact carcinoma had intermediate labelling intensity. These findings are consistent with human studies, such as the report by Vella et al. (2001), who showed that IGF-1 and its receptor are overexpressed in thyroid cancer, suggesting that IGF-1R is activated in an autocrine/paracrine manner. The simultaneous increase of IGF-1 and IGF-1R expression in the stroma (fibroblasts and endothelial cells) supports the existence of crosstalk between these cell types; this can lead to the activation of proliferation signals and/or facilitate nutrient access, thus contributing to tumour growth (Bissell and Radisky, 2001; Gribben et al., 2010). These factors were expressed at an intermediate level in follicular-compact carcinomas, which is consistent with the degree of differentiation of this type of tumour compared with compact carcinoma. Indeed, we have recently shown (Castillo et al., 2016) that thyroid follicular compact carcinomas had a greater time to recurrence than compact carcinomas in dogs.

In the present study, we showed that the pattern of expression of VEGF was similar to that of IGF-1/IGF-1R in the different groups, as demonstrated by the upregulation of VEGF expression in fibroblasts and endothelial cells of compact carcinoma. The upregulation of VEGF in endothelial cells in compact carcinoma when compared to the healthy thyroid tissue was consistent with the findings of our previous study (Pessina et al., 2014). This is in agreement with Campos et al. (2014) that suggested that VEGF may play an important role in the progression of canine thyroid cancer. Our present results showed that FGF-2 expression was higher in endothelial cells of compact carcinoma than in those of healthy glands or follicular-compact glands. These data were consistent with the pattern of VEGF expression in the same cell type, and support the fact that VEGF stimulates endothelial cells to produce FGF-2, which further enhances angiogenesis (Pallares et al., 2006). Overall, data suggest a positive feedback loop between VEGF and FGF-2 that contributes to tumour progression, despite the higher efficacy of the VEGF system for neovascularization compared to FGF-2 as reported previously (Giavazzi et al., 2003). In the present study, no differences in follicular cell expression of IGF-1/IGF-1R, VEGF and FGF-2 were found among groups, whereas the expression of these factors in stromal cells differed. Tumour progression is promoted by crosstalk between the tumour and its surrounding supporting tissue either via cell-to-cell contact, or mediated by secreted molecules (Bouziges et al., 1991). Indeed, the stroma itself can trigger tumour development (Bissell and Radisky, 2001), and one hypothesis on oncogenesis is based on stromal cell functionality, despite the fact that the mechanisms by which tumour and stromal cells co-evolve remain unclear (Gribben et al., 2010).

The expression of RARα and RXR in healthy thyroid glands and thyroid carcinomas in dogs has not been reported previously. In humans, the expression of these retinoic receptors in healthy thyroid tissue, thyroid cell lines, and in thyroid adenomas and carcinomas has been reported (Hoftijzer et al., 2009); however, the expression of these receptors in dogs has only been described in lymphoma, melanoma and osteosarcoma (Miyajima et al., 2006; Ohashi et al., 2006; de Mello Souza et al., 2010, 2014). In the present study, RARα expression in follicular cells did not differ in carcinomas and healthy thyroid glands. However, endothelial cells of compact carcinomas showed higher expression of RARα than those of the other groups (healthy and follicular-compact carcinomas), and further studies are needed to help our understanding of the role of this receptor in carcinoma progression. Retinoic receptor expression in thyroid carcinoma is consistent with our recent study (Castillo et al., 2016) in which isotretinoin 9-cis (RA9-cis) treatment increased time of recurrence and survival time in dogs with follicular-compact and compact thyroid carcinoma when compared to doxorubicin after surgery. Miyajima et al. (2006) showed that in canine masts cells, RARα expression was positively correlated with response to retinoic acid treatment. Because the present study did not test all isoforms of RXR, these data should be considered preliminary. Indeed, Haugen et al. (2004) showed that while RXRγ was expressed in different cell lines of thyroid human tumours, it was not expressed in normal thyroid tissue. Moreover, none of the RXR isoforms are expressed in canine non-tumoural lymphocytes, whereas RXRγ is expressed in 78% of tumour T cells (de Mello Souza et al., 2014).

In conclusion, factors related to proliferation and angiogenesis were expressed at higher levels in fibroblasts and/or endothelial cells of compact carcinomas than in those of healthy glands, with mostly intermediate expression in follicular-compact carcinomas, suggesting a role of stromal cells in tumour progression.

Acknowledgements

We gratefully acknowledge the technical assistance of Lic. Claudia Menezes and Rosina Sánchez for immunohistochemical evaluation of samples. This work was supported in part by Project No. 277 CSIC-UdelaR (Uruguay).

Conflict of interest

The authors declare that there is not conflict of interest.

References

Barber, L.G. 2007. Thyroid tumors in dogs and cats. Vet. Clin. North Am. Small Anim. Pract. 37(4), 755-773.

Bissell, M.J. and Radisky, D. 2001. Putting tumors in context. Nat. Rev. Cancer 1(1), 46-54.

Boelaert, K., McCabe, C.J., Tannahill, L.A., Gittoes, N.J., Holder, R.L., Watkinson, J.C., Bradwell, A.R., Sheppard, M.C. and Franklyn, J.A. 2003. Pituitary tumor transforming gene and fibroblast growth factor-2 expression: potential prognostic indicators in differentiated thyroid cancer. J. Clin. Endocrinol. Metab. 88(5), 2341-2347.

Boos, A., Meyer, W., Schwarz, R. and Grunert, E. 1996. Immunohistochemical assessment of oestrogen receptor and progesterone receptor distribution in biopsy samples of the bovine endometrium collected throughout the oestrous cycle. Anim. Reprod. Sci. 44, 11-21.

Bouziges, F., Simo, P., Simon-Assmann, P., Haffen, K. and Kedinger, M. 1991. Altered deposition of basement membrane molecule in co-culture of colonic cancer cells and fibroblast. Int. J. Cancer 48(1), 101-108.

Buishand, F.O., van Erp, M.G., Groenveld, H.A., Mol, J.A., Kik, M., Robben, J.H., Kooistra, H.S. and Kirpensteijn, J. 2012. Expression of insulin-like growth factor-1 by canine insulinomas and their metastases. Vet. J. 191(3), 334-340.

Campos, M., Peremans, K., Vandermeulen, E., Duchateau, L., Bosmans, T., Polis, I. and Daminet, S. 2012. Effect of Recombinant Human Thyrotropin on the Uptake of Radioactive Iodine (123I) in Dogs with Thyroid Tumors. PLoS ONE 7(11): e50344. doi:10.1371/journal.pone.0050344.

Campos, M., Ducatelle, R., Kooistra, H.S., Rutteman, G., Duchateau, L., Polis, I. and Daminet, S. 2014. Immunohistochemical expression of potential therapeutic targets in canine thyroid carcinoma. J. Vet. Intern. Med. 28(2), 564-570.

Carmeliet, P. and Jain, R.K. 2000. Angiogenesis in cancer and other diseases. Nature 407, 249-257.

Castillo, V.A., Giacomini, D., Páez-Pereda, M., Stalla, J., Labeur, M., Theodoropoulou, M., Holsboer, F., Grossman, A.B., Stalla, G.K. and Arzt, E. 2006. Retinoic Acid as a Novel Medical Therapy for Cushing's Disease in Dogs. Endocrinology 147(9), 4438-4444.

Castillo, V.A. and Gallelli, M.F. 2010. Corticotroph adenoma in the dog: pathogenesis and new therapeutic possibilities. Res. Vet. Sci. 88(1), 26-32.

Castillo, V., Pessina, P., Hall, P., Blatter, M.F., Miceli, D., Arias, E.S. and Vidal, P. 2016. Postsurgical treatment of thyroid carcinoma in dogs with retinoic acid 9 cis improves patient outcome. Open Vet. J. 6(1), 6-14.

Ciampolillo, A., De Tullio, C., Perlino, E. and Maiorano, E. 2007. The IGF-I axis in thyroid carcinoma. Curr. Pharm. Des. 13(7), 729-735.

de Araujo-Filho, V.J., Alves, V.A., de Castro, I.V., Lourenço, S.V., Cernea, C.R., Brandão, L.G. and Ferraz, A.R. 2009. Vascular endothelial growth factor expression in invasive papillary thyroid carcinoma. Thyroid 19(11), 1233-1237.

de Mello Souza, C.H., Valli, V.E., Selting, K.A., Kiupel, M. and Kitchell, B.E. 2010. Immunohistochemical detection of retinoid receptors in tumors from 30 dogs diagnosed with cutaneous lymphoma. J. Vet. Inter. Med. 24(5), 1112-1117.

de Mello Souza, C.H., Valli, V.E. and Kitchell, B.E. 2014. Detection of retinoid receptors in non-neoplastic canine lymph nodes and in lymphoma. Can. Vet. J. 55(1), 1219-1224.

Giavazzi, R., Sennino, B., Coltrini, D., Garofalo, A., Dossi, R., Ronca, R., Tosatti, M.P. and Presta, M. 2003. Distinct role of fibroblast growth factor-2 and vascular endothelial growth factor on tumor growth and angiogenesis. Am. J. Pathol. 162(6), 1913-1926.

Gribben, J., Rosenwald, A., Gascoyne, R. and Lenz, G. 2010. Targeting the microenvironment. Leuk. Lymphoma 51 Suppl. 1, 34-40. doi: 10.3109/10428194.2010.500072.

Haugen, B.R., Jensen, D.R., Sharma, V., Pulawa, L.K., Hays, W.R., Krezel, W., Chambon, P. and Ecke, R.H. 2004. Retinoid X receptor gamma-deficient mice have increased skeletal muscle lipoprotein lipase activity and less weight gain when fed a high-fat diet. Endocrinology 145(8), 3679-3685.

Hoftijzer, H.C., Liu, Y.Y., Morreau, H., van Wezel, T., Pereira, A.M., Corssmit, E.P., Romijn, J.A. and Smit, J.W. 2009. Retinoic acid receptor and retinoid X receptor subtype expression for the differential diagnosis of thyroid neoplasms. Eur. J. Endocrinol. 160(4), 631-638.

Holmgren, L., O'Reilly, M.S. and Folkman, J. 1995. Dormancy of micrometastases: balance proliferation and apoptosis in the presence of angiogenesis suppression. Nat. Med. 1(2), 149-153.

Jones, J.I. and Clemmons, D.R. 1995. Insulin-like growth factors and their binding proteins: biological actions. Endocr. Rev. 16(1), 3-34.

Kasimanickam, V.R., Kasimanickam, R.K. and Rogers, H.A. 2013. Immunolocalization of retinoic acid receptor-alpha, -beta, and -gamma, in bovine and canine sperm. Theriogenology 79(6), 1010-1018.

Klein, M.K., Powers, B.E., Withrow, S.J., Curtis, C.R., Straw, R.C., Ogilvie, G.K., Dickinson, K.L., Cooper, M.F. and Baier, M. 1995. Treatment of thyroid carcinoma in dogs by surgical resection alone: 20 cases (1981-1989). J. Am. Vet. Med. Assoc. 206(7), 1007-1009.

Kondo, T., Zheng, L., Liu, W., Kurebayashi, J., Asa, S.L. and Ezzat, S. 2007. Epigenetically controlled fibroblast growth factor receptor 2 signaling imposes on the RAS/BRAF/mitogen activated protein kinase pathway to modulate thyroid cancer progression. Cancer Res. 67(11), 5461-5470.

LeRoith, D. and Roberts, C.T. 2003. The insulin-like growth factor system and cancer. Cancer Lett. 195(2), 127-137.

Lin, J.D. and Chao, T.C. 2005. Vascular endothelial growth factor in thyroid cancers. Cancer Biother. Radiopharm. 20(6), 648-661.

Liu, J. and Brown, R.E. 2011. Immunohistochemical expressions of fatty acid synthase and phosphorylated c-Met in thyroid carcinomas of follicular origin. Int. J. Clin. Exp. Pathol. 4(8), 755-764.

Liu, Y.J., Qiang, W., Shi, J., Lv, S.Q., Ji, M.J. and Shi, B.Y. 2013. Expression and significance of IGF-1 and IGF-1R in thyroid nodules. Endocrine 44(1), 158-164.

Malaguarnera, R., Morcavallo, A. and Belfiore, A. 2012. The insulin and igf-I pathway in endocrine glands carcinogenesis. J. Oncol. 2012:635614. doi: 10.1155/2012/635614.

Maniscalco, L., Iussich, S., Morello, E., Martano, M., Gattino, F., Miretti, S., Biolatti, B., Accornero, P., Martignani, E., Sánchez-Céspedes, R., Buracco, P. and De Maria, R. 2014. Increased expression of insulin-like growth factor-1 receptor is correlated with worse survival in canine appendicular osteosarcoma. Vet. J. 205(2), 272-280.

Miller, W.H.Jr. 1998. The emerging role of retinoids and retinoic acid metabolism blocking agents in the treatment of cancer. Cancer 83(8), 1471-1482.

Miyajima, N., Watanabe, M., Ohashi, E., Mochizuki, M., Nishimura, R., Ogawa, H., Sugano, S. and Sasaki, N. 2006. Relationship between retinoic acid receptor a gene expression and growth-inhibitory effect of all-trans retinoic acid on canine tumor cells. J. Vet. Intern. Med. 20(2), 348-354.

Nadeau, M. and Kitchell, B.E. 2011. Evaluation of the use of chemotherapy and other prognostic variables for surgically excised canine thyroid carcinoma with and without metastasis. Can. Vet. J. 52(9), 994-998.

Nishida, N., Yano, H., Nishida, T., Kamura, T. and Kojiro, M. 2006. Angiogenesis in Cancer. Vasc. Health Risk Manag. 2(3), 213-219.

Ohashi, M., Miyajima, N., Nakagawa, T., Takahashi, T., Kagechika, H., Mochizuki, M., Nishimura, R. and Sasaki, N. 2006. Retinoids induce growth inhibition and apoptosis in mast cell tumor cell lines. J. Vet. Med. Sci. 68(8), 797-802.

Pallares, J., Rojo, F., Iriarte, J., Morote, J., Armadans, L.I. and de Torres, I. 2006. Study of microvessel density and the expression of the angiogenic factors VEGF, bFGF and the receptors Flt-1 and FLK-1 in benign, premalignant and malignant prostate tissues. Histol. Histopathol. 21(8), 857-865.

Patnaik, A.K. and Lieberman, P.H. 1991. Gross, histologic, cytochemical, and immunocytochemical study of medullary thyroid carcinoma in sixteen dogs. Vet. Pathol. 28(3), 223-233.

Pessina, P., Castillo, V., Sartore, I., Borrego, J. and Meikle, A. 2014. Semiquantitative immunohistochemical marker staining and localization in canine thyroid carcinoma and normal thyroid gland. Vet. Comp. Oncol. 14(3), e102-12. doi: 10.1111/vco.12111.

Ramos-Vara, J.A., Miller, M.A., Johnson, G.C. and Pace, L.W. 2002. Immunohistochemical detection of thyroid transcription factor-1, thyroglobulin, and calcitonin in canine normal, hyperplastic, and neoplastic thyroid gland. Vet. Pathol. 39(4), 480-487.

Redler, A., Di Rocco, G., Giannotti, D., Frezzotti, F., Bernieri, M.G., Ceccarelli, S., D'Amici, S., Vescarelli, E., Mitterhofer, A.P., Angeloni, A. and Marchese, C. 2013. Fibroblast growth factor receptor-2 expression in thyroid tumor progression: potential diagnostic application. PLoS One. 8(8), e72224. doi: 10.1371/journal.pone.0072224.

Restucci, B., Maiolino, P., Paciello, O., Martano, M., De Vico, G. and Papparella, S. 2003. Evaluation of angiogenesis in canine seminomas by quantitative immunohistochemistry. J. Comp. Pathol. 128(4), 252-259.

Sarfstein, R., Pasmanik-Chor, M., Yeheskel, A., Edry, L., Shomron, N., Warman, N., Wertheimer, E., Maor, S., Shochat, L. and Werner, H. 2012. Insulin-like growth factor-I receptor (IGF-IR) translocates to nucleus and autoregulates IGF-IR gene expression in breast cancer cells. J. Biol. Chem. 287(4), 2766-2776.

Tlsty, T.D. and Coussens, L.M. 2006. Tumor stroma and regulation of cancer development. Annu. Rev. Pathol. 1, 119-150.

Vella, V., Sciacca, L., Pandini, G., Mineo, R., Squatrito, S., Vigneri, R. and Belfiore, A. 2001. The IGF system in thyroid cancer: new concepts. Mol. Pathol. 54(3), 121-124.

White, S.D., Rosychuk, R.A., Scott, K.V., Trettien, A.L., Jonas, L. and Denerolle, P. 1993. Use of isotretinoin and etretinate for the treatment of benign cutaneous neoplasia and cutaneous lymphoma in dogs. J. Am. Vet. Med. Assoc. 202(3), 387-391.

Wucherer, K.L. and Wilke, V. 2010. Thyroid cancer in dogs: An update based on 638 cases (1995-2005). J. Am. Anim. Hosp. Assoc. 46(4), 249-254.

8

Tear production and intraocular pressure in canine eyes with corneal ulceration

David L. Williams[*] and Philippa Burg

Department of Veterinary Medicine, University of Cambridge, Madingley Road, Cambridge, CB3 0ES, UK

Abstract

This study aimed to evaluate changes in lacrimation and intraocular pressure (IOP) in dogs with unilateral corneal ulceration using the Schirmer tear test (STT) and rebound (TonoVet®) tonometry. IOP and STT values were recorded in both ulcerated and non-ulcerated (control) eyes of 100 dogs diagnosed with unilateral corneal ulceration. Dogs presented with other ocular conditions as their primary complaint were excluded from this study. The mean ± standard deviation for STT values in the ulcerated and control eyes were 20.2±4.6 mm/min and 16.7±3.5 mm/min respectively. The mean ± standard deviation for IOP in the ulcerated and control eyes were 11.9±3.1 mmHg and 16.7±2.6 mmHg respectively. STT values were significantly higher (p<0.000001) in the ulcerated eye compared to the control eye while IOP was significantly lower (p<0.0001). There is an increase in lacrimation and a decrease in IOP in canine eyes with corneal ulceration. The higher tear production in ulcerated eyes shows the importance of measuring STT in both eyes in cases of corneal ulceration, since this increased lacrimation may mask an underlying keratoconjunctivitis sicca only evident in the contralateral eye. The lower IOP in ulcerated eyes is likely to relate to mild uveitic change in the ulcerated eye with a concomitant increase in uveoscleral aqueous drainage. While these changes in tear production and IOP in ulcerated eyes are widely recognised in both human and veterinary ophthalmology, it appears that this is the first controlled documented report of these changes in a large number of individuals.

Keywords: Corneal ulcer; Dog, Intraocular pressure, Tear production.

Introduction

Despite being widely accepted that corneal ulceration causes an increase in tear production and a decrease in intraocular pressure (IOP) as evidenced by the values from the Schirmer tear test (STT) and tonometric measurements, there appear to be few if any reports documenting these changes in ulcerated eyes in the human or canine population. This study seeks to fill this lacuna in the ophthalmic literature by comparing the tear production and IOP of eyes with ulcerated corneas compared with the control fellow eye in dogs with unilateral corneal ulceration.

The cornea serves a major refractive function while maintaining a protective barrier between the eye and the environment (Gilger et al., 2008). Despite being exposed to environmental hazards, the cornea maintains the integrity of its outer surface by continual replacement of its surface epithelium and through the provision a protective covering of the surface tear-film by the lacrimal glands. Corneal ulceration is one of the most common ocular disorders encountered in veterinary practice and a major cause of ocular pain through exposure of free trigeminal nerve endings in the superficial stroma and blindness either due to excessive scarring or through subsequent perforation of the cornea. (Gilger et al., 2008).

Tear secretion is controlled by the lacrimal functional unit consisting of the ocular surface (cornea, conjunctiva, accessory lacrimal glands, and meibomian glands), the main lacrimal gland and the interconnecting innervation (sensory afferent and autonomic efferent nerves) (Stern et al., 2004; Williams, 2008).

The sensory nerves derived from the ophthalmic branch of the trigeminal nerve in the cornea activate the efferent parasympathetic and sympathetic nerves originating in the parasympathetic motor nucleus of the facial nerve but travelling with the trigeminal nerve to the lacrimal gland (Marfurt et al., 2001; Situ and Simpson, 2010). The functional unit regulates the major components of the tear film in order to protect the ocular surface. Painful stimulation of the eye is known to result in tear secretion and other reflexes to prevent the eye from potential damage (Unger, 1990; Belmonte et al., 1997; Situ and Simpson, 2010) but there is little in the literature to show a direct link of increased tear secretion with corneal ulceration.

The IOP occurs through a balance between the production of aqueous humour and its drainage through the iridiocorneal angle (conventional outflow) and through the uveoscleral pathways (unconventional outflow) (Reinstein et al., 2009).

*Corresponding Author: David L. Williams. Department of Veterinary Medicine, University of Cambridge, Madingley Road, Cambridge, CB3 0ES, UK. Email: dlw33@cam.ac.uk

It has been previously documented that after an initial rise in IOP following ocular surface injury, a prolonged reduction in IOP is usually found (Unger, 1990). An antidromal trigeminal reflex arc is considered to be responsible for this hypotony, predominantly caused by a prostaglandin induced increase in unconventional aqueous outflow (Camras *et al.*, 1977; Fine *et al.*, 2007). Despite this understanding of the mechanism of such a change in IOP there appear to be few is any reports in the literature, just as with tear secretion, to show a direct link between corneal ulceration and decreased IOP in the dog.

Materials and Methods

This prospective study aims to determine tear production using the STT I method and IOP by rebound tonometry using the TonoVet® (ICare, Helsinki, Finland) in canine eyes with unilateral corneal ulcers to establish the difference in the values between the ulcerated and the fellow control eye. The second eye in the same animal was used as a control to eliminate any diurnal variations of time of sampling or effects of age, gender or weight of the patient (Berger and King, 1998; Gelatt and MacKay, 1998; Hartley *et al.*, 2006).

This study was undertaken over 12 months at the Queen's Veterinary Hospital, Department of Veterinary Medicine, University of Cambridge and at 14 first opinion clinics visited by the senior author in an ambulatory referral clinic. The study was conducted in line with the regulations of the UK Veterinary Surgeons' Act 1966 and was approved by the Ethics and Welfare Committee of the Department of Veterinary Medicine.

One hundred dogs with unilateral corneal ulcers as their presenting complaint were selected for this study in order to compare values between the ulcerated eye and the non-ulcerated fellow eye acting as a control. For each subject, the breed, sex, age, duration and depth of the ulcer were recorded. Any dogs with bilateral corneal ulceration or other conditions as a presenting complaint were excluded as were animals in which either eye had significant additional pathology at presentation.

Corneal ulceration was diagnosed on the basis of a full ocular examination including the use of direct and indirect ophthalmoscopy and slit lamp biomicroscopy, with ulceration confirmed by fluorescein staining undertaken after the STT and IOP values had been obtained. Ulceration was scored as superficial (i.e. a corneal epithelial erosion), mid-stromal (extending no deeper than half stromal thickness, or deep (extending deeper than half the thickness of the stroma) but not including descmetocoeles or perforating corneal lesions. Signs of mild ocular inflammation (conjunctival hyperaemia, aqueous flare, miosis but without profound cellular infiltrative change in the eye) were recorded where present and scored as mild,

moderate or severe. Tear production was measured in both eyes using the Schirmer I test which measures aqueous production over one minute in an unanaesthetised eye, therefore measuring basal and reflex tear production (Gelatt *et al.*, 1975). Standard STT strips (Eaglevision™, Schering-Plough, Memphis TN, USA) with the same batch number were used to measure tear production. IOP was measured in both eyes using the TonoVet® rebound tonometer (Icare, Helsinki, Finland) on calibration setting D (used when evaluating iop in the dog) and without the need for topical anaesthesia of the corneal surface (Leiva *et al.*, 2006).

All statistical analyses were undertaken using SPSS v19 (IBM, Armonk, USA). STT and IOP data obeyed the three sigma rule and were thus considered normally distributed, this confirmed using the Kolmogorov-Smirnov test which yielded values of $Z=1.239$, $P=0.093$ for IOP and $Z=0.886$ $P=0.413$ for STT. Values for the ulcerated eye were compared with those for the control fellow eye using a Students' T test with significance deemed to have been reached at $P=0.05$. A cumulative logit model was used to investigate the relationship between STT and IOP and ulcer depth. This model is valuable when analysing ordered categorical data (such as ulcer depth scored as 0, 1, 2 or 3) with the reduced amount of information that such data sets contain (Lee, 1992).

Each eye was entered as an individual data point, with dog ID included as a subject effect to take non-independence into account. Ulcer depth was entered as an ordinal variable from 0 (no ulcer) to 3 (deep ulcer), with STT and IOP as covariates. Given the mean value of 20 ± 3 mm/min from normal dogs in one paper from the senior author's research group (Hartley *et al.*, 2006) and 20 ± 1 mm/min in a paper from another group (Giannetto *et al.*, 2009) a power calculation showed that detecting a 3mm/min difference between ulcerated and control eyes with a statistical power of 0.8 and significance at 0.05 would require 30 cases. Similarly detecting a difference of 5mmHg in dogs with a mean and standard deviation of 19 ± 6 mmHg, a figure derived from a previous published large sample of normal dogs (Giannetto *et al.*, 2009), would require a sample size of 36 dogs. We examined 100 dogs to ensure sufficient power of the study.

Results

Signalment of cases, ulcer depth and duration, are shown in Table (1). STT results and measurements of IOP for both the ulcerated and the control contralateral eye are given in Table (2) together with scoring of conjunctival hyperaemia, a summary score of signs of intraocular inflammation (aqueous flare, iris swelling, iris hyperaemia, hypopyon) and degree of miosis, all semi-quantitatively assessed from 0 (not present) to 3 (severe).

Table 1. Signalment and ulcer characteristics of dogs involved in study.

Case	Breed	Gender	Age	Ulcer duration (days)	Ulcer type
1	Boxer	fn	7	6	superficial
2	CKCS	mn	13	14	mid stromal
3	Cross bred	me	12	21	mid stromal
4	Cocker spaniel	mn	5	1	superficial
5	WHWT	mn	12	21	mid stromal
6	Shih Tzu	mn	5	14	superficial
7	Labrador retriever	me	0.2	2	deep stromal
8	Pug	fe	0.8	3	deep stromal
9	French bulldog	fe	4	21	superficial
10	French bulldog	me	6	12	superficial
11	Boxer	me	5	7	superficial
12	Jack Russell terrier	me	8	21	superficial
13	English springer spaniel	me	7	14	mid stromal
14	Boxer	me	12	7	superficial
15	Pug	fn	8	4	mid stromal
16	Pug	fe	0.8	2	pinpoint mid stromal
17	Boxer	mn	8	14	superficial
18	Cross bred	mn	7	12	superficial
19	English springer spaniel	mn	8	21	superficial
20	Pug	fe	6	10	pinpoint mid-stromal
21	Pug	fn	7	7	central mid stromal
22	Cross bred	mn	9	7	superficial
23	German shepherd dog	mn	11	14	superficial
24	Cairn terr	fn	13	21	superficial
25	Yorkshire terrier	mn	12	7	superficial
26	Yorkshire terrier	mn	11	7	mid stromal
27	CKCS	fn	11	7	superficial
28	Cross bred	fn	10	21	mid stromal
29	Yorkshire terrier	fn	11	7	superficial
30	Boxer	mn	12	21	superficial
31	CKCS	fn	8	7	punctuate mid-stromal
32	Pug	mn	6	5	superficial
33	SBT	mn	6	21	superficial
34	Pug	mn	4	5	superficial
35	Boxer	me	8	6	superficial
36	Shih-tzu	mn	5.5	14	superficial
37	SBTx	mn	9	7	superficial
38	Boxer	fn	7.5	10	superficial
39	Cross bred	fn	1.5	4	superficial
40	Boxer	fn	10	21	superficial
41	SBT	fn	8	28	superficial
42	Boxer	mn	8	21	superficial
43	Yorkshire terrier	fn	10	28	superficial
44	CKCS	fn	10	28	superficial
45	Sharpei	mn	3	14	superficial
46	Boxer	fn	10	21	superficial
47	SBT	fn	8	28	superficial
48	SBT	mn	7.6	100	deep stromal
49	Pug	fn	6	14	mid stromal
50	Cross bred	me	12	7	superficial
51	WHWT	Fn	8	28	sup epith + KCS
52	Pug	Fe	7.6	100	deep stromal

Table 1. Signalment and ulcer characteristics of dogs involved in study (*Cont.*).

Case	Breed	Gender	Age	Ulcer duration (days)	Ulcer type
53	Cross-bred	Mn	6	14	mid stromal
54	Boxer	Mn	12	7	sup ep
55	Cross-bred	Fn	13	7	mid stromal
56	CKCS	Fe	7	14	mid stromal
57	Boxer	Mn	8	21	superficial
58	SBT	Fn	10	14	mid stromal
59	Boxer	Mn	4	10	superficial
60	Pug	Fn	2	10	mid stromal
61	Boxer X	Me	9	7	superficial
62	Bulldog	Me	4	21	superficial
63	Labrador	Mn	7	21	mid stromal
64	Boxer	Mn	8	28	superficial
65	Chihuahua	Fn	3	12	mid stromal
66	Lhasa Apso	Fn	5	14	mid stromal
67	Sharpei	Fe	6	7	superficial
68	Yorkshire terrier	Mn	4	5	deep stromal
69	Boxer	Mn	8	12	superficial
70	Boxer	Mn	7	21	superficial
71	Cross bred	Me	9	28	superficial
72	Chihuahua	Fn	10	5	superficial
73	Boxer cross	Mn	11	14	superficial
74	Pug	Mn	5	7	deep stromal
75	Cross-bred	Me	12	14	superficial
76	Rotweiler	Fn	7	5	deep stromal
77	Miniature Schnauzer	Fe	6	7	superficial
78	Lhasa Apso	Fe	7	7	superficial
79	German Shepherd dog	Mn	12	14	superficial
80	Short-haired pointer	Mn	9	21	superficial
81	Boxer	Mn	8	35	superficial
82	Cross-bred	Fn	6	14	deep stromal
83	Finnish laphund	Fn	4	10	deep stromal
84	CKCS	Fe	6	6	deep stromal
85	Cocker spaniel	Fn	12	35	superficial
86	Pembroke Corgi	Me	6	5	mid stromal
87	Boxer	Mn	8	21	superficial
88	Pekingese	Me	5	2	deep stromal
89	Cross-bred	Fe	6	28	superficial
90	Boxer	Mn	8	21	superficial
91	French bulldog	Mn	5	21	deep stromal
92	Cross-bred	Fe	7	28	superficial
93	Dalmatian	Fn	9	12	superficial
94	Alaskan Malamute	Fn	7	18	superficial
95	WHWT	Mn	8	21	superficial
96	English Springer spaniel	Mn	9	25	superficial
97	Boxer	Fn	8	12	superficial
98	Yorkshire terrier	Fn	5	18	superficial
99	German shepherd dog	Fn	8	14	superficial
100	Boxer	Me	12	56	superficial

(CKCS): Cavalier King Charles Spaniel; (SBT): Staffordshire Bull Terrier; (WHWT): West Highland white terrier; (me): male entire; (mn): male neutered; (fe): female entire; (fn): female neutered.

Table 2. Intraocular pressure (IOP) and tear production measured at Schirmer tear test (STT) in ulcerated eye and normal fellow eye together with clinical data on presence (1) or absence (0) of ocular hyperaemia, clinical signs of inflammation and miosis.

Case	IOP ulcerated eye	IOP normal eye	STT ulcerated eye	STT normal eye	Conjunctival hyperaemia	Intraocular inflammation	Miosis
1	14	17	19	16	0	0	0
2	9	14	22	18	0	0	1
3	13	18	19	15	0	0	0
4	10	21	21	14	0	0	3
5	7	13	22	19	0	0	0
6	13	14	16	10	0	0	0
7	7	15	25	23	1	1	1
8	8	16	10	14	1	1	1
9	12	16	17	16	0	0	0
10	8	13	22	17	0	0	0
11	12	18	24	19	0	0	0
12	13	15	27	22	1	0	0
13	12	17	24	20	1	0	1
14	14	16	22	19	0	0	0
15	8	13	24	17	0	0	1
16	10	15	22	19	0	0	1
17	12	15	26	23	0	0	0
18	14	18	15	13	0	0	0
19	12	22	24	19	1	0	0
20	13	16	14	16	0	0	0
21	9	16	18	14	0	0	1
22	12	15	19	15	1	0	0
23	9	15	22	18	1	0	0
24	12	17	19	15	1	0	0
25	8	16	22	17	1	0	0
26	18	21	24	9	1	0	0
27	15	17	20	12	1	1	0
28	11	15	18	15	1	0	1
29	13	14	14	11	1	1	0
30	4	11	22	16	0	0	0
31	4	11	0	12	0	0	0
32	15	9	19	8	0	0	0
33	12	15	24	6	1	0	0
34	15	11	28	9	0	0	0
35	13	25	20	27	0	0	0
36	12	18	17	14	0	0	0
37	15	13	19	23	0	0	0
38	13	23	15	13	0	0	0
39	13	17	15	7	0	0	0
40	12	17	22	16	0	0	0
41	17	15	13	17	0	0	0
42	9	24	18	21	1	1	0
43	14	15	22	20	0	0	0
44	15	16	18	15	0	0	0
45	11	15	32	21	0	0	0
46	27	14	18	22	1	0	1
47	12	15	0	15	1	1	0
48	10	20	22	18	1	0	0
49	7	14	22	18	1	1	1
50	15	21	18	14	0	0	0
51	14	16	19	16	0	0	0
52	12	16	15	13	1	1	1

Table 2. Intraocular pressure (IOP) and tear production measured at Schirmer tear test (STT) in ulcerated eye and normal fellow eye together with clinical data on presence (1) or absence (0) of ocular hyperaemia, clinical signs of inflammation and miosis (*Cont.*).

Case	IOP ulcerated eye	IOP normal eye	STT ulcerated eye	STT normal eye	Conjunctival hyperaemia	Intraocular inflammation	Miosis
53	13	18	20	17	1	1	1
54	11	16	21	17	0	0	0
55	12	18	18	16	1	0	0
56	11	17	19	17	1	0	1
57	12	15	22	18	1	0	1
58	13	20	21	16	0	0	1
59	11	16	18	15	0	0	0
60	14	16	18	17	0	0	0
61	12	17	16	16	0	1	0
62	13	19	19	18	1	1	0
63	13	18	22	18	1	0	0
64	10	16	18	19	0	0	0
65	14	16	26	22	0	1	1
66	15	18	21	18	0	0	0
67	13	16	25	21	1	0	0
68	13	17	27	17	0	0	1
69	13	18	24	21	1	0	0
70	8	14	18	18	1	0	0
71	13	16	24	23	1	1	0
72	7	17	17	16	0	1	0
73	14	17	19	15	0	1	1
74	12	18	22	17	1	0	1
75	15	18	24	18	0	0	0
76	13	17	21	18	0	0	0
77	14	19	27	21	1	0	0
78	7	19	22	18	0	1	0
79	6	17	19	17	0	1	1
80	8	19	19	16	0	1	1
81	13	17	15	13	0	1	1
82	11	19	20	17	1	0	0
83	14	19	26	19	1	0	0
84	7	20	22	16	1	0	0
85	14	18	21	19	0	1	1
86	12	18	23	15	1	0	0
87	8	18	25	19	0	0	0
88	13	15	22	15	1	1	1
89	13	19	24	19	0	0	Miosis
90	14	17	22	17	0	0	0
91	12	18	25	21	0	0	0
92	10	15	17	13	1	0	0
93	12	16	19	17	0	0	0
94	13	15	21	16	0	0	0
95	12	17	22	17	1	0	0
96	14	17	18	14	0	0	0
97	8	16	19	18	1	1	0
98	9	15	21	19	0	1	1
99	13	18	18	16	0	1	0
100	14	17	22	17	1	0	0

The mean (± standard deviation) of STT values are shown in Table (3) and the mean (± standard deviation) of IOP values are shown in Table (4). Both tables also show the values for eyes with superficial, mid stromal and deep stromal corneal ulcers and significance of differences between ulcerated and control eyes.

Table 3. Mean ± Standard Deviation of Schirmer tear test (STT) values in the ulcerated and non-ulcerated eyes categorised according to the depth of the ulcer as superficial, mid stromal or deep and significance of difference in STT between ulcerated and normal eyes.

Category	Mean±Standard Deviation STT (mm/min)		Significance of difference
	Ulcerated	Non-ulcerated	
All ulcers (100)	20.8±4.6	16.7±3.5	P<0.000001
Superficial (68)	20.2±5.1	16.6±6.2	p<0.0001
Mid Stromal (18)	19.9±2.9	16.4±3.27	p<0.001
Deep (13)	19.0±7.9	16.7±3.9	p<0.001

Table 4. Mean ± Standard Deviation of intraocular pressure (IOP) values in the ulcerated and non-ulcerated eyes categorised according to the depth of the ulcer as superficial, mid stromal or deep and significance of difference in IOP between ulcerated and normal eyes.

Category	Mean±Standard Deviation IOP (mmHg)		Significance of difference
	Ulcerated	Normal	
All Ulcers (50)	12.8±7.7	16.1±3.3	p<0.0001
Superficial (37)	12.7±2.8	16.6±2.7	p<0.00001
Mid Stromal (10)	14.1±3.8	16.2±2.2	p<0.0001
Deep (3)	7.9±1.1	17.0±1.9	p<0.0001

Mean (± standard deviation) STT values in the ulcerated eye compared to the non-ulcerated fellow eye were 20.8±4.6 and 16.7±3.5 respectively, this difference being highly statistically significant at p<0.000001. Mean (± standard deviation) values for IOP in the ulcerated eye compared to the control eye were 11.8±3.0 mmHg and 16.7±2.6 mmHg respectively, these being statistically significantly different at $P=0.0001$. Both IOP and STT were significant predictors of ulcer depth, with IOP significantly different at x^2 (chi squared) = 11. 25 p<0.00001 and STT significantly different at x^2 (chi squared) = 8.28 p<0.00001. Variations in duration of ulceration did not predict differences in IOP or STT.

Discussion

The results of this study show an increased tear production and decreased IOP to occur in eyes with corneal ulceration in the dog. An increase in tear production has been noted in the literature with reference to ocular pain (Belmonte *et al.*, 1997). One previous paper has documented that the STT in dogs with corneal epithelial defects is significantly greater when compared to the contralateral unaffected eyes (Murphy *et al.*, 2001), a result confirmed in this study, but in that report the change in tear production was but a marginal note in a larger study of superficial epithelial erosions: here we extend the investigation to a greater number of ulcerated eyes with ulcers of different types and depths. The most likely cause of increased tear production in corneal ulceration is the interaction of corneal nociceptive stimulation and subsequent lacrimal secretion (Unger, 1990).

The cornea is one of the most richly innervated tissues in the body receiving dense innervation by sensory nerves predominantly originating from neurons located in the ipsilateral trigeminal ganglion and modest sympathetic innervation from the superior cervical ganglion. The peripheral axons of the neurons terminate throughout the corneal epithelium as free nerve endings (Marfurt *et al.*, 2001). A previous study investigating the relationship between the stimulation of corneal sensory nerves and efferent output of the lacrimal functional unit determined by tear secretion showed that tear secretion increased almost linearly with the increase of stimulus intensity (Situ and Simpson, 2010). When noxious stimuli activate sensory afferents in the functional unit, a series of co-ordinated reflexes, including reflex tearing, are triggered to protect the eye from potential damage.

The current study supports previous findings that ocular pain, in this case resulting from corneal ulceration, will cause an increase in tear production due to stimulation of the lacrimal functional unit. It is possible that noxious stimuli causing the ulceration were also responsible for generating inflammation, but the ulcerated eyes did not show clinical signs of marked external inflammation which one would expect were this to be the cause of the changes in tear production and hypotony. There were no significant differences between eyes with signs of mild inflammation, as noted above, and those without.

The study makes the assumption that there is no significant difference in STT or IOP between the right and left eyes, this based on the fact that previous studies have not shown a difference between STT values of left and right eyes in normal dogs (Wyman *et al.*, 1995), and similarly IOP values have not been shown to differ between eyes (Giannetto *et al.*, 2009) so we feel confident that differences between ulcerated and control eyes here are highly likely to be related to the ulceration and not a random difference between eyes.

One limitation of this study was to only perform the Schirmer I test which measures both basal and reflex tear production. Further studies could evaluate use of the Schirmer II test to measure changes in basal tear production in corneal ulceration, by eliminating reflex tear production. It might also be argued that for completeness the study should have evaluated the ocular aqueous outflow tract by gonioscopy, but since IOP was normal or reduced and not increased in these eyes, such an additional diagnostic step was not considered essential. It will be noted that a significant number of animals (24%) had one or both eyes in which the STT was less than 15mm/min. While impossible to prove with the current data set, it is conceivable that animals with subnormal tear production are predisposed to corneal ulceration; such a hypothesis would merit further study evaluating STT values in age and breed-matched populations with and without corneal ulceration. A decrease in IOP is well recognised in association with ocular inflammation (Fine *et al.*, 2007) but not previously associated with corneal ulceration in dogs, or indeed in any other species to these authors' knowledge. It has been noted above that IOP is formed due to a balance between the production of aqueous humour and its drainage through the uveoscleral outflow and iridocorneal angle.

Prostaglandins (PGs) are regarded as mediators of the inflammatory process and are also present in ocular tissues. Studies have shown that during ocular inflammation PG concentration in the aqueous humour is higher than that found in normal aqueous humour (Camras *et al.*, 1977). It has been shown that PGs reduce IOP in a number of animal species including dogs, cats, nonhuman primates and rabbits by increasing uveoscleral aqueous humour outflow (Nilsson *et al.*, 1989; Weinreb *et al.*, 2002).

Thus we postulate that the trigeminal antidromic reflex occurring after exposure of free stromal and intra-epithelial nerve endings following corneal ulceration results in a prostaglandin production in the anterior segment of the eye, increased unconventional aqueous outflow and a hypotony, as demonstrated in the majority of cases here. It is conceivable that changes in the ulcerated cornea such as corneal oedema alter the elasticity of the tissues and thus invalidate the rebound tonometry but recent studies suggest that such changes are small and not clinically significant (Smedowski *et al.*, 2014). The present study documents that corneal ulceration in the dog is associated with an increase in tear production and a decrease in IOP. We would suggest that the ulceration is a cause of increased lacrimation through trigeminal stimulation and reduced IOP through prostaglandin-related increase in uveoscleral outflow, but clearly these postulates cannot be proven in such an observational study. This would require an experimental protocol in which corneal ulceration was caused and lacrimation and unconventional outflow measured before and after ocular surface injury. The welfare compromise of animals used in such an investigation would be

considerable and would preclude it under UK law, but we hope that this study on eyes with spontaneous corneal ulceration has provided useful data on the ocular changes associated with corneal ulceration.

This study shows the importance of measuring tear production in both eyes of dogs with corneal ulceration since the higher tear production in the ulcerated eye may produce an apparently normal STT reading and mask an underlying case of KCS. In the cuirrent series of animals cases 6, 18, 21, 26, 27, 29, 31, 32, 33, 34 and 39 all had suboptimal STT values in the normal eye although the raised STT in the ulcerated eye would have made it appear that they did not have any deficit in tear production if only that eye had been tested. It is impossible to know if a low tear production was involved in the development of ulceration before trigeminal stimulation in the ulcerated cornea increased the STT but we consider that this may be possible. The reduction in IOP suggests a mild intraocular inflammatory process in many if not all eyes with corneal ulceration which should be documented by tonometry in any eye with an ulcerated cornea and addressed therapeutically if severe. Many facts in veterinary ophthalmology, as in many other areas of veterinary medicine, are widely accepted but without any firm data to back them up. That eyes with corneal ulceration have increased lacrimation and decreased IOP is one of these unquestioned truths. It is hoped that this study has provided some evidence to support these assumptions and also suggested areas of further research to elucidate the mechanisms by which these ocular changes occur.

Conflict of interest:

The authors declare that there is no conflict of interest.

References

Belmonte, C., Garcia-Hirschfield, J. and Gallar, J. 1997. Neurobiology of ocular pain. Prog. Retin. Eye Res. 16, 117-156.

Berger, S.L. and King, V.L. 1998. The fluctuation of tear production. J. Am. Anim. Hosp. Assoc. 34(1), 79-83.

Camras, C.B., Bito, L.Z. and Eakins, K.E. 1977. Reduction of intraocular pressure by prostaglandins applied topically to the eyes of conscious rabbits. Invest. Ophthalmol. Vis. Sci. 16(12), 1125-1134.

Fine, H.F., Biscette, O., Chang, S. and Schiff, W.M. 2007. Ocular hypotony: a review. Compr. Ophthalmol. Update 8(1), 29-37.

Gelatt, K.N., Peiffer, R.L., Erickson, J.L. and Gum, G.G. 1975. Evaluation of tear formation in the dog, using a modification of the Schirmer tear test. J. Am. Vet. Med. Assoc. 166(4), 368-370.

Gelatt, K.N. and MacKay, E.O. 1998. Distribution of intraocular pressure in dogs. Vet. Ophthalmol. 1(2-3), 109-114.

Giannetto, C., Piccione, G. and Giudice, E. 2009. Daytime profile of the intraocular pressure and tear production in normal dog. Vet. Ophthalmol. 12(5), 302-305.

Gilger, B.C., Ollivier, F.J. and Bentley, E. 2008. Diseases and surgery of the canine cornea and sclera. In: Essentials of veterinary ophthalmology, 2nd edn (ed. Gelatt KN). Blackwell Publishing, Iowa, pp: 119-154.

Hartley, C., Williams, D.L. and Adams, V.J. 2006. Effect of age, gender, weight, and time of day on tear production in normal dogs. Vet. Ophthalmol. 9(1), 53-57.

Lee, J. 1992. Cumulative logit modelling for ordinal response variables: applications to biomedical research. Comput. Appl. Biosci. 8(6), 555-562.

Leiva, M., Naranjo, C. and Peña, M.T. 2006. Comparison of the rebound tonometer (ICare) to the applanation tonometer (Tonopen XL) in normotensive dogs. Vet. Ophthalmol. 9(1), 17-21.

Marfurt, C.F., Murphy, C.J. and Florczak, J.L. 2001. Morphology and neurochemistry of canine corneal innervation. Invest. Ophthalmol. Vis. Sci. 42(10), 2242-2251.

Murphy, C.J., Marfurt, C.F., McDermott, A., Bentley, E., Abrams, G.A., Reid, T.W. and Cambell, S. 2001. Spontaneous chronic corneal epithelial defects (SCCED) in dogs: Clinical features, innervation, and effect of topical SP, with or without IGF-1.

Invest. Ophthalmol. Vis. Sci. 42(10), 2252-2261.

Nilsson, S.F., Samuelson, M., Bill, A. and Stjernschantz, J. 1989. Increased uveoscleral outflow as a possible mechanism of ocular hypotension caused by prostaglandin F2α-1-isopropylester in the Cynomolgus monkey. Exp. Eye Res. 48(5), 707-716.

Reinstein, S., Rankin, A. and Allbaugh, R. 2009. Canine glaucoma: pathophysiology and diagnosis. Compend. Contin. Educ. Vet. 31(10), 450-452.

Situ, P. and Simpson, T.L. 2010. Interaction of corneal nociceptive stimulation and lacrimal secretion. Invest. Ophthalmol. Vis. Sci. 51(11), 5640-5645.

Stern, M.E., Gao, J., Siemasko, K.F., Beuerman, R.W. and Pflugfeilder, S.C. 2004. The role of the lacrimal functional unit in the pathophysiology of dry eye. Exp. Eye Res. 78(3), 409-416.

Unger, W.G. 1990. Mediation of the ocular response to injury. J. Ocul. Pharmacol. 6(4), 337-353.

Weinreb, R.N., Toris, C.B., Gabelt, B.'A.T., Linsey, J.D. and Kaufman, P.L. 2002. Effects of prostaglandins on the aqueous humor outflow pathway. Surv. Ophthalmol. 47(Suppl. 1), S53-64.

Williams, D.L. 2008. Immunopathogenesis of keratoconjunctivitis sicca in the dog. Vet. Clin. North Am. Small Anim. Pract. 38(2), 251-268.

Wyman, M., Gilger, B., Mueller, P., Norrýs, K., 1995. Clinical evaluation of a new Schirmer tear test in the dog. Vet. Comp. Ophthalmol. 5, 211-214.

9

Splenophrenic portosystemic shunt in dogs with and without portal hypertension: can acquired and congenital porto-caval connections coexist?

M. Ricciardi*

"Pingry" Veterinary Hospital, via Medaglie d'Oro 5, Bari Italy

Abstract

The possible existence of the same pattern of porto-caval connection in dogs having a single congenital portosystemic shunt (CPSS) and in dogs having multiple acquired portosystemic shunt (MAPSS) secondary to portal hypertension (PH) was evaluated. Retrospective evaluation of all CT examinations of patients having portosystemic shunt (PSS) was performed in a 4-year time period. All anomalous *porto-caval connections* were assessed for anatomical pattern and compared with published veterinary literature. Records of 25 dogs were reviewed. 16 dogs had a single CPSS (CPSS group), and 9 dogs had multiple acquired PSS secondary to PH (APSS group). The splenophrenic shunt pattern was found in 3 dogs of the CPSS group as a single congenital anomaly without PH and in 2 dogs of the APSS group associated with MAPSS and ascites due to different hepatic diseases causing PH. These findings corroborate two hypotheses: 1) Splenophrenic PSS should be considered as a classical CPSS but if this is not sufficient to alleviate a PH developed after birth because of eventual hepatic or portal diseases, in this case ascites and acquired portal collaterals may develop. In this case, MAPSS and CPSS may coexist. 2) The pattern of splenophrenic PSS, classically described among CPSS, may develop as acquired portal collateral in dogs with PH and it should also be included in the category of APSS. These preliminary findings may be helpful in reconsidering the classical haemodynamics of porto-caval diseases, enrich the classification of APSS in dogs and refine the imaging evaluation of patients with PH.

Keywords: Computed tomography, Dog, Portal hypertension, Portosystemic shunt.

Introduction

Extrahepatic portosystemic shunts (PSS) are abnormal vascular connections between the portal and caval venous systems at the level of their major trunks or secondary branches (Watson and Herrtage, 1998; Nelson and Nelson, 2011). Based on their development and appearances, PSS are classically considered to be distinct, with congenital PSS (CPSS) deriving from embryogenetic errors in the development of vitelline and cardinal venous systems (Ferrell *et al.*, 2003), and acquired PSS (APSS) deriving from recanalization of pre-existing, vestigial embryonic vascular connections between portal and caval systems in the case of portal hypertension (PH) (Fossum, 2002; Szatmàri *et al.*, 2004; Bertolini, 2010a).

In patients with CPSS, clinical signs are related to the mixing of portal blood, which bypasses the hepatic sinusoids, with peripheral venous circulation and include hepatic encephalopathy, stunted growth, cystic calculi, vomiting, and diarrhea (Watson and Herrtage, 1998; Agg, 2006; Kraun *et al.*, 2014). In APSS, clinical signs may be related to the primary underlying disease causing portal flow obstruction with PH or may be due only to PH such as ascites, which is often, but not always, associated (Buob *et al.*, 2011).

Differences in treatment options and prognoses between patients having CPSS and those with APSS make it essential to distinguish between these two conditions but, unfortunately, this cannot be made only on the basis of clinicopathologic findings (Adam *et al.*, 2012).

In this context, non-invasive vascular imaging techniques such as ultrasonography, computed tomography, and magnetic resonance angiography play an important role in detecting pathologic porto-caval connections and defining their origins (Lamb, 1996; Bertolini *et al.*, 2006; Bertolini 2010a, 2010b; Bruehschwein *et al.*, 2010; Nelson and Nelson, 2011; Fukushima *et al.*, 2014).

APSS and CPSS have been described and classified in dogs from an anatomical point of view, using computed tomography angiography (CTA), taking into account their size, origin, course, and termination between portal and caval venous systems (Bertolini *et al.*, 2006; Bertolini, 2010a, 2010b; Nelson and Nelson, 2011; Fukushima *et al.*, 2014; Ricciardi *et al.*, 2014).

It has been reported that in dogs the most consistently observed route of APSSs are left splenogonadal shunt and splenophrenic varices (Szatmàri *et al.*, 2004; Bertolini, 2010a; Ricciardi *et al.*, 2014) while splenocaval, splenophrenic and splenoazygos PSS pattern are reported more frequently among CPSSs (Szatmàri *et al.*, 2004; Bertolini *et al.*, 2006; Nelson and Nelson, 2011; Fukushima *et al.*, 2014).

*Corresponding Author: Mario Ricciardi. "Pingry" Veterinary Hospital, via Medaglie d'Oro 5, 70126 Bari, Italy.
Email: ricciardi.mario@alice.it*

In the last few years, different, repeatable but always distinct, vascular patterns have been observed within each category without any overlapping of anatomical pathway between APPS and CPPS. These differences in the course of congenital and acquired PSS allow for their categorization during an angiographic study. To date, few descriptions on the coexistence of APSS and CPSS in the same patient have been published in dogs (Ferrell et al., 2003; Hunt, 2004) but unfortunately they lack a detailed categorization of the shunt phenotype according to the actual anatomical classifications of the of CPSS and APSS. Hence, at present, the coexistence of CPSS in patients having PH, with secondary multiple APSS and ascites, is not fully accepted and still is debated (Ferrell et al., 2003; Szatmári, 2003).

The aim of this retrospective study is to evaluate the possible simultaneous coexistence of the same anatomical pattern of porto-caval connection in dogs having a single CPSS and those having MAPSS.

Material and Methods

The medical records of all cases of PSS in dogs presented at the "Pingry" Veterinary Hospital in Bari, Italy, between September 2011 and August 2015 were reviewed. Dogs were eligible for inclusion in the study if they fulfilled the following criteria:

1) Complete physical examination, blood count, biochemical profile and urinalysis;
2) Exclusion of right-sided heart failure or severe hypoproteinemia for dogs having ascites;
3) Computed tomography angiography (CTA) of the thoracic and abdominal regions;
4) Confirmation of the vascular anomaly during surgery (for single PSS) and a histopathologic or surgical confirmation of the cause of PH (for patients with multiple PSS).

Multidetector Computed Tomography examination protocol

All CTA were acquired using a 16-slice multidetector computed tomography (MDCT) scanner (Somatom Emotion, Siemens, Forchheim, Germany) before and after the manual injection of iodinate contrast medium (640 mg I/kg; Iopamigita® Insight Agents GmbHR, Heildeberg, Germany). Scanning and reconstruction parameters were as follows: helical modality, 0.6 - 1 sec/gantry rotation, 1 mm slice thickness; 180 kV, 110 mAs; soft tissue reconstruction algorithm.

MDCT image analysis

For selected patients, MDCT data were retrieved and restored from picture archiving and communication systems (PACS) (Marcel van Herk, "Conquest DICOM software." Online Available: http://ingenium.home.xs4all.nl/dicom.html.), and carefully assessed by the author for thoracic and abdominal vascular anomalies. Multiplanar reformatted images and volume rendered angiographic reconstructions were obtained from native CT images, using a dedicated post-processing software (OsiriX DICOM-viewer; Pixmeo, Geneva, Switzerland). Information extracted from CTA of each dog included in the study comprised number of PSS (single or multiple), size (large shunt or varices), pattern of PSS (according to the major classifications of CPSS (Szatmàri et al., 2004; Bertolini, 2010b; Nelson and Nelson, 2011; Fukushima et al., 2014) and APSS (Bertolini, 2010a), presence/absence of abdominal effusion (ascites), and presence of macroscopic structural cause of portal flow obstruction.

Histopathologic evaluation

All liver biopsy samples in dogs, with suspected PH, were obtained by exploratory laparotomy. Specimens were sent for histopathologic evaluation in a certified veterinary laboratory (San Marco Veterinary Laboratory, Padova, Italy). All histopathological evaluations were made by board certified pathologists.

Results

The medical records of 25 dogs with PSS matched the inclusion criteria and were reviewed.

16 dogs had a single PSS shunt without abdominal effusion. Regarding the anatomical pattern there were 7 splenocaval, 4 right gastric-caval, 2 splenoazygos and 3 splenophrenic PSS.

In Table 1, clinical signs, hematobiochemical and urinalysis abnormalities, and PSS pattern are summarized individually for each dog of this group. The final diagnosis for all these dogs was single congenital PSS.

Nine dogs had multiple PSS. In this group, 8 dogs had concomitant abdominal effusion and no structural nor attenuation changes of the liver were evident on CT images. In one dog, CT showed multiple hepatic masses suggestive of diffuse hepatic neoplasia, absence of abdominal effusion, and multiple large porto-caval connections. Two large vessels, originating respectively from the pancreaticoduodenal vein and from splenic vein, ran ventro-caudally and joined in a single vessel draining into the caudal vena cava at level of right gonadal vein (Table 2 – Fig. 1, dog 5).

The other porto-caval connection was a left splenogonadal shunt (Fig. 2). Hepatic lesions were diagnosed histopathologically as histiocytic sarcoma. One dog with multiple PSS had a large shunt between portal vein and cranial vena cava via left internal thoracic vein (Table 2 – Fig. 3, dog 1). In one dog multiple tangled large shunts were found between the main trunk of portal vein at level of splenic vein insertion and the pre-hepatic segment of the caudal vena cava (Table 2 – Fig. 4, dog 7).

All dogs had a final diagnosis of PH with multiple APSS based on clinical, CT and histopathologic findings. In 8 dogs PH was due to hepatic microvascular or parenchymal disorder based on evaluation of liver biopsy samples.

Table 1. Signalment, clinical signs, major hematobiochemical and urinalysis abnormalities and shunt pattern in dogs with CPSS.

n	Signalment	Clinical signs	Pattern of CPSS evident on CTA	Major hematobiochemical and urinalysis abnormalities
1	9-years-old, female, Yorkshire Terrier	Abnormal mentation; vomiting	Right gastric-caval shunt	ALT (UI/L): 150 (20-70); UBA (mmol/L): 157 (1-12.5)
2	10-years-old, male, Yorkshire Terrier	Seizures; abnormal mentation; vomiting	Left gastric-azygos shunt	UBA (mmol/L): 70 (1-12.5)
3	1-year-old, male, Mongrel	Abnormal mentation; vomiting	Spleno-caval shunt	ALT (UI/L): 86 (20-70); UBA (mmol/L): 98 (1-12.5)
4	5-years-old, female, Pinscher	Abnormal mentation; mild hematuria	Splenophrenic shunt	AST (UI/L): 179 (20-50); ALT (UI/L): 230 (20-70); Albumin (g/dL): 2.4 (2.5-4.0); UBA (mmol/L): 400 (1-12.5)
5	5-years-old, female, Beagle	Polyuria and polydipsia; hematuria.	Right gastric-caval shunt	UBA (mmol/L): 336 (1-12.5)
6	8-months-old, female, Yorkshire Terrier	Seizures; disappetence	Splenophrenic shunt	AST (UI/L): 135 (20-50); ALT (UI/L): 112 (20-70); UBA (mmol/L): 27 (1-12.5)
7	11-years-old, male, Shih-tzu	Abnormal mentation	Right gastric-caval shunt	Albumin (g/dL): 2.0 (2.5-4.0); UBA (mmol/L): 363 (1-12.5)
8	1-year-old, female, Pinscher	Seizures; abnormal mentation; depression	Spleno-caval shunt	Albumin (g/dL): 1.6 (2.5-4.0); UBA (mmol/L): 144 (1-12.5)
9	3-years-old, female, Yorkshire Terrier	Abnormal mentation; disappetence; vomiting	Spleno-caval shunt	Albumin (g/dL): 2.0 (2.5-4.0); UBA (mmol/L): 213 (1-12.5)
10	2-years-old, male, Chihuahua	Abnormal mentation; lethargy	Splenophrenic shunt	UBA (mmol/L): 30 (1-12.5)
11	4-years-old, female, Yorkshire Terrier	Hematuria; disappetence; vomiting	Left gastric-azygos shunt	Albumin (g/dL): 2.1 (2.5-4.0); UBA (mmol/L): 161 (1-12.5)
12	6-months-old, male, Mongrel	Abnormal mentation; depression; vomiting;	Spleno-caval shunt	Albumin (g/dL): 2.0 (2.5-4.0); UBA (mmol/L): 182 (1-12.5)
13	3-months-old, female, Florence Spitz	Abnormal mentation; vomiting	Spleno-caval shunt	UBA (mmol/L): 102 (1-12.5)
14	5-months-old, female, Pinscher	Vomiting; lethargy	Right gastric-caval shunt	ALT (UI/L): 90 (20-70); UBA (mmol/L): 159 (1-12.5)
15	1-year-old, male, Mongrel	Abnormal mentation	Spleno-caval shunt	UBA (mmol/L): 49 (1-12.5)
16	7-months-old, male, Mongrel	Seizures; depression; vomiting	Spleno-caval shunt	Albumin (g/dL): 2.2 (2.5-4.0); UBA (mmol/L): 173 (1-12.5)

In one dog the increased portal flow and subsequent PH was due to a large extra-hepatic arteriovenous fistula in which the hepatic artery joined the portal vein. In each dog with acquired portal collaterals there were both large PSS and small varices. Clinical signs, hematobiochemical and urinalysis abnormalities, histopathologic findings and APSS patterns are summarized in Table 2.

Five dogs had a large porto-caval connection between the left gastric vein and the post hepatic segment of caudal vena cava at the phrenic vein level. In 3 of these 5 patients (Table 1: dog 4, 6, 10) the extrahepatic splenophrenic PSS was found as a single porto-caval connection and no abdominal effusion was present (Fig. 5). In the other two dogs (Table 2: dog 1, 2) the extrahepatic splenophrenic PSS was associated with multiple APSS and ascites (which developed as a consequence of PH due to primary liver disease i.e.

primary hypoplasia of the portal vein and lobular dissecting hepatitis) (Fig. 6 and 7).

Discussion

In veterinary literature simultaneous congenital and acquired PSS have been reported in three dogs (Ferrell *et al.*, 2003; Hunt, 2004). In two of these cases the vascular anomalies and their anatomical pattern were not assessed (Ferrell *et al.*, 2003) and not available for review (Hunt, 2004). In one of these 3 dogs the coexistence of CPSS and APSS has been hypothesized because of the presence of a large venous connection between splenic vein and post-hepatic caudal vena cava, multiple porto-caval collaterals near the left kidney and histologic liver findings similar to those found with congenital shunts (Ferrell *et al.*, 2003). However, this condition is not fully accepted by veterinary specialists and is still debated. (Szatmári, 2003).

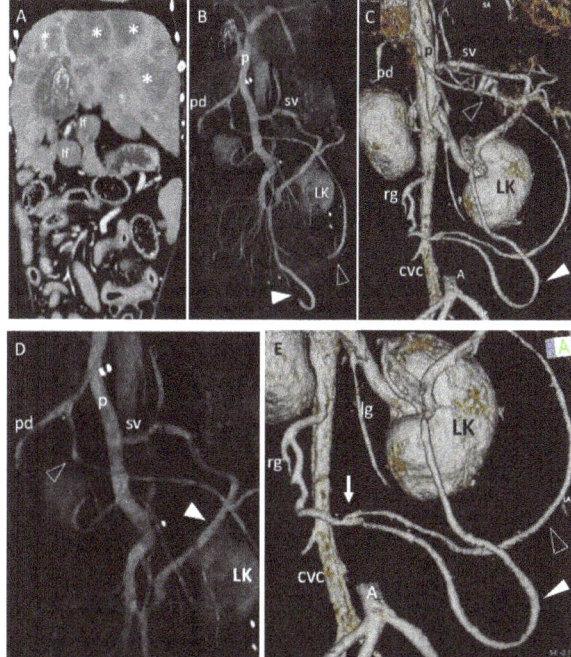

Fig. 1. Dog 5 of PH group. (A) Dorsal contrast-enhanced multiplanar reformatted CT image of the abdomen. There are multiple hepatic neoformations (asterisks) ipoattenuating to hepatic parenchyma, periportal lymph nodes enlargement (lf) and no abdominal effusion. (B,C,D,E) Three-dimensional volume rendered image of the portal vein (p) and caudal vena cava (CVC) – ventral views. Two large vessels (empty and full arrowheads) originate respectively from the pancreaticoduodenal vein (pd) and from splenic vein (sv), run caudally and join in a single vessel draining into the caudal vena cava at level of right gonadal vein (rg). (B) whole portal vein, ventral view; (C) detail of the entire PSS from its double portal origin to its caval termination; (D) detail of origins of the anomalous vessels from pancreaticoduodenal vein (empty arrowhead) and splenic vein (full arrowhead); (E) detail of connection (arrow) of the two shunts in one vessel which enters caudal vena cava at level of right gonadal vein. These vessels appeared suggestive of APSS because they were associated with a visible cause of PH (diffuse hepatic neoplasia) and other classical APSS (see Fig. 5). The absence of ascites could be explained by a complete effectiveness of these APSS in alleviating portal pressure. LK, left kidney; lg, left gonadal vein; A, caudal abdominal aorta (sectioned and partially removed).

The possibility of the coexistence of congenital and acquired PSS in the same patient is considered unlikely for different reasons:

1) APSS may be small tortuous vessels, defined as varices, but may also be found as large vessels (Bertolini, 2010a; Ricciardi *et al.*, 2014). Hence, if a large PSS is found together with other multiple small tortuous porto-caval connections, it is conceivable that all these abnormal vessels might be acquired PSS.

2) According to hemodynamic principles the presence of a CPSS, in a dog with portal flow obstruction at level of the liver, would bypass portal blood in the systemic (caval) circulation that presents the lowest resistance, making development of PH unlikely (Szatmári, 2003). The presence of ascites should be considered incompatible with a CPSS (Wrigley *et al.*, 1987; Szatmari and Rothuizen, 2002) and such a finding, in non-cardiac, non-hypoalbuminemic patients, should prompt recognition of a likely diagnosis of APSS secondary to PH (Adam *et al.*, 2012).

3) Histopathologic liver changes may be identical in case of primary diseases causing PH (idiopathic non-cirrhotic PH, portal venous hypoplasia, hepatic microvascular dysplasia and congenital arterioportal fistula) or in the case of reduced portal perfusion (congenital PSS). Thus differentiation between APSS due to primary liver disease and CPSS may not be possible based on liver histopathologic findings (Van den Ingh *et al.*, 1995a, 1995b; Center, 1996; Bunch *et al.*, 2001).

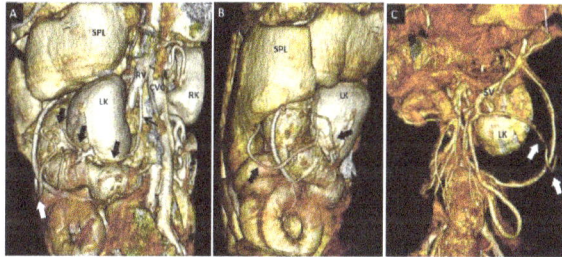

Fig. 2. Dog 5 of PH group. Three-dimensional volume-rendered CT angiography of the left splenogonadal PSS. (A) dorso-lateral view; (B) left lateral view; (C) ventral view. From left gonadal vein (A, black arrow) a tortuous vessel (thick arrows) runs in caudo-ventro-lateral direction to join the splenic vein (SV). As shown in Fig. 1, splenic vein drained into right gonadal vein. SPL, spleen; LK, left kidney; RK, right kidney. This dog had both classified and unclassified APSS.

It has been demonstrated that signalment, clinical signs, and results of biochemical analysis would be unlikely to enable differentiation between dogs with congenital and acquired PSS (Hunt, 2004; Adam *et al.*, 2012). Currently, advanced diagnostic imaging and physical examination (detection of ascites) are considered the most reliable means of discrimination between acquired and congenital PSS in dogs (Szatmári, 2003). In major classifications of APSS and CPSS different patterns have been codified using MDCT angiography and their morphology appear constant and repeatable in all the different reported cases (Szatmàri *et al.*, 2004; Bertolini, 2010a, 2010b; Nelson and Nelson, 2011; Fukushima *et al.*, 2014; Ricciardi *et al.*, 2014).

Table 2. Clinical, imaging, hematobiochemical/urinalysis and histopathologic findings in dogs with PH and APSS. Asterisks indicate unclassified APSS patterns.

n	Signalment	Clinical signs	Abdominal effusion	Pattern of APSS evident on CTA according to major classification [4]	Hematobiochemical and urinalysis abnormalities	Histopathologic diagnosis
1	6-months-old, female, Rottweiler	Abdominal distension; inappetence	Pure transudate	- Gastro-phrenic varices; - Large shunt between colic vein and right internal iliac vein; - Large shunt between portal vein and left internal thoracic vein*; - Large shunt between left gastric vein and phrenic vein* (Splenophrenic shunt)	AST (UI/L): 77 (20-50); ALP (UI/L): 4797 (50-200); Albumin (g/dL): 2.4 (2.5-4.0) UBA (mmol/L): 160 (1-12.5)	PHPV (primary hypoplasia of the portal vein)
2	1-year-old, male, Maltese	Abdominal distension; inappetence	Pure transudate	- Gastro-phrenic varices; - Mesenteric collaterals (Large shunt between left colic vein and left gonadal vein); - Large shunt between left gastric vein and phrenic vein* (Splenophrenic shunt)	AST (UI/L): 226 (20-50); ALT (UI/L): 175 (20-70); UBA (mmol/L): 160 (1-12.5)	Lobular dissecting hepatitis
3	4-months-old, male, Mongrel	Abdominal distension; Drowsiness; Vomiting; Diarrhea	Pure transudate	Gastro-phrenic varices	AST (UI/L): 46 (20-50); ALT (UI/L): 231 (20-70); Albumin (g/dL): 1.9 (2.5-4.0) UBA (mmol/L): 82 (1-12.5)	PHPV
4	7-months-old, female, Mongrel	Abdominal distension	Pure transudate	- Gastro-phrenic varices; - Left splenogonadal shunt (large shunt between splenic vein and left gonadal vein)	AST (UI/L): 79 (20-50); UBA (mmol/L): 89 (1-12.5)	PHPV
5	12-years-old, female, Mongrel	Weight loss; Vomiting; Diarrhea	None	- Left splenogonadal shunt; - Large shunt between pancreaticoduodenal vein, splenic vein and right gonadal vein*	ALT (UI/L): 320 (20-70); ALP (UI/L): 938 (50-200); Fibrinogen (mg/dL): 145 (152-184) FSPs (µg/mL): 17 (0.11-2.84)	Diffuse hepatic neoplasia (histiocytic sarcoma)
6	2-years-old, female, German shepherd	Weight loss; Abdominal distension; Abnormal mentation; inappetence	Pure transudate	- Gastro-phrenic varices; - Left splenogonadal shunt	AST (UI/L): 109 (20-50); ALT (UI/L): 214 (20-70); UBA (mmol/L): 133 (1-12.5)	PHPV
7	4-months-old, male, Great dane	Weight loss; Abdominal distension; inappetence	Pure transudate	- Gallbladder varices; - Gastro-phrenic varices; - Left splenogonadal shunt; - multiple, tangled, large shunts between portal vein (main trunk at level of splenic vein insertion) and caudal vena cava (main trunk – pre-hepatic segment)*	AST (UI/L): 93 (20-50); ALT (UI/L): 342 (20-70); Albumin (g/dL): 2.4 (2.5-4.0) UBA (mmol/L): 166 (1-12.5)	Large extra-hepatic artero-portal fistula
8	1-year-old, female, Pit Bull Terrier	Weight loss; Abdominal distension	Pure transudate	- Gastro-phrenic varices - Left splenogonadal shunt (large shunt between splenic vein and left gonadal vein)	AST (UI/L): 1081 (20-50); ALT (UI/L): 1645 (20-70); Albumin (g/dL): 1.5 (2.5-4.0) UBA (mmol/L): 1282.4 (1-12.5)	PHPV
9	9-months-old, male, Mongrel	Abdominal distension	Pure transudate	- Gastro-phrenic varices - Colic varices - Left splenogonadal shunt	AST (UI/L): 57 (20-50); UBA (mmol/L): 339 (1-12.5)	End-stage chronic hepatitis

To date, codified CPSS patterns have not been reported in dogs with PH and, vice versa, codified APSS patterns have never been reported as single shunt without ascites. Thus, the evaluation of the size, number and anatomical pattern of a PSS as seen on CT images, along with the presence or absence of abdominal effusion, may be helpful for the categorization of the PSS type (Szatmàri et al., 2004; Bertolini, 2010a, 2010b; Nelson and Nelson, 2011; Fukushima et al., 2014; Ricciardi et al., 2014).

The clinical relevance of the differentiation between CPPS and APSS patterns derives from the necessity to distinguish patients with underlying PH (testified by the presence of MAPSS), for which shunt closure is not indicated and that require further investigations in order to diagnose the cause of the hypertensive disorder, from patients with congenital porto-caval connections which require surgical closure.

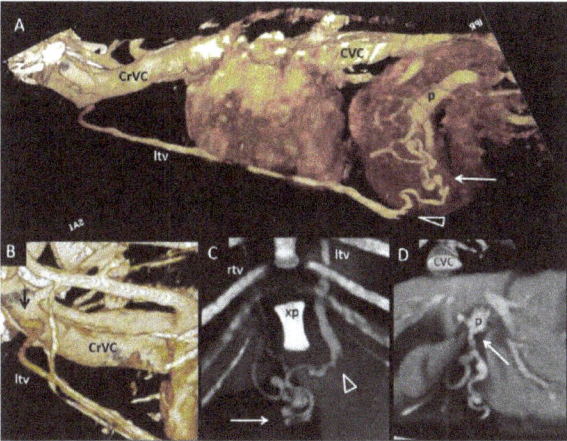

Fig. 3. Dog 1 of PH group; APSS from portal vein to cranial vena cava via left internal thoracic vein. (A) Three-dimensional volume-rendered CT angiography of cranial abdomen and thorax. A Tortuous vessel (long arrow) originates from the portal vein (p) before its intra-hepatic branches, courses ventrally and joins the left internal thoracic vein (ltv) to reach cranial vena cava (CrVC). (B) Three-dimensional volume-rendered detail of left internal thoracic vein origin (ltv) (black arrow) from cranial vena cava (CrVC). (C) Ventral three-dimensional volume-rendered image at level of xiphoid process of the sternum (xp) showing in detail the point of connection (arrowhead) between the PSS (long arrow) and left internal thoracic vein (ltv). (D) Transverse three-dimensional volume-rendered image at level of portal vein just before its intrahepatic division. The long arrow points to the PSS origin from the portal vein. rtv, right internal thoracic vein; CVC, caudal vena cava.

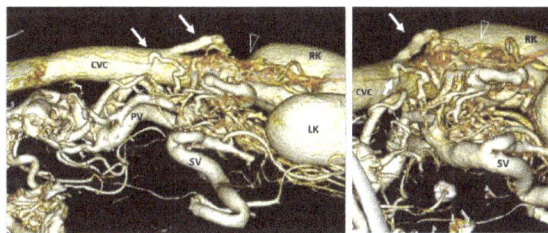

Fig. 4. Dog 7 of PH group. APSS of unclassified pattern. Three-dimensional volume-rendered CT angiography of portal vein and caudal vena cava. (A) Left lateral view; (B) detail of caudal vena cava (CVC) - dorso-cranial view. Two large vessels (arrows) originating at different points from portal vein (PV) drained into main trunk of caudal vena cava just cranially to the kindeys. Gastrophrenic varices are also evident (arrowheads). LK, left kidney; RK, right kidney.

Among the cases examined in this study, 5 dogs had a large extrahepatic PSS attributable to the splenophrenic pattern. This shunt type has been classified among CPSS (Bertolini, 2010b, Nelson and Nelson, 2011) and in a study on 178 cases of congenital extra-hepatic PSS it has been described as one of the most common anatomical patterns (Fukushima *et al.*, 2014). However, a splenophrenic PSS pattern has never been reported among APSS (Bertolini, 2010a).

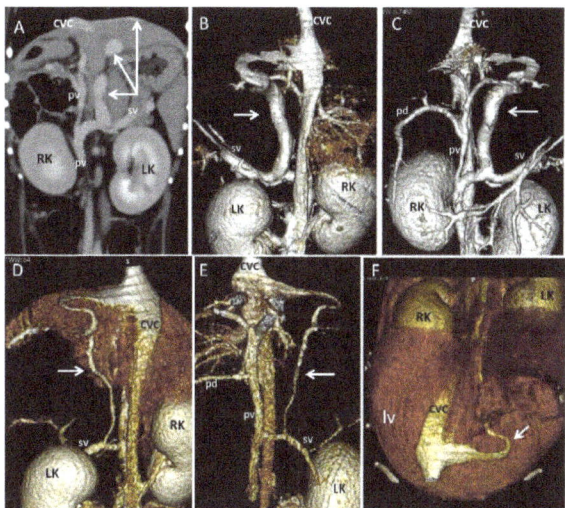

Fig. 5. Splenophrenic PSS in dog 4 (A, B, C) and dog 10 (D, E, F) of CPSS group. (A) Dorsal multiplanar reformatted CT image of the abdomen at level of kidneys. A Splenophrenic PSS is evident (arrows) between splenic vein (sv) and post-hepatic segment of caudal vena cava (CVC). No varices nor abdominal effusion are evident. Three-dimensional volume-rendered CT angiography of portal system and caudal vena cava in dogs 4 and 10. (B, D – Dorsal views; C,E - ventral views; F - dorso-cranial view at level of hepatic surface.). On three-dimensional volume-rendered CT angiography of portal system and caudal vena cava of both dogs the splenophrenic PSS (arrows) had same anatomical pattern seen in dogs with PH of Fig. 1 and 2. These PSS were assumed to be congenital because appear as single porto-caval connections not associated with ascites or varices, and no structural causes of portal flow obstruction were evident on CT images.

In three out of 5 of our dogs the splenophrenic PSS was single and not associated with ascites so it was considered most likely a CPSS. However, in the other two of these 5 dogs the splenophrenic PSS was associated with PH, due to PHPV (Table 2 - dog 1) and lobular dissecting hepatitis (Table 2 - dog 2), with multiple APSS and abdominal effusion.

Based on these findings, for both cases two hypothesis were made:

1) Coexistence of CPSS of splenophrenic pattern and multiple APSS in these two patients with PH. In this case, a CPSS may be not sufficient to alleviate PH caused by primary diffuse intrahepatic microvascular or parenchymal disease. Consequently, APSS and ascites develop (Szatmári, 2003). This hypothesis would disavow the theory that development of PH is unlikely in the presence of a CPSS, as previously reported (Szatmári, 2003), and would help refine imaging evaluation of patients with PH.

2) The splenophrenic PSS may also be a pattern of APSS until now unreported, which regains patency if PH develops. The portal vein in the normal dog

has at least three embryonic connections with the systemic venous system, which usually are not, or only minimally perfused. One of these connects the phrenic vein with small branches of the portal vein (Huntington and Mcclure, 1920; Bertolini, 2010a). Such embryonic pathways of porto-caval connection may develop in splenophrenic APSS when PH occurs.

explained by the complete effectiveness of the APSS in alleviating portal pressure. However, in cases of primary microvascular or parenchymal hepatic disorders macroscopically undetectable on imaging evaluation (such as PHPV), the possible absence of ascites and the presence of a single acquired splenophrenic shunt (without other MAPSS) may disorient the presumptive diagnosis of PH.

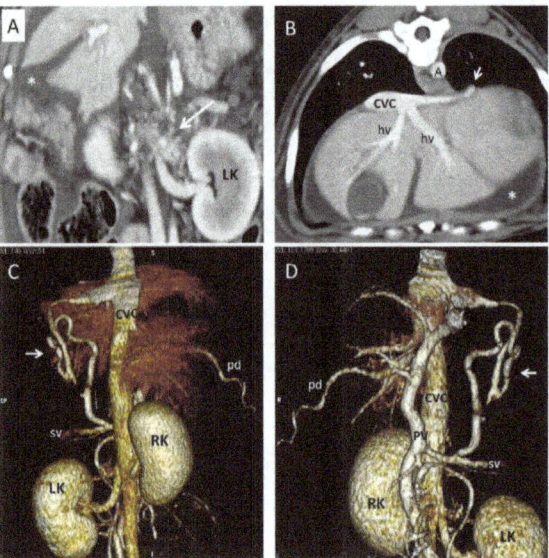

Fig. 6. Dog 1 of PH group. (A) Dorsal multiplanar reformatted CT image of abdomen at level of kidneys. Gastrophrenic varices (long arrow) are visible medially to the left kidney (LK). Large amount of fluid (ascites) is evident in background (asterisk). (B) Transverse multiplanar reformatted CT image of abdomen at level of liver and insertion of phrenic vein. Short arrow indicates insertion of a PSS in caudal vena cava (CVC). (C) Dorsal and (D) ventral three-dimensional volume-rendered CT angiography of portal system and caudal vena cava. Short arrows point to splenophrenic shunt. A, aorta; RK, right kidney; PV, portal vein; pd, pancreaticoduodenal vein; sv, splenic vein.

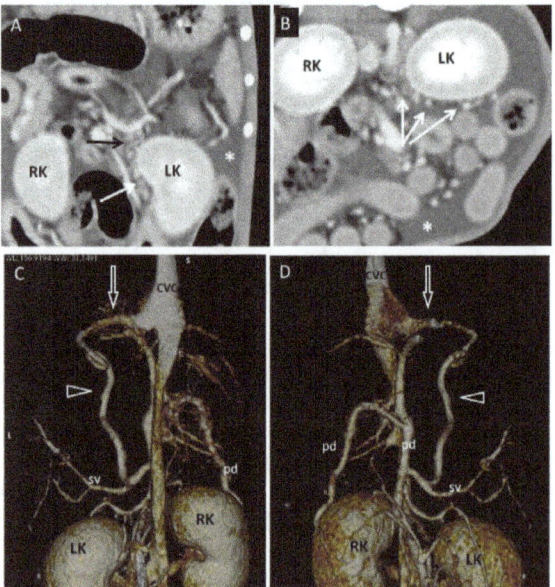

Fig. 7. Dog 2 of PH group. (A) Dorsal and (B) transverse multiplanar reformatted CT images of abdomen at level of kidneys. Gastrophrenic varices (long arrows) are visible medially and ventrally to the left kidney (LK). Large amount of fluid (ascites) is evident in background (asterisks). (C) Dorsal and (D) ventral three-dimensional volume-rendered CT angiography of portal system and caudal vena cava. A splenophrenic PSS (arrowheads) connects splenic vein (sv) and caudal vena cava (CVC) at level of insertion of phrenic vein (empty arrows). RK, right kidney; PV, portal vein; pd, pancreaticoduodenal vein.

If splenophrenic PSS represents a pattern shared by both APSS and CPSS, categorization of the vascular anomaly based only on imaging findings may be challenging. In this case diagnosis may be influenced by the presence or absence of abdominal effusion as a frequent distinctive hallmark between PH or congenital vascular anomaly. Interestingly, in one dog with PH secondary to diffuse hepatic histiocytic sarcoma (Table 2, dog 5), CT showed multiple large porto-caval connections (of both classified and unclassified anatomical patterns) but no abdominal effusion (Fig. 1 and 2). In this dog the presence of multiple portal collaterals with one left splenogonadal shunt (which until now has never been reported among CPSS) and imaging findings compatible with diffuse hepatic neoplasia, suggested a presumptive diagnosis of PH with APSS. In this case the absence of ascites could be

Unfortunately the retrospective nature of this study did not allowed to demonstrate this eventuality in the three patients of CPSS group having a single splenophrenic shunt without ascites, due to the lack of liver histopathology. However, in the author's opinion, this eventuality would deserve to be considered in further studies. It has been demonstrated that the development of ascites in humans is inconstant or uncommon in major diseases showing PH such as cirrhosis (incidence of ascites: 50%) and idiopathic portal hypertension (IPH) (incidence of ascites: 10%) (Gines *et al.*, 1987; Sarin and Kapoor, 2002; Sarin *et al.*, 2007). Furthermore, one study on congenital and acquired PSS in dogs showed a prevalence of 45% for ascites in patients with APSS (Adam *et al.*, 2012). Actually, among CTA of dogs with PH reviewed in this paper, only one imaging findings was shared: the presence of more than one porto-caval vascular connections. In seven out of 9 cases multiple large shunt and varices were found. One out of 9 dogs had only varices and one out of 9 had two large PSS and severe hepatic structural disorder (diffuse hepatic neoplasia). Although considered a rare phenomenon, multiple CPSS have also been described in dogs (Johnson *et al*., 1987; Wilson *et al*., 1997; Morandi *et al*., 2005; Leeman *et al*., 2013); in all cases however, large porto-caval or porto-azygous vascular connections were reported without varices. Also, in the author's opinion, the possibility that dogs 1 and 2 of PH-group had all CPSS (including the splenophrenic) is considered less likely because the majority of the PSS patterns found in these dogs were codified in (and seemed typical of) different classifications of MAPSS (Bertolini, 2010a; Ricciardi *et al*., 2014) (Table 2 – dogs 1 and 2). Furthermore, it would be unlikely that multiple CPSS (even large ones) are all together (i.e. working simultaneously) insufficient to alleviate PH, so that ascites would develop, like in our dogs 1 and 2.

Finally, from an anatomical point of view, besides splenophrenic shunt, several unclassified patterns of large porto-caval vascular connections were observed in the group of dogs with PH (Table 2, asterisks). They connected various portal branches (eg. Splenic vein, pre-hepatic portal branches, pancreaticoduodenal vein) with caval circulation at different points, such as right gonadal vein (Fig. 1), main trunk of caudal vena cava (Fig. 4) or even cranial vena cava via internal thoracic veins (Fig. 3). These PSS have never been previously classified among APSS but in our cases they were considered acquired portal collaterals because they were associated with ascites, other porto-caval connections, and a confirmed cause of PH.

In summary, the results of this study corroborate two hypotheses: 1) acquired and congenital PSS may share the same anatomical pattern of porto-caval connection (in the case of splenophrenic pattern). Hence large shunts previously classified as congenital may be expected in patients with PH or, otherwise, 2) in the same dog with PH, large portal collaterals and splenophrenic PSS, we can consider the possibility of the coexistence of APSS and CPSS.

PSS pattern and the presence or absence of ascites did not permit in any case differentiation between congenital vascular disease and acquired portal collaterals secondary to PH. Indeed, the number of PSS (single vs. multiple porto-caval connections), presence/absence of varices and macroscopic structural cause of portal flow disturbance seem to be more useful in distinguishing congenital from acquired conditions.

This study is limited by the scarcity of dogs examined due to the low incidence of such vascular diseases. Further studies are needed in order to evaluate if other PSS patterns, besides splenophrenic, may be found as

both congenital and acquired vascular disorders and to correlate them with other signs of PH, such as ascites. Lastly, from the analysis of APSS in the group of dogs with PH, three new anatomical patterns of acquired porto-caval connection were seen:
1) portal vein—right gonadal vein;
2) portal vein—caudal vena cava (main trunk);
3) portal vein—left internal thoracic vein.

Conflict of Interests
The Author declare that there is no conflict of interest.

Acknowledgments
The authors wish to thank all the staff of the "Pingry" Veterinary Hospital of Bari, Italy for their assistance with data collection.

References
Adam, F.H., German, A.J., McConnell, J.F., Trehy, M.R., Whitley, N., Collings, A., Watson, P.J. and Burrow, R.D. 2012. Clinical and clinicopathologic abnormalities in young dogs with acquired and congenital portosystemic shunts: 93 cases (2003-2008). J. Am. Vet. Med. Assoc. 241, 760-765.

Agg, E.J. 2006. Acquired extrahepatic portosystemic shunts in a young dog. Can. Vet. J. 47, 697-699.

Bertolini, G. 2010a. Acquired portal collateral circulation in the dog and cat. Vet. Radiol. Ultrasound. 51, 25-33.

Bertolini, G. 2010b. MDCT for abdominal vascular assessment in dogs: MDCT basics, CT-angiography, normal anatomy and congenital anomalies. LAMBERT Academic Publishing, Saarbrucken, Germany.

Bertolini, G., Rolla, E.C., Zotti, A. and Caldin, M. 2006. Three-dimensional multislice helical computed tomography techniques for canine extra-hepatic portosystemic shunt assessment. Vet. Radiol. Ultrasound. 47, 439-443.

Bruehschwein, A., Foltin, I., Flatz, K., Zoellner, M., Matis, U. 2010. Contrast-enhanced magnetic resonance angiography for diagnosis of portosystemic shunts in 10 dogs. Vet. Radiol. Ultrasound. 51, 116-121.

Bunch, S.E., Johnson, S.E. and Cullen, J.M. 2001. Idiopathic noncirrhotic portal hypertension in dogs: 33 cases (1982-1998). J. Am. Vet. Med. Assoc. 218, 392-399.

Buob, S., Johnston, A.N. and Webster, C.R. 2011. Portal hypertension: pathophysiology, diagnosis, and treatment. J. Vet. Intern. Med. 25, 169-186.

Center, S.A. 1996. Hepatic Vascular Diseases, In: Strombeck's Small Animal Gastroenterology. 3rd ed. W.B. Saunders Company, Philadelphia, pp: 802-846.

Ferrell, E.A., Graham, J.P., Hanel, R.S., Randell, S., Farese, J.P. and Castleman, W.L. 2003. Simultaneous congenital and acquired extrahepatic portosystemic shunts in two dogs. Vet. Radiol. Ultrasound. 44, 38-42.

Fossum, T.W. 2002. Small Animal Surgery, 2nd ed., Mosby, St. Louis, pp: 457-468.

Fukushima, K., Kanemoto, H., Ohno, K.M., Takahashi, R., Fujiwara, R., Nishimura, R. and Tsujimoto, H. 2014. Computed tomographic morphology and clinical features of extrahepatic portosystemic shunts in 172 dogs in Japan. Vet. J. 199, 376-381.

Gines, P., Quintero, E., Arroyo, V., Terés, J., Bruguera, M., Rimola, A., Caballería, J., Rodés, J. and Rozman, C. 1987. Compensated cirrhosis: natural history and prognostic factors. Hepatology 7, 122-128.

Hunt, G.B. 2004. Effect of breed on anatomy of portosystemic shunts resulting from congenital diseases in dogs and cats: a review of 242 cases. Aust. Vet. J. 82, 746-749.

Huntington, G.S. and Mcclure, C.F.W. 1920. The development of the veins in the domestic cat (Felis domestica) with especial reference, (1) to the share taken by the supracardinal veins in the developmentof the postcava and azygos veins and (2) to the interpretation of the variant conditions of the postcava and its tributaries as found in the adult. Anat. Rec. 20, 1-30.

Johnson, C.A., Armstrong, P.J. and Hauptman, J.G. 1987. Congenital portosystemic shunts in dogs: 46 cases (1979-1986). J. Am. Vet. Med. Assoc. 191, 1478-1483.

Kraun, M.B., Nelson, L.L., Hauptman, J.G. and Nelson, N.C. 2014. Analysis of the relationship of extrahepatic portosystemic shunt morphology with clinical variables in dogs: 53 cases (2009-2012). J. Am. Vet. Med. Assoc. 245, 540-549.

Lamb, C.R. 1996. Ultrasonographic diagnosis of congenital portosystemic shunts in dogs: Results of a prospective study. Vet. Radiol. Ultrasound. 37, 281-288.

Leeman, J.J., Kim, S.E., Reese, D.J., Risselada, M. and Ellison, G.W. 2013. Multiple congenital PSS in a dog: case report and literature review. J. Am. Anim. Hosp. Asso. 49, 281-285.

Morandi, F., Cole, R.C., Tobias, K.M., Berry, C.R., Avenell, J. and Daniel, G.B. 2005. Use of 99mTCO4(-) trans-splenic portal scintigraphy for diagnosis of portosystemic shunts in 28 dogs. Vet. Radiol. Ultrasound. 46, 153-161.

Nelson, N.C. and Nelson, L.L. 2011. Anatomy of extrahepatic portosystemic shunts in dogs as determined by computed tomography angiography. Vet. Radiol. Ultrasound. 52, 498-506.

Ricciardi, M., Martino, R. and Assad, E.A. 2014. Imaging diagnosis--celiacomesenteric trunk and portal vein hypoplasia in a pit bull terrier. Vet. Radiol. Ultrasound. 55, 190-194.

Sarin, S.K. and Kapoor, D. 2002. Non-cirrhotic portal fibrosis: current concepts and management. J. Gastroenterol. Hepatol. 17, 526-34.

Sarin, S.K., Kumar, A., Chawla, Y.K., Baijal, S.S., Dhiman, R.K., Jafri, W., Lesmana, L.A., Guha Mazumder, D., Omata, M., Qureshi, H., Raza, R.M., Sahni, P., Sakhuja, P., Salih, M., Santra, A., Sharma, B.C., Sharma, P., Shiha, G. and Sollano, J. 2007. Noncirrhotic portal fibrosis/idiopathic portal hypertension: APASL recommendations for diagnosis and treatment. Hepatol. Int. 1, 398-413.

Szatmári, V. 2003. Simultaneous congenital and acquired extrahepatic portosystemic shunts in two dogs. Vet. Radiol. Ultrasound. 44, 486-487.

Szatmari, V. and Rothuizen, J. 2002. How can you tell with ultrasound that a patient with high blood ammonia has a congenital or acquired portosystemic shunt or no shunt at all? In the Proceedings of the 27th Congress of the World Small Animal Veterinary Association, October 3-6, Granada, Spain, pp: 42.

Szatmàri, V., Rothuizen, J., van den Ingh, T.S., van Sluijs, F. and Voorhout, G. 2004. Ultrasonographic findings in dogs with hyperammonemia: 90 cases (2000-2002). J. Am. Vet. Med. Assoc. 224, 717-727.

Van den Ingh, T.S., Rothuizen, J. and Meyer, H.P. 1995a. Circulatory disorders of the liver in dogs and cats. Vet. Q. 17, 70-76.

Van den Ingh, T.S., Rothuizen, J. and Meyer, H.P. 1995b. Portal hypertension associated with primary hypoplasia of the hepatic portal vein in dogs. Vet. Rec. 137, 424-427.

Watson, P.J. and Herrtage, M.E. 1998. Medical management of congenital portosystemic shunts in 27 dogs—a retrospective study. J. Small Anim. Pract. 39, 62-68.

Wilson, K., Scrivani, P. and Léveillé, R. 1997. Veterinary medicine today "What is your diagnosis?". J. Am. Vet. Med. Assoc. 21, 415-416.

Wrigley, R.H., Konde, L.J., Park, R.D. and Lebel, J.L. 1987. Ultrasonographic diagnosis of portacaval shunts in young dogs. J. Am. Vet. Med. Assoc.191, 421-424.

10

Calcitonin-negative primary neuroendocrine tumor of the thyroid (nonmedullary) in a dog

E.A. Soler Arias[1,*], V.A. Castillo[1] and M.E. Caneda Aristarain[2]

[1]*Hospital Escuela, Unidad de Endocrinología, Area de Clínica Médica de Pequeños Animales, Fac. de Ciencias Veterinarias, UBA, Av. Chorroarín 280, Ciudad Autónoma de Buenos Aires, Argentina*
[2]*Alumna de Programa de Investigación. Fac. de Ciencias Veterinarias, UBA, Chorroarín 280, Ciudad Autónoma de Buenos Aires, Argentina*

Abstract

The Calcitonin-negative neuroendocrine tumor of the thyroid (CNNET) or "nonmedullary" in humans is a rare tumor that arises primarily in the thyroid gland and may be mistaken for medullary thyroid carcinoma; it is characterized by the immunohistochemical (IHC) expression of neuroendocrine markers and the absence of expression for calcitonin. An Argentine dogo bitch showed a solid, compact thyroid tumor, which was IHC negative for the expression of calcitonin, carcinoembryonic antigen, thyroglobulin and S100 protein, and positive for synaptophysin and cytokeratin AE1-AE3. The Ki-67 proliferation index was low. We cite this case not only because it is the first case report of calcitonin-negative primary neuroendocrine tumor of the thyroid in dogs but also because we want to highlight the diagnostic importance of IHC in this regard.

Keywords: Calcitonin-negative, Immunohistochemistry, Ki-67, Medullary thyroid carcinoma, Neuroendocrine.

Introduction

With the exception of the medullary thyroid carcinoma (MTC), other neuroendocrine tumors (NETs) can rarely be seen in the human thyroid gland (Nakazawa *et al.*, 2014); among these tumors we can cite the paraganglioma (Pg), the hyalinising trabecular tumor, the metastatic neuroendocrine tumor to the thyroid gland and the intrathyroid parathyroid adenoma or tumor. Several reports have recently postulated a rare calcitonin-negative NET of the thyroid or nonmedullary (CNNET) as a new entity based on its IHC features: negative staining for calcitonin (CT) and carcinoembryonic antigen (CEA) and positive staining for neuroendocrine markers Chromagranin A (CGA) and Synaptophysin (Syn) (Ismi *et al.*, 2014; Kim *et al.*, 2015; Chernyavsky *et al.*, 2011; Zengguang *et al.*, 2016).

These tumors pose a challenge in terms of diagnosis due to their histopathological similarities to MTC and the corresponding IHC expression of neuroendocrine markers. Several reports on MTC in dogs have been published (Campos *et al.*, 2014; Patnaik *et al.*, 2002). However, as per the best knowledge of authors, this would be the first CNNET case to have ever been published.

Case details

A 8-year old spayed, Argentine dog was presented to the Endocrinology Service Unit at our hospital. The patient presented a cervical region tumor, located in the left thyroid lobe's projection area. The ultrasound revealed a 7 x 4.5 cm hyperechoic, well-defined, multi-lobed mass with moderate peripheral and intratumoral vascularization; the right thyroid lobe had preserved shape and size with a slightly increased heterogeneous echogenicity. The regular blood test and the endocrine/biochemical testing (TSH: 0.22 ng/ml, reference value 0.03 - 0.35 ng/ml; T4f: 0.98 ng/dl, reference value 0.6 - 1.6 ng/dl; PTH: 1.7 pmol/l, reference value 0.6 −3.55 pmol/l) showed all results within the reference values, with the exception of the alkaline phosphatase: 635UI/l (Reference value up to 250UI/l).

The exact nature of mass could not be determined by cytology, however, it was indicative of malignant. A left hemithyroidectomy was performed under suspicion of thyroid carcinoma, after ruling out other thoracic and abdominal neoplasias by means of X-rays and ultrasonography. The clinical stage of the thyroid gland tumor (TNM) was: T3b (>5cm, fixed), N0 (no evidence of regional lymph node involvement), M0 (no evidence of distant metastasis) (Owen, 1980). During the surgery, local extension of the tumor to sternothyroid muscle and the esophagus wall was observed. No evidence of invasion to the regional lymph node was detected (Fig. 1A). The neoplastic cells were arranged in nests surrounded by a moderate fibrovascular stroma with large nuclei and abundant, slightly acidophilic cytoplasm. At that moment, the histological diagnosis of neoplasia was thyroid carcinoma subclassified as the solid, compact type.

Corresponding Author: Elber Alberto Soler Arias. Area de Clínica Médica de Pequeños Animales, Fac. de Ciencias Veterinarias, UBA, Av. Chorroarín 280, Ciudad Autónoma de Buenos Aires, Argentina. Email: *mveterinario@yahoo.es*

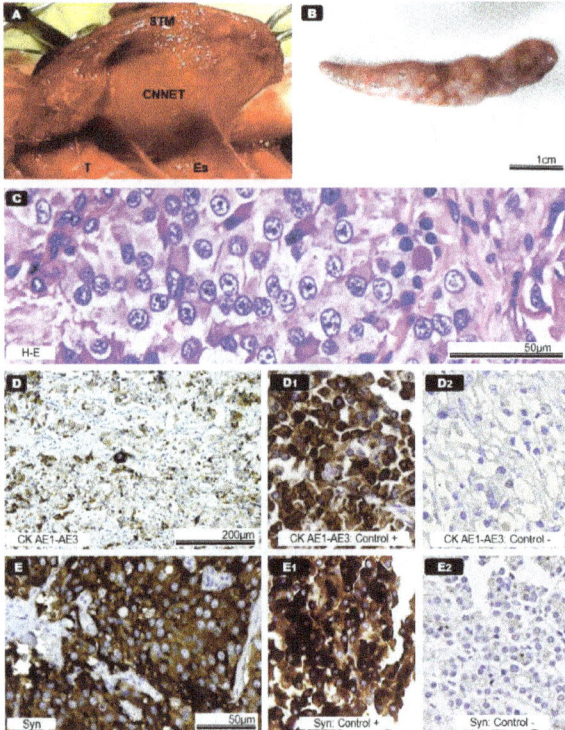

Fig. 1. (A-E): Calcitonin-negative primary neuroendocrine tumor of the thyroid (CNNET). (A): CNNET aspect during surgery with invasion to esophagus (Es) and sternothyroid muscle (STM); T: trachea. (B): Right thyroid lobe (necropsy); notice the whitish, mottled look. (C): CNNET microscopic aspect with hematoxylin and eosin staining (H-E). Bar = 50μm. (D): CNNET immunohistochemical positive staining for cytokeratin (CK AE1-AE3). Bar = 200μm. (D1): CK AE1-AE3 positive control (Liver tissue). (D2): CK AE1-AE3 negative control (Liver tissue). (E): CNNET immunohistochemical positive staining for synaptophysin (Syn). Bar = 50μm. (E1): Syn positive control (medullar thyroid carcinoma). (E2): Syn negative control (thyroid follicular cells).

Tumor cells stained positive for cytokeratin (CK) AE1-AE3 and for the neuroendocrine marker Syn, and they stained negative for thyroglobulin (Tg), CT, CEA and S100 protein (S100). The Ki 67 proliferation index was low. Based on IHC results it was conclude that mass was neuroendocrine tumor of thyroid gland. The postsurgical evolution was as satisfactory as the biochemical and imagining follow-ups performed eight and sixteen weeks after the surgery.

Regrettably, the animal developed gastric dilation-volvulus and died. The necropsy revealed no evidence of tumors. The right thyroid lobe, with preserved shape and size, displayed several whitish foci, which were firm when dissected (Fig. 1B) and histopathological examinations revealed similar features to those of the thyroid tumor located in the left lobe. In conclusion, the patient showed a calcitonin-negative primary neuroendocrine tumor of the thyroid.

Immediately after the surgery, the surgical specimen was fixed in 10% buffered formalin and embedded in paraffin blocks. 3μm-thin sections were cut and stained with hematoxylin and eosin.

The IHC staining and control (Table 1) were perfomed by means of the Avidin-Biotin Complex (ABC) and the 3.3'-diaminobenzidine chromogen (DAB). The images were taken with a Leica DC160 digital camera connected to a trinocular microscope (Leica DM4000B led).

Quantification of the staining IHC was performed semi-quantitatively through the percentage of tumor cells stained positively/cells per field. Staining intensity was subjectively classified as mild, moderate and intense.

Macroscopically, the entire left lobe of the thyroid was affected by neoplasia, which was well-defined by a moderately vascularized, thin capsule. The cutting surface showed solid-cystic features with hard, yellowish consistency and dark-colored, doughy areas. Histologically, the tumor was surrounded a thin capsule fibrous peripheral.

In some sections, the invasion of neoplastic cells into the striated muscle was visible. Adittionaly, atrophic thyroid follicles were observed, as well as a few healthy follicles trapped in neoplasia. The tumor was composed of polyhedral cells with moderate pleomorphism and anaplasia, large and round nuclei, prominent nucleoli and acidophilic cytoplasm. No mitotic figures were discerned. The cells were arranged in the form of solid nests supported in by a moderate fibrovascular stroma (Fig. 1C). IHC data is summarized in Table 2.

The cytoplasm of tumor cells (20 % of the field) was moderately positive for CK AE1-AE3 (Fig. 1D), whereas 100 % of the cells were intensely positive for Syn (Fig. 1E). "With the exception of a few healthy follicles trapped in neoplasia," it stained negative for Tg (Fig. 2A), CT (Fig. 2B), CEA and S100. The determination of the nuclear antigen Ki-67 was 3%, which is deemed as low (Fig. 2C).

Discussion

This report depicts the contribution of IHC to the definitive diagnosis of a rare NET, which primarily arises in the thyroid gland, and of which, to the authors' knowledge, there are no prior references in veterinary bibliography. Upon review of human literature, some case reports were found displaying similar IHC features. Those cases were initially referred to as "atypical medullary thyroid carcinoma" (Schmid and Ensinger, 1998), then, "calcitonin-negative medullary thyroid carcinoma" (Wang et al., 2008) and finally, "Calcitonin-negative neuroendocrine tumor of the thyroid" or nonmedullary (CNNET) (Chernyavsky et al., 2011). The use of Syn helped determining the neuroendocrine origin of our case. The procedure can also be performed by means of CGA or Neuron-specific enolase (ENS), even though the latter is less specific.

Table 1. Antibodies used in immunohistochemistry.

Primary antibody	Type of antibody	Dilution	Positive control	Negative control
Tg	Mouse monoclonal Santa Cruz Biotechnology	1:50	Normal thyroid follicular cells in dogs	MTC parafollicular cells in dogs.
CT	Rabbit polyclonal Biolaboratorio Dako	1:400	MTC (previously reported)	Normal thyroid follicular cells in dogs.
CEA	Mouse monoclonal Biolaboratorio Dako	1:50	Colon (epithelial cells)	Colon (epithelial cells).
Syn	Mouse monoclonal Santa Cruz Biotechnology	1:50	MTC parafollicular cells in dogs	Normal thyroid follicular cells in dogs
CK AE1–AE3	Mouse monoclonal Biolaboratorio Dako	1:100	Liver tissue	Liver tissue.
S100	Rabbit polyclonal Biolaboratorio Dako	1:200	Peripheral Nervous Tissue	Peripheral nervous tissue.
MIB-1	Mouse monoclonal Biolaboratorio Dako	1:75	Nodal lymphoma	Non tumoral thyroid tissue.

Table 2. Immunohistochemical profile of calcitonin-negative neuroendocrine tumor of the thyroid, previously reported.

Author	Immunohistochemistry								Nomenclature
	Tg	CT	CEA	Syn	CGA	S100	CK	MIB-1	
Chernyavsky et al., 2011	+	-	Np	+	W	Np	+	Np	Calcitonin-negative neuroendocrine tumor of the thyroid.
Ismi et al., 2014	-	-	-	+	+	-	Np	70 %	Calcitonin-negative neuroendocrine tumor of the thyroid.
Kim et al., 2015	+	-	-	+	+	Np	-	Np	Calcitonin-negative neuroendocrine tumor of the thyroid with follicular cell origin.
Zengguang et al., 2016	-	-	Np	+	+	Np	Np	40%	Thyroid neuroendocrine cancer accompanied with papillary carcinoma.
Gonzalez Alcolea et al., 2015	-	-	Np	+	Np	Np	Np	Np	Calcitonin-negative nonmedullary neuroendocrine tumor of the thyroid.
Nakazawa et al., 2014	-	-	-	+	+	Np	+	2%	C-cell-derived calcitonin-free neuroendocrine carcinoma of the thyroid ●CGRP.
Soler et al., 2016*	-	-	-	+	Np	-	+	3%	Calcitonin-negative primary nonmedullary neuroendocrine tumor of the thyroid

W: Weak.
Np: Not performed.
*: This report.
●CGRP: positive for the calcitonin gene-related peptide (CGRP).

Regarding the NETs that may affect the thyroid gland, the MTC certainly is the most prevalent tumor both in dogs and in humans (Campos et al., 2014; Kim et al., 2015).

However, its highly variable histological features call for the use of IHC with its most specific marker, the CT, coupled with CEA. The latter is not specific, it has a major role in the diagnosis of poorly differentiated MTC, though. (Ismi et al., 2014; Schmid, 2015). In our case, the tumor cells were negative for CT and CEA. Consequently, MTC was ruled out.

The other NETs rarely affect the thyroid. Even though it has not been deemed as a primary thyroid tumor, among the rare NETs we find the Pg (Nakazawa et al., 2014), which is typically composed of two cell types: the principal cells, which stain positive for neuroendocrine markers but negative for CKAE1/AE3, Tg, CT, CEA and PTH; and the sustentacular cells, which stain positive for S100 protein and are located at the periphery of tumor nests (Yu et al., 2013). Therefore, the lack of S100 expression and the presence of CK expression in our patient ruled out the Pg.

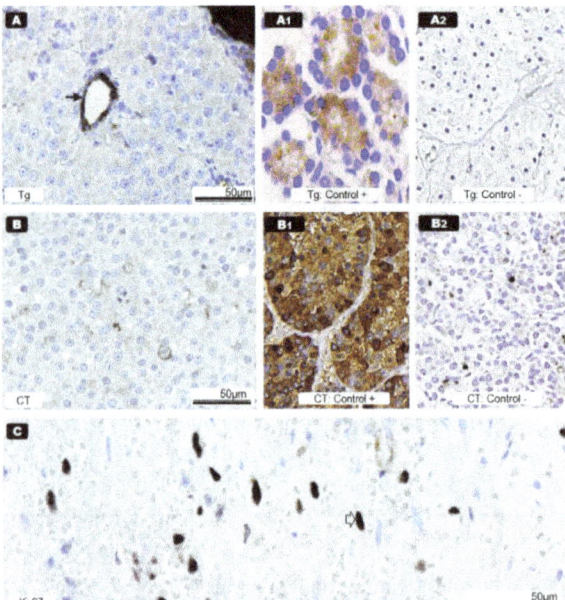

Fig. 2. (A): CNNET immunohistochemical negative staining for thyroglobulin (Tg); thyroid follicle trapped in neoplasia with positive staining for Tg (arrow). (A1): Tg positive control (Thyroid follicular cells). (A2): Tg negative control (Thyroid parafollicular cells-medullar thyroid carcinoma). (B): Immunohistochemical negative staining for calcitonin (CT). (B1): CT positive control (medullary thyroid carcinoma). (B2): CT negative control (thyroid follicular cells). (C): Nuclear antigen Ki-67 staining in tumor cells with the monoclonal antibody MIB I (arrow); proliferation index of 3%. Bar=50µm.

Nevertheless, S100 has been described in a rare type of MTC referred to as *"MTC like-paraganglioma"* (Schmidt, 2015; Yu *et al.*, 2013). In the dog, S100 was also expressed in five MTC (Patnaik and Lieberman, 1991).

The hyalinizing trabecular tumor is another human thyroid tumor with relative neuroendocrine staining. However, these tumors are also positive for Tg and present a unique membranous expression of Ki-67. Thus, it was easily ruled out from our case (Brunas *et al.*, 2005; Yu *et al.*, 2013).

The intrathyroid parathyroid adenoma and carcinoma are NETs (Li *et al.*, 2014) whose initial diagnosis is established by means of the concentrations elevated the plasmatic PTH (primary hyperparathyroidism), being both the histopathology as the IHC merely confirmatory (Li *et al.*, 2014). In connection with our case, we were not able to carry out the PTH staining. The clinical and biochemical diagnosis of primary hyperparathyroidism had already been excluded, though.

All the other types of thyroid NETs having been ruled out, there is only one option left: the metastasis of an unknown primary tumor, which human medicine calls "neuroendocrine tumor of unknown primary site"

(Gonzalez Alcolea *et al.*, 2015). The data gathered from the necropsy concluded that it was a primary NET of the thyroid and that it affected both lobes of the thyroid. Hence, our final diagnosis was: calcitonin-negative primary neuroendocrine tumor of the thyroid (nonmedullary), an entity described by Chernyavsky *et al.* (2011), which had not been reported in dogs so far. Other cases of similar IHC features have arisen in human medicine in the recent years (Table 2). Only two reports stated that the tumor had also been positive for Tg. Thus, their authors implied that those tumors might have a follicular origin (Kim *et al.*, 2015; Chernyavsky *et al.*, 2011).

Nakazawa *et al.* (2014) described a CNNET with positive staining for the calcitonin gene-related peptide (CGRP), which proved it originated in parafollicular cells, where both CGRP and CT are coexpressed. This confirms the existence of an unusual type of MTC. In a study performed in dogs, six MTC were positive for CGRP and only four of them showed positivity for CT. These findings indicate that CGRP may be a better marker for the diagnosis of MTC in dogs than CT (Leblanc *et al.*, 1991). In that study, CEA levels were not measured. While in one of the cases the expression of CGRP was only observed in the parafollicular cells trapped in neoplasia, in the second case the expression was mild. Consequently, we suggest CGRP measurements should be made in a larger group of MTC cases in dogs.

Regarding neoplasia malignancy, the presence of local invasion to the capsule, soft tissues and striated muscle were sufficient evidence to confirm its malignant behavior. Nevertheless, both the low Ki-67 and mitotic index matched a low-grade neuroendocrine tumor of the thyroid in histopathology (Klimstra *et al.*, 2010). This fact highlights the importance of linking the findings deriving from surgery, histopathology and IHC so as to properly stage the tumor.

In conclusion, many of the thyroid tumors cannot be correctly diagnosed without the routine use of IHC. The implementation of CGRP and CEA markers to differentiate atypical MTC from CNNET is highly recommended. The direct effect of specific identification and differentiation of each type of thyroid carcinoma, as well as the search for new molecular markers with a therapeutic targets will facilitate the provision of more realistic prognosis, based on recurrence and survival rates applicable to upcoming cases.

Conflict of interest

The authors declare that there is no conflict of interest.

References

Brunas, O., García, M.G., Sarancone, S., Novelli, J.L. 2005. Adenoma trabecular hialinizante: un tumor poco frecuente de la glandula tiroides. Glán Tir

Paratir 14:35-38.

Campos, M., Ducatelle, R., Rutteman, G., Kooistra, H.S., Duchateau, L., Rooster, de H., Peremans, K. and Daminet, S. 2014. Clinical Pathologic, and Immunohistochemical Prognostic Factors in Dogs with Thyroid Carcinoma. J. Vet. Intern. Med. 28, 1805-1813.

Chernyavsky, V.S., Farghani, S., Davidov, T., Ma, L., Barnard, N., Amorosa, L.F. and Trooskin, S.Z. 2011. Calcitonin-negative neuroendocrine tumor of the thyroid: a distinct clinical entity. Thyroid 21, 193-196.

Gonzalez Alcolea, N., Artés Caselles, M., Laiz Diez, B., Jiménez Cubedo, E., Calvo Espino, P., González Plo, D., Rivera Bautista, J.A. and Sánchez Turrión, V. 2015. Carcinoma neuroendocrino de tiroides calcitonina-negative (No medular). A propósito de un caso. Cir Esp, 93 (Espec congr), 322.

Ismi, O., Arpaci, R.B., Berkesoglu, M., Dag, A., Sezer, E., Bal, K.K. and Vayisoglu, Y. 2014. Calcitonin-negative neuroendocrine tumor of thyroid gland mimicking anaplastic carcinoma: an unusual entity. Gland surg. 4(4), 344-349.

Kim, G.Y., Park, C.Y., Cho, C.H., Park, J.S., Jung, E.D. and Jeon, E.J. 2015. A Calcitonin-Negative Neuroendocrine Tumor Derived from Follicular Lesions of the Thyroid. Endocrinol. Metab. 30, 221-225.

Klimstra, D.S., Modlin, I., Coppola, D., Lloyd, R.V. and Suster, S. 2010. The Pathologic Classification of Neuroendocrine Tumors A Review of Nomenclature, Grading, and Staging Systems. Pancreas 39, 707-712.

Leblanc, B., Parodi, A.L., Lagadic, M., Hurtrel, M. and Jobit, C. 1991. Immunocytochemistry of Canine Thyroid Tumors. Vet. Pathol. 28, 370-380.

Li, J., Chen, W. and Liu, A. 2014. Clinicopathologic features of parathyroid carcinoma: a study of 11 cases with review of literature. Zhonghua Bing Li Xue Za Zhi. 43(5), 296-300.

Nakazawa, T., Teijeiro, C., Vinagre, J., Soares, P., Rousseau, E., Eloy, C. and Sobrinho-Simões, M. 2014. C-cell-Derived Calcitonin-Free Neuroendocrine Carcinoma of the Thyroid: The diagnostic Importance of CGRP Immunoreactivity. Int. J. Surg. Pathol. 22(6), 530-535.

Owen, L.N. 1980. TNM Classifications of tumor in domestic animals. World Health Organization, Veterinary Public Health Unit WHO, Collaborating Center for Comparative Oncology. First Edition Geneve, pp: 51-52.

Patnaik, A.K., Ludwig, L.L. and Erlandson, R.A. 2002. Neuroendocrine carcinoma of the Nasopharynx in a dog. Vet. Pathol. 39, 496-500.

Patnaik, A.K. and Lieberman, P.H. 1991. Gross, Histologic, Cytochemical, and Immunocytochemical Study of Medullary Thyroid Carcinoma in Sixteen Dogs. Vet. Pathol. 28, 223-233.

Schmid, K.W. and Ensinger, C. 1998. "Atypical" medullary thyroid carcinoma with little or no calcitonin expression. Virchows Arch. 433, 209-215.

Schmid, K.W. 2015. Histopathology of C cells and Medullary Thyroid Carcinoma. Recent Results Cancer Res. 204, 41-60.

Wang, T.S., Ocal, I.T., Sosa, J.A., Cox, H. and Roman, S. 2008. Medullary thyroid carcinoma without marked elevation of calcitonin: a diagnostic and surveillance dilemma. Thyroid 18, 889-894.

Yu, B.H., Sheng, W.Q. and Wang, J. 2013. Primary paraganglioma of thyroid gland: A clinicopathologic and immunohistochemical analysis of three cases with a review of the literature. Head Neck Pathol. 7, 373-380.

Zengguang, L., Jin, M., Su, C., Ren, J., Wan, F., Guan, Q., Miao, Z., Chen, G. and Wang, G. 2016. Thyroid neuroendocrine cancer accompanied with multiple papillary thyroid carcinomas: a case report. Int. J. Clin. Exp. Pathol. 9(2), 2396-2401.

11

Fibrosarcoma of the eyelid in two sibling Czech wolfdogs

Laura Nordio[1,*], Sabina Fattori[2] and Chiara Giudice[1]

[1]Department of Veterinary Medicine, Università di Milano, via Celoria 10, 20133, Milano (MI), Italy
[2]Studio veterinario associato di Fattori Sabina e Gasparini Emanuele, Via Gabrielli Gabrielangelo 85, 61032, Fano (PU), Italy

Abstract
Most canine tumors of the eyelid are tumors generally encountered in the skin. They are most commonly of epithelial origin and benign. In this report, we describe the cases of two sibling Czech wolfdogs presented, one year apart, with a subcutaneous mass involving the left eyelid. Both lesions were histologically consistent with a diagnosis of subcutaneous fibrosarcoma. Immunohistochemical analyses of the tumors revealed a mild positivity for vimentin and negativity for GFAP, desmin, αSMA, myoglobin, S100, PNL2 and calponin, excluding all differential diagnosis (i.e. peripheral nerve sheath tumor, melanoma, perivascular sarcoma, myofibroblastic sarcoma, rhabdomyosarcoma). To the best of authors' knowledge, this is the first report of canine eyelid fibrosarcoma. Since this rare tumor has been observed in two full siblings, we could speculate the existence of some genetic predisposition to sarcoma, however the present data did not allow any definite conclusion on the etiopathogenesis or genetic basis of these tumors.
Keywords: Dog, Eyelid tumor, Sarcoma, Siblings.

Introduction
Most tumors affecting canine eyelids are tumors generally encountered in the skin. They include melanocytic tumors, sebaceous gland adenomas, histiocytic and mast cell tumors, squamous papillomas and carcinomas, trichoblastomas and trichoepitheliomas (Krehbiel and Langham, 1975; Dubielzig, 2002). Benign tumors are more common than malignant ones, the latter being rare and usually not metastasizing, and epithelial tumors are considered more common than mesenchymal ones (Krehbiel and Langham, 1975). In the present report the authors described two unusual cases of mesenchymal tumors of the eyelids (fibrosarcomas) presenting in two sibling Czech wolfdogs.

Case details
Case 1
A 10-year-old male spayed Czech wolfdog was presented to a private veterinary practice in November 2014 for a bulging on the lower lid of the left eye. The owners reported that the lesion had grown over several months and currently caused a slight closure of the palpebral fissure. There was no history of trauma, of previous ocular or systemic health problems.
Menace responses, palpebral reflexes, dazzle and direct and consensual pupillary light responses were present in both eyes (OU). Ophthalmic examination, slit-lamp biomicroscopy, indirect ophthalmoscopy, and applanation tonometry were carried out under general anesthesia due to the aggressive behavior of the dog.
In the lower left eyelid, a subcutaneous mass, not ulcerated and not adherent to the skin, was detected, causing mild epiphora and mild conjunctival hyperemia OS (left eye).
The cornea was fluorescein stain negative OU, intraocular pressure (IOP) was within normal limits and fundus examination was normal.
A skull x-ray and an ultrasound of the mass and of the abdomen were performed as ancillary tests. A skyline projection showed that the orbital bone was not affected. At ultrasound the mass was dense and mildly vascularised. Thoracic X-ray and abdominal ultrasounds were unremarkable.
Complete blood count and serum chemistry results, included as pre-operative diagnostics, were within normal limits.
The mass, which rested on the orbital bone, without infiltrating it, was surgically removed. Nine months later (August 2015), the dog presented to emergency with severe hemoperitoneum due to rupture of a splenic hematoma. The dog was humanely euthanized. No recurrence of the eyelid mass was recorded at that time. Necropsy was proposed but declined by the owner.

Case 2
An 11-years-old female Czech wolfdog, sibling of case 1, was presented in October 2015 with a bulging in the left eye lower eyelid causing deformation of the eyelid profile (Fig. 1A).
At ophthalmic examination, carried out using an E-collar due to the aggressive behavior of the dog, menace responses, palpebral reflexes, dazzle and direct and consensual pupillary light responses were present.

*Corresponding Author: Laura Nordio. Department of Veterinary Medicine, Università di Milano, via Celoria 10, 20133, Milano (MI), Italy. Email: laura.nordio@unimi.it

A large subcutaneous mass, not ulcerated and not adherent to the skin, causing closure of the palpebral fissure was present in the lower eyelid OS. Other investigations (slit-lamp bio microscopy, indirect ophthalmoscopy, and applanation tonometry) were carried out under general anesthesia and the findings were within normal limits.

Abdominal ultrasounds were performed and a small splenic nodular lesion was detected. FNA cytology of the splenic lesion was consistent with splenic hematoma. Complete blood count and serum chemistry panel were within normal limits.

The eyelid mass was surgically removed and submitted for histology.

In February 2016 the dog showed recurrence of the eyelid neoplasia, presenting at this time as a large mass extending to the orbit and causing exophthalmos. At ultrasound examination, compression and distortion of the eye globe without scleral invasion were observed. Complete blood count and serum chemistry panel were within normal limits and clinical staging was negative. Orbital exenteration was surgically performed, and all tissues removed were submitted for histology.

In June 2016 the dog presented with a further recurrence of the tumor within the orbital cavity, with swelling of the eyelid suture, and with difficult mouth opening. Due to the severe deterioration of general conditions, the owner elicited for euthanasia. Necropsy was not accepted.

Histopathology

All samples were fixed in 10% buffered formalin and routinely processed for histology. Microtomic section were obtained and stained with hematoxylin and eosin for histopathological examination.

In case 1, a 2.5 cm bilobate expansile subcutaneous mass, partially circumscribed by a fibrous capsule and focally extending to the cut borders, was observed. The neoplasia had two distinct cell populations with different growth patterns. The first component consisted of large interlacing bundles of amorphous fibrillar material (collagen) with scarce interspersed spindle cells characterized by mild atypia and less than 1 mitosis in 10 HPF.

The second component consisted of long, irregular, densely cellular bundles of spindle cells with indistinct borders, oval vesicular nuclei with marginated chromatin and scant eosinophilic cytoplasm. Anisocytosis and anisokaryosis were moderate and mitoses ranged from 0 to 3 per HPF (mitotic activity index 0.7) (Fig. 2). A large necrotic center and hemosiderin deposits were also observed. A diagnosis of subcutaneous fibrosarcoma (grade 2) was posed. Differential diagnosis included poorly differentiated peripheral nerve sheath tumor (PNST), perivascular wall tumor (PWT), myofibroblastic sarcoma, amelanotic melanoma and rhabdomyosarcoma.

In case 2, a bilobate neoplastic mass infiltrated the eyelid subcutaneous tissue. The neoplasia was partially enclosed by a pseudocapsule, and, where the capsule lacked, infiltrated muscular layers and extended to the cut borders. Neoplastic cells were spindle-shaped, arranged in interlacing bundles or occasionally in whorls circumscribing blood vessels and were characterized by indistinct cell borders, high nuclear/cytoplasmic ratio, scarce eosinophilic cytoplasm with occasional vacuolation, and oval nucleus with finely granular chromatin and one or two small nucleoli.

Anisocytosis and anisokaryosis were moderate and mitoses ranged from 0 to 4 per HPF (mitotic activity index 1.7). Large multifocal areas of necrosis were also present. A diagnosis of poorly differentiated subcutaneous fibrosarcoma (grade 3) was posed. Differential diagnoses considered were the same as listed for case 1.

Recurrence of neoplasia in case 2 was a 6,5 cm mass expanding the subcutaneous tissue and invading skeletal muscles, adipose tissue and salivary glands (Fig. 1B).

The neoplasia was densely cellular, poorly demarcated and un-encapsulated, with cells variably arranged in long interwoven bundles, whorls or herringbone. Cells were spindle-shaped with moderate fibrillary cytoplasm and oval nuclei with grossly granular chromatin and no evident nucleoli. Anysocytosis and anysokaryosis were moderate and mitoses ranged 0 to 1 per HPF (mitotic activity index 0.1).

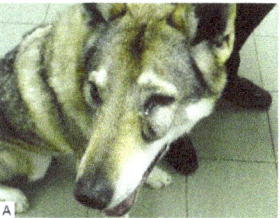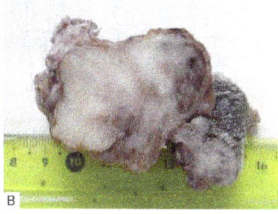

Fig. 1. (A): External view of the neoplastic mass *in situ,* case 2 at first presentation. **(B):** Longitudinal section of the formalin-fixed mass, case 2 recurrence.

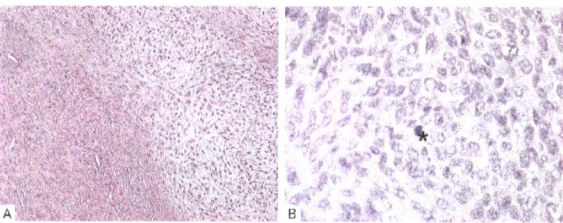

Fig. 2. (A): Fibrosarcoma composed by two cellular populations consisting in large interlacing bundles of amorphous fibrillar material with scarce interspersed spindle cells (on the right) and long densely cellular bundles of spindle cells (on the left) (H&E, 10X). **(B):** Neoplastic cells exhibited moderate anisocytosis and anisokaryosis. A mitotic figure is present (*) (H&E, 40X).

Multifocal hemorrhages and deposits of hematoidin pigment were also present. A diagnosis of subcutaneous fibrosarcoma (grade 2) was posed. The eye globe was unremarkable, characterized by diffuse blood vessels hyperemia and a small aggregate of mature lymphocytes in the episcleral area adjacent to the limbus.

Immunohistochemistry

Serial microtomic sections of all tumors were obtained, mounted on polylysine coated slides (Menzel-Gläser, Braunschweig, Germany) and immunostained with the standard ABC method using a panel of monoclonal and polyclonal antibodies. Details of antibodies used, dilutions, retrieval methods and positive controls are listed in Table 1. DAB (3,3'-diaminobenzidine) or AEC (3-amino-9-ethylcarbazole) substrate-chromogen kit (Vector Laboratories, Burlingame, USA) were used as chromogen, sections were counterstained with Mayer's hematoxylin. Negative controls were prepared by replacing the respective primary antibody with normal rabbit or mouse serum (non-immune serum, Dakocytomation).

Consistent immunohistochemical results were obtained in all tumors (case 1, case 2, case 2 recurrence): in all cases, neoplastic cells were moderately, diffusely, intracytoplasmically labelled with vimentin (Fig. 3). GFAP, desmin, αSMA, myoglobin, S100, PNL2 and calponin were always negative. Specifically PNL2 and S100 negative staining excluded melanocytic origin; desmin, αSMA, myoglobin and calponin negativity excluded myofibroblastic sarcoma, PWT and rhabdomyosarcoma, and S100 and GFAP negativity excluded PNST. On this basis, the diagnosis of fibrosarcoma was confirmed.

Discussion

This case report describes the clinical and histopathological features of eyelid fibrosarcoma occurring in two full sibling Czech wolfdogs. To the best of the authors' knowledge, this is the first report of this type of eyelid tumor in the canine species and the first report describing the occurrence of eyelid fibrosarcoma in sibling dogs.

Canine eyelid sarcomas are infrequent: generally, eyelid epithelial neoplasms outnumber the mesenchymal ones by a ratio of 5 to 1 and benign neoplasm outnumber malignant ones by a ratio of 3 to 1 (Stades and van der Woerdt, 2013). The tumors described in this case report presented as subcutaneous eyelid masses that were histologically consistent with a diagnosis of fibrosarcoma, characterized respectively by an intermediate or high grade of morphological malignancy (grade 2 and 3).

An aggressive behavior was confirmed in case 2 by the early recurrence of the lesion. Immunohistochemical staining excluded poorly differentiated forms of neurogenic, muscular and melanocytic neoplasia. In dogs, palpebral fibrosarcoma has not been reported so far.

Recently two cases of periocular extracranial cutaneous meningiomas have been reported. Eyelid meningiomas exhibited spindle to epithelioid cells, and were characterized by lobular arrangement and positivity to S100 immuno-labelling (Teixeira *et al.*, 2014). Meningioma was not initially considered among our differentials, however S100 immunohistochemical staining was consistently negative in all our samples, excluding a possible meningeal origin of neoplastic cells in our cases.

Table 1. Immunohistochemical examination: details of antibodies used, dilutions, retrieval methods and positive controls.

IHC marker	Antigen retrieval	Primary antibody	Positive control
Vimentin	Microwave oven, citrate buffer pH 6.0 (10', 500W)	Clone 3B4; dilution 1:1000, Dako, Carpinteria, USA	Internal: dermal fibrocytes
Desmin	Pepsin enzymatic digestion*	Clone NCL-L-DES-DERII dilution 1:150, Leica Biosystem, Nussloch, Germany	Internal: muscle of arterial wall
αSMA	None	Clone 1A4, dilution 1:2000, Dako, Carpinteria, USA	Internal: muscle of arterial wall
Myoglobin	None	Polyclonal, dilution 1:10, Dako, Carpinteria, USA	Internal: skeletal muscles
GFAP	None	Polyclonal, dilution 1:3000, Dako, Carpinteria, USA	Internal: peripheral nerves
PNL2	Microwave oven, EDTA buffer pH 8.5 (10', 500W)	Clone PNL2, dilution 1:50, Monosan, Uden, Netherlands	Section of canine melanoma
S100	None	Polyclonal, dilution 1:100, Dako, Carpinteria, USA	Internal: peripheral nerves
Calponin	Proteinase K (37°C 10') + Microwave oven, citrate buffer pH 6.0 (10', 500W)	Clone hCP, dilution 1:2000, Sigma-Aldrich, Saint Louis, MI, USA	Internal: muscle of arterial wall

*Digest-All Invitrogen, Thermo Fisher Scientific, Carlsbad, USA.

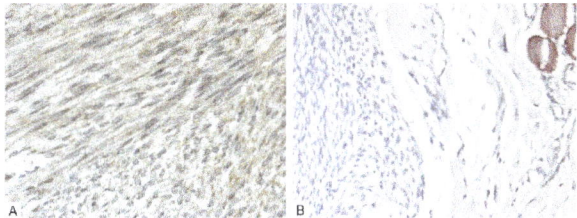

Fig. 3. (A): Immunohistochemistry anti-vimentin, intracytoplasmic positivity of neoplastic cells (DAB chromogen, 40X). **(B):** Immunohistochemistry anti-desmin, negativity of neoplastic cells (on the left) with positive skeletal muscle as internal control (AEC chromogen, 20X).

Most reports of canine eyelid sarcoma in the literature at a closer view are actually extension of orbital sarcomas presenting as eyelid swelling. For example, orbital embryonal rhabdomyosarcoma, typically diagnosed in young patients, may clinically presents as eyelid enlargement but it should be considered a primary orbital tumor (Plowman, 2007; Kato et al., 2012).

In our cases initial presentation was restricted to the eyelid subcutis, without orbital involvement. Moreover, markers of muscle differentiation were always negative in the present cases.

Although not previously described in the literature in this anatomic location, based on histological features observed, canine perivascular wall tumors (specifically angioleiomyosarcoma) was also considered as a possible differential diagnosis for the tumors described in the present report. Angioleiomyosarcoma can be negative to αSMA immune-labelling, but they are positive for calponin staining (Avallone et al., 2007). The immunohistochemical staining for αSMA and calponin were both negative in our cases and these results excluded the perivascular origin of the tumors.

Eyelid sarcomas are also rare in species other than dog. In man, palpebral angiosarcoma, Kaposi's sarcoma and malignant peripheral nerve sheath tumor have been described (Pe'er, 2016).

Palpebral lymphangiosarcomas and hemangiosarcomas have been reported in horses (Serena et al., 2006; Gerding et al., 2015), liposarcoma in guinea pigs (Quinton et al., 2013), hemangiosarcomas and peripheral nerve sheath tumors in cats (Newkirk and Rohrbach, 2009).

Interestingly, the two dogs presented in this case report were full-siblings with lesions similar in location, gross and histological morphology.

In human medicine there are proved evidences of tumors arising on genetic bases. Different inherited genetic syndromes increase the risk for sarcoma development, such as neurofibromatosis (NF1), Li-Fraumeni syndrome (LFS), and Retinoblastoma (Rb) (Burningham et al., 2012; Thomas et al., 2012). NF1 derives from an autosomal dominant event and

increases the risk of developing malignant peripheral nerve sheath tumor (Evans et al., 2012); LFS results from germline mutations in the tumor suppressor gene TP53 and it is strongly related to the early development of a wide variety of tumors (eg., breast cancer, soft tissue sarcoma, brain tumor, adrenocortical carcinoma) (Gonzalez et al., 2009); Rb leads to a greater risk of developing secondary tumors, particularly osteosarcoma (Wong et al., 1997).

In the veterinary literature there are sparse reports of tumors affecting littermates (Teske et al., 1994; Shaw et al., 2010; Munday et al., 2012), in which the role of an undetermined underlying genetic predisposition has been hypothesized, and few studies have investigated the possible genetic risk factors in carcinogenesis, like a recent wide-genome study in canine mammary tumors (Melin et al., 2016).

The available data regarding the two Czech wolfdogs described in the present report and the current knowledge are not sufficient to speculate of a genetic bases underlying the etiopathogenesis of these sarcomas. However, the occurrence in two full-sibling dogs of exceedingly uncommon eyelid fibrosarcomas, similar for location, age of onset, clinical and pathological features leads to hypothesize that carcinogenesis may have been influenced by shared undetermined genetic and environmental factors.

The study of familial tumors in dogs is a field of interest that would be worth of deeper investigations.

Conclusion

To the best of authors' knowledge this is the first report of fibrosarcoma of the eyelids in the canine species. Moreover eyelid fibrosarcomas in the present report were observed in two full-sibling dogs, leading to the speculation that a possible genetic factors may played a role in the carcinogenesis of these tumors.

Conflict of interests

The Author declare that there is no conflict of interest.

References

Avallone, G., Helmbold, P., Caniatti, M., Stefanello, D., Nayak, R.C. and Roccabianca, P. 2007. The spectrum of canine cutaneous perivascular wall tumors: morphologic, phenotypic and clinical characterization. Vet. Pathol. 44, 607-620.

Burningham, Z., Hashibe, M., Spector, L. and Schiffman, J.D. 2012. The epidemiology of sarcoma. Clin. Sarcoma Res. 2, 14.

Dubielzig, R.R. 2002. Tumors of the eye. In: Meuten, D.J., ed. Tumors in domestic animals. Ed. Blackwell publishing, Ames, pp: 739-754.

Evans, D.G., Huson, S.M. and Birch, J.M. 2012. Malignant peripheral nerve sheath tumours in inherited disease. Clin. Sarcoma Res. 2(1), 17.

Gerding, J.C., Gilger, B.C., Montgomery, S.A. and Clode, A.B. 2015. Presumed primary ocular lymphangiosarcoma with metastasis in a miniature horse. Vet. Ophthalmol. 18, 502-509.

Gonzalez, K.D., Noltner, K.A., Buzin, C.H. Gu, D., Wen-Fong, C.Y., Nguyen, V.Q., Han, J.H., Lowstuter, K., Longmate, J., Sommer, S.S. and Weitzel, J.N. 2009. Beyond Li Fraumeni Syndrome: clinical characteristics of families with p53 germline mutations. J. Clin. Oncol. 27, 1250-1256.

Kato, Y., Notake, H., Kimura, J., Murakami, M., Hirata, A., Sakai, H. and Yanai, T. 2012. Orbital embryonal rhabdomyosarcoma with metastasis in a young dog. J. Comp. Path. 147, 191-194.

Krehbiel, J.D. and Langham, R.F. 1975. Eyelid neoplasms of dogs. Am. J. Vet. Res. 36(1), 115-119.

Melin, M., Rivera, P., Arendt, M., Elvers, I., Murén, E., Gustafson, U., Starkey, M., Borge, K.S., Lingaas, F., Häggström, J., Saellström, S., Rönnberg, H. and Lindblad-Toh, K. 2016. Genome-Wide Analysis Identifies Germ-Line Risk Factors Associated with Canine Mammary Tumours. PLoS Genetics 12:e1006029.

Munday, J.S., Aberdein, D., Cullen, G.D. and French, A.F. 2012. Ménétrier disease and gastric adenocarcinoma in 3 Cairn terrier littermates. Vet. Pathol. 49, 1028-1031.

Newkirk, K.M. and Rohrbach, B.W. 2009. A retrospective study of eyelid tumors from 43 cats. Vet. Pathol. 46, 916-927.

Pe'er, J. 2016. Pathology of eyelid tumors. Indian J. Ophthalmol. 64, 177-190.

Plowman, P.N. 2007. Eyelid tumours. Orbit. 26, 207-213.

Quinton, J.F., Ollivier, F. and Dally, C. 2013. A case of well-differentiated palpebral liposarcoma in a Guinea pig (Cavia porcellus). Vet. Ophthalmol. 16, 155-159.

Serena, A., Joiner, K.S. and Schumacher, J. 2006. Hemangiopericytoma in the eyelid of a horse. Vet. Pathol. 43, 576-578.

Shaw, T.E., Harkin, K.R., Nietfeld, J. and Gardner, J.J. 2010. Aortic body tumor in full-sibling English bulldogs. J. Am. Anim. Hosp. Assoc. 46, 366-370.

Stades, F.C. and van der Woerdt, A. 2013. Diseases and surgery of the canine eyelid. In: Gelatt, K.N., ed. Veterinary ophthalmology. Wiley-Blackwell, Hoboken, pp: 832-893.

Teixeira, L.B., Pinkerton, M.E. and Dubielzig, R.R. 2014. Periocular extracranial cutaneous meningiomas in two dogs. J. Vet. Diagn. Invest. 26, 575-579.

Teske, E., de Vos, J.P., Egberink, H.F. and Vos, J.H. 1994. Clustering in canine malignant lymphoma. Vet. Q. 16, 134-136.

Thomas, D.M., Savage, S.A. and Bond, G.L. 2012. Hereditary and environmental epidemiology of sarcomas. Clin. Sarcoma Res. 2, 13.

Wong, F.L., Boice, J.D. Jr, Abramson, D.H., Tarone, R.E., Kleinerman, R.A., Stovall, M., Goldman, M.B., Seddon, J.M., Tarbell, N., Fraumeni, J.F. Jr. and Li, F.P. 1997. Cancer incidence after retinoblastoma. Radiation dose and sarcoma risk. JAMA 278, 1262-1267.

12

Thoracic duct lymphography by subcutaneous contrast agent injection in a dog with chylothorax

T. Iwanaga[1], S. Tokunaga[1,2] and Y. Momoi[3,*]

[1]*Veterinary Teaching Hospital, Joint Faculty of Veterinary Medicine, Kagoshima University, Korimoto 1-21-24, Kagoshima 890-0065, Japan*
[2]*Department of Environmental and Radiological Health Sciences, College of Veterinary Medicine and Biomedical Sciences, Colorado State University, Fort Collins, CO, 80523, USA*
[3]*Department of Clinical Medical Science, Joint Faculty of Veterinary Medicine, Kagoshima University, Korimoto 1-21-24, Kagoshima 890-0065, Japan*

Abstract

A 4-year-old male Japanese Shiba Inu presented with recurrent chylothorax. The thoracic duct was successfully imaged using computed tomography after the injection of an iodine contrast agent into the subcutaneous tissue surrounding the anus. The thoracic duct was successfully ligated and pericardectomy performed via an open thoracotomy. Pleural effusion improved but relapsed a week after the surgery. A second lymphography revealed a collateral thoracic duct that was not detected during the first lymphography. The collateral duct was ligated and chylothorax was resolved after the second surgery. The lymphography applied in this study was minimally-invasive and easily provided images of the thoracic duct in a dog with chylothorax.

Keywords: Chylothorax, Computed tomography, Lymphography, Thoracic duct.

Introduction

Chylothorax in dogs can be caused by thoracic damage such as that from traumatic injury or inflammation. Accumulation of chylous pleural effusion often causes dyspnoea and requires periodic removal or a curative approach. Thoracic duct ligation and pericardectomy has been reported as a treatment for chylothorax in dogs (Carobbi *et al.*, 2008; da Silva and Monnet, 2011; Mayhew *et al.*, 2012). Pre-operative thoracic duct imaging may reveal the cause of disruption of the thoracic duct (Naganobu *et al.*, 2006; Johnson *et al.*, 2009) or aid in surgical planning.

Recently, minimally invasive imaging methods have been reported in experimental settings. These methods involved imaging the thoracic duct using computed tomography (CT) after the injection of an iodine contrast agent into the superficial lymph nodes (i.e., popliteal lymph nodes) or subcutaneous tissue (Enwiller *et al.*, 2003; Naganobu *et al.*, 2006; Johnson *et al.*, 2009; Millward *et al.*, 2011; Singh *et al.*, 2011; Ando *et al.*, 2012).

In this report, we applied this method to a dog with chylothorax and found it helpful for imaging the thoracic duct in cases with primary and relapsed chylothorax.

Case Details

A 4-year-old male Japanese Shiba Inu weighing 4.08 kg was referred to Kagoshima University Veterinary Teaching Hospital. The dog had been injured in a traffic accident 2 years previously and presented with repeated dyspnoea caused by pleural effusion. Based on the diagnosis of chylothorax, the dog had been treated with low-fat diet therapy and rutin administration, as well as repeated thoracocentesis at another veterinary hospital. On initial examination, the dog exhibited mild respiratory distress (respiration rate of 52 breaths per min) and auscultation revealed a heart rate of 100 beats per min with sinus arrest observed at a frequency of one arrest per 30 beats. The dog had a body condition score of 2/5, although appetite and activity levels were normal.

The results of a complete blood cell count were within the normal ranges, but serum biochemistry showed elevation of C-reactive protein (61.0 mg/L: reference range 0–10 mg/L) and alkaline phosphatase activity (537 IU/L: reference range 104–239 IU/L). Thoracic radiography showed pleural effusion and a mass-like lesion with soft tissue opacity around the middle lobe. No abnormal findings were observed during echocardiography. Ultrasound-guided thoracocentesis was performed. Pleural fluid was chylous and hypertriglyceridemic (500 mg/dL), typical findings of chylothorax. Computed tomography revealed pleural effusion and collapse of the middle right lung lobe. Based on these findings and the patient's history, chylothorax secondary to a traffic accident was

*****Corresponding Author:** Yasuyuki Momoi. Department of Clinical Medical Science, Joint Faculty of Veterinary Medicine, Kagoshima University, Korimoto 1-21-24, Kagoshima 890-0065, Japan. Email: *momoi@agri.kagoshima-u.ac.jp*

suspected. Thoracic duct imaging with CT was performed according to a previous publication (Ando *et al.*, 2012), with minor modifications. A water-soluble contrast medium (iopamidol, OIPALOMIN 370 Inj., Konica Minolta, Tokyo, Japan), warmed to body temperature, was injected subcutaneously into four sites surrounding the dog's anus at a total dosage of 0.6 ml/kg using a 25-G 5/8 inch needle.

The sites was massaged for 2 min. The time was shortened from 5 min in the original report (Ando *et al.*, 2012) to obtain earlier CT images. Images were obtained with a multi-detector helical CT scanner (Aquilion™ LB, TOSHIBA MEDICAL SYSTEMS, Tochigi, Ootawara, Japan) at 2, 8, 10 and 15 min after the injection. The timing of the scanning was also changed from the original study (Ando *et al.*, 2012). The contrast medium reached the mediastinal lymph nodes at 10 min after injection and leakage of the contrast agent was detected at the anterior mediastinal lesion (Fig. 1).

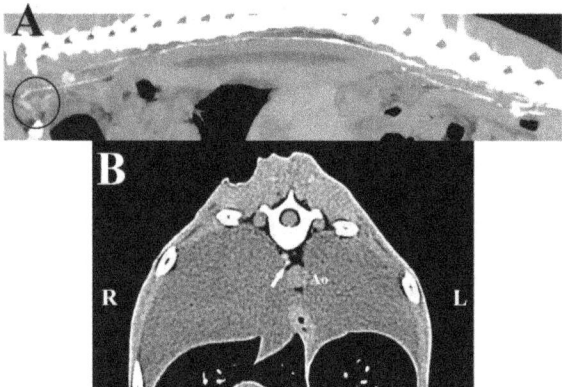

Fig. 1. Computed tomograph (CT)-generated lymphography of the thoracic duct prior to surgery. Imaging was performed using a multi-detector helical CT scanner 10 min after iopamidol injection into the subcutaneous tissue around the anus. (A) The lymphatic duct was identifiable in both the thoracic and abdominal cavities in the sagittal plane. The contrast agent blurred around the mediastinal lymph nodes (ellipse), indicating a leak into the thoracic cavity. (B) In the transverse plane at the eighth thoracic vertebra, a lymphatic duct (arrow) passing between the aorta (Ao) and azygos vein (asterisk) could be identified.

Thoracic duct ligation was planned at the eighth-ninth vertebrae, as the collateral of the thoracic duct was not observed in this lesion. The thoracic duct was approached via a right intercostal thoracotomy performed at the eighth intercostal space. Indocyanine green was injected into the subcutaneous tissue around the anus to allow visualization of the thoracic duct in the surgical field. The thoracic duct was ligated using vascular clips.

A pericardectomy was performed because the increased systemic venous pressure caused by a thickened

pericardium may impede the drainage of chyle via the lymphatic venous communications (Fossum *et al.*, 2004). A thoracostomy tube was inserted to allow the drainage of pleural fluid. Although the volume of chylous fluid initially decreased to 10 mL per day by 3 days after surgery, it subsequently increased. On day 7 post-surgery, 78 mL of pleural fluid was removed from the thoracostomy tube. A second lymphography was scheduled to clarify the cause of the relapse. During the second lymphography, the thoracic duct was completely ligated with vascular clips at the eighth thoracic vertebra. However, a collateral thoracic duct running along the left-hand side of the ligated duct was found (Fig. 2).

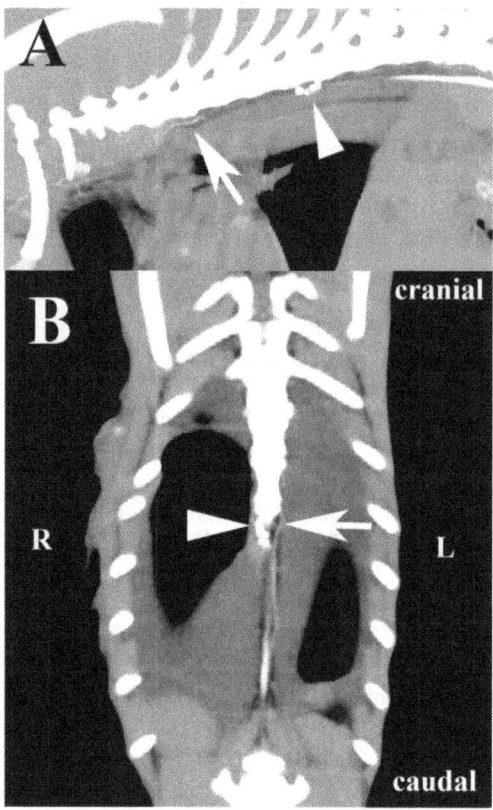

Fig. 2. Lymphography 7 days after thoracic duct ligation. Computed tomography imaging was performed 15 min after iopamidol injection into the subcutaneous tissue around the anus. (A) In the sagittal plane, the vascular clips used to ligate the thoracic duct during the first surgery can be seen (arrowheads). Thoracic tracts cranial to the vascular clips were also observed, indicating the incomplete blockade of lymph flow (arrows). (B) In the coronal plane, the collateral lymphatic duct (arrows) passing through the left side of the vascular clips (arrowheads) could be identified near the eighth vertebra.

This collateral thoracic duct was not detected at the first lymphography. A second surgery was performed via a left intercostal thoracotomy and the collateral thoracic duct was ligated using vascular clips. Small volumes of pleural effusion were drained after the second surgery, but the fluid was not chylous nor hypertriglyceridemic. The thoracostomy tube was removed on day 5 after the second surgery. At 17 months after the surgery (at the time of writing), the dog was living without detectable pleural effusion.

Discussion

In this case report, a method of lymphography described by Ando et al. (2012) was successfully applied to a clinical case to aid planning of the surgical procedure. The injection of indocyanine green during the thoracotomy was helpful to visualize the thoracic duct in the surgical field. The indocyanine green is usually injected into the popliteal or mesenteric lymph nodes or cisterna chyli (Radlinsky et al., 2002; Enwiller et al., 2003; Hayashi et al., 2005; Sicard and Mcanulty, 2005; Macdonald, 2008; Leasure et al., 2011; McAnulty, 2011; Mayhew et al., 2012).

The injection into perianal tissue is easier than into the popliteal nodes and less invasive than into the mesenteric lymph nodes, as there is no need for laparotomy. Adverse events caused by the injection were not observed in this case, other than local swelling and redness at the injection sites. The reaction was mild and relieved within 72 hrs (3 days). We applied this method to another case with chylothorax and delineated the thoracic duct successfully (data not shown). Because this method is easy to perform, it can be a technique of choice for thoracic duct imaging in chylothorax cases. The chylothorax relapsed after the first surgery and a second lymphography revealed the presence of a collateral lymphatic duct.

The recurrence of chylothorax has been reported in 0%–30 % of cases receiving thoracic duct ligation and pericardectomy (Fossum et al., 2004; Carobbi et al., 2008; Allman et al., 2010; da Silva and Monnet, 2011). Recurrence often occurs several months to a year after surgery and the development of a collateral lymphatic duct is thus thought to be a cause of recurrence (Kerpsack et al., 1995; Hayashi et al., 2005; Carobbi et al., 2008; da Silva and Monnet, 2011; McAnulty, 2011; Staiger et al., 2011; Mayhew et al., 2012).

In one case report, multiple collateral lymphatic ducts were detected by lymphography 50 days after thoracic duct ligation (Kerpsack et al., 1995). As there was only a single collateral duct (not multiple) and recurrence occurred soon after the first surgery, the hidden collateral lymphatic duct may have already existed at the time of the first surgery in this case. It may be worthwhile to try lymphography during surgery after thoracic duct ligation to detect hidden collateral lymphatic ducts to reduce the recurrence rate, if intraoperative CT is available.

In conclusion, CT-based lymphography involving the injection of a contrast agent into the perianal subcutaneous tissue is a minimally invasive and easy method of imaging the thoracic duct. It enabled the necessary imaging to be obtained for surgical treatment of a case of chylothorax. The method was also useful in the identification of the cause of recurrence after surgery with minimal invasion.

Conflict of interest

The authors declare that there is no conflict of interest.

References

Allman, D.A., Radlinsky, M.G., Ralph, A.G. and Rawlings, C.A. 2010. Thoracoscopic thoracic duct ligation and thoracoscopic pericardectomy for treatment of chylothorax in dogs. Vet. Surg. 39, 21-27.

Ando, K., Kamijyou, K., Hatinoda, K., Shibata, S., Shida, T. and Asari, M. 2012. Computed tomography and radiographic lymphography of the thoracic duct by subcutaneous or submucosal injection. J. Vet. Med. Sci. 74, 135-140.

Carobbi, B., White, R.A. and Romanelli, G. 2008. Treatment of idiopathic chylothorax in 14 dogs by ligation of the thoracic duct and partial pericardiectomy. Vet. Rec. 163, 743-745.

da Silva, C.A. and Monnet, E. 2011. Long-term outcome of dogs treated surgically for idiopathic chylothorax: 11 cases (1995-2009). J. Am. Vet. Med. Assoc. 239, 107-113.

Enwiller, T.M., Radlindky, M.G., Mason, D.E. and Roush, J.K. 2003. Popliteal and mesenteric lymph node injection with methylene blue for coloration of the thoracic duct in dogs. Vet. surg. 32, 359-364

Fossum, T.W., Mertens, M.M., Miller, M.W., Peacock, J.T., Saunders, A., Gordon, S., Pahl, G., Makarski, L.A., Bahr, A. and Hobson, P.H. 2004. Thoracic duct ligation and pericardectomy for treatment of idiopathic chylothorax. J. Vet. Intern. Med. 18, 307-310.

Johnson, E.G., Wisner, E.R., Kyles, A., Koehler, C. and Marks, S.L. 2009. Computed tomographic lymphography of the thoracic duct by mesenteric lymph node injection. Vet. Surg. 38, 361-367.

Kerpsack, S.J., Smeak, D.D. and Birchard, S.J. 1995. Progressive lymphangiectasis and recurrent chylothorax in a dog after thoracic duct ligation. J. Am. Vet. Med. Assoc. 207, 1059-1062.

Hayashi, K., Sicard, G., Gellasch, K., Frank, J.D., Hardie, R.J. and McAnulty, J.F. 2005. Cisterna chyli ablation with thoracic duct ligation for chylothorax: results in eight dogs. Vet. Surg. 34, 519-523.

Leasure, C.S., Ellison, G.W., Roberts, J.F., Coomer, A.R. and Choate, C.J. 2011. Occlusion of the thoracic duct using ultrasonically activated shears in six dogs. Vet. Surg. 40, 802-810.

Macdonald, N.J. 2008. Efficacy of en bloc ligation of the thoracic duct: Descriptive study in 14 dogs. Vet. Surg. 37, 696-701.

Mayhew, P.D., Culp, W.T., Mayhew, K.N. and Morgan, O.D. 2012. Minimally invasive treatment of idiopathic chylothorax in dogs by thoracoscopic thoracic duct ligation and subphrenic pericardiectomy: 6 cases (2007-2010). J. Am. Vet. Med. Assoc. 241, 904-909.

McAnulty, J.F. 2011. Prospective comparison of cisterna chyli ablation to pericardectomy for treatment of spontaneously occurring idiopathic chylothorax in the dog. Vet. Surg. 40, 926-934.

Millward, I.R., Kirberger, R.M. and Thompson, P.N. 2011. Comparative popliteal and mesenteric computed tomography lymphangiography of the canine thoracic duct. Vet. Radiol. Ultrasound. 52, 295-301.

Naganobu, K., Ohigashi, Y., Akiyoshi, T., Hagio, M., Miyamoto, T. and Yamaguchi, R. 2006. Lymphography of the thoracic duct by percutaneous injection of iohexol into the popliteal lymph node of dogs: experimental study and clinical application. Vet. Surg. 35, 377-381.

Radlinsky, M.G., Mason, D.E., Biller, D.S. and Olsen, D. 2002. Thoracoscopic visualization and ligation of the thoracic duct in dogs. Vet. Surg. 31, 138-146.

Sicard, G.K. and Mcanulty, J.F. 2005. The effect of cisterna chyli ablation combined with thoracic duct ligation on abdominal lymphatic drainage. Vet. Surg. 34, 64-70.

Singh, A., Brisson, B.A, Nykamp, S. and O'Sullivan, M.L. 2011. Comparison of computed tomographic and radiographic popliteal lymphangiography in normal dogs. Vet. Surg. 40, 762-767.

Staiger, B.A., Stanley, B.J. and McAnulty, J.F. 2011. Single paracostal approach to thoracic duct and cisterna chyli: experimental study and case series. Vet. Surg. 40, 786-794.

13

TGF-β1 serum concentrations and receptor expressions in the lens capsular of dogs with diabetes mellitus

Stephan Neumann[1,*], Jens Linek[2], Gerhard Loesenbeck[3], Julia Schüttler[1] and Sonja Gaedke[1]

[1]*Institute of Veterinary Medicine, University of Goettingen, Burckhardtweg 2, D-37077 Goettingen, Germany*
[2]*Veterinary specialists, Hamburg, Germany*
[3]*Laboklin GmbH&CO.KG, Bad Kissingen, Germany*

Abstract

Tissue fibrosis as complication of diabetes mellitus is known in humans. Because TGF-β1induces fibrosis and is elevated in humans suffering from diabetes mellitus we measured this growth factor in serum of dogs with diabetes mellitus and compared it with healthy dogs and those with fibrotic diseases. Further we measured the expression of TGF-β1receptor on lens capsule to investigate possible association between diabetes mellitus and cataract associated alterations. TGF-β1 was measured in serum of 12 dogs with diabetes mellitus, 20 healthy controls and 12 dogs with fibrotic diseases. Dogs with diabetes mellitus and fibrotic diseases have significantly increased TGF-β1 serum concentrations compared to healthy controls. Some dogs with diabetes mellitus showed increased expression of TGF-β1 receptor in lens capsule. Based on our observations we can conclude that TGF-β1 elevation in dogs with diabetes mellitus may induces complications of the disease and may participates on lens alteration.

Keywords: Cataracts, Diabetes mellitus, Dogs, TGF-β1.

Introduction

Diabetes mellitus is one important endocrine disease in humans as well as in dogs. Clinical complications of diabetes mellitus influence functions in different organs and can induce on this way beside others neuropathy, retinopathy and glomerulopathy (Gangwani *et al.* 2016; Juster-Switlyk and Smith, 2016; Leung *et al.*, 2016). All these diseases are described as microvascular complications of diabetes mellitus (Gilbert, 2013). The underlying mechanism was firstly described in the sixties and includes fibrosis of extracellular matrix (Siperstein *et al.*, 1968; Tsilibary, 2003). Compared to humans dogs with hyperglycemia also develop microvascular alterations (Gardiner *et al.*, 1994). Because fibrosis is part of the pathogenesis of diabetic complications we hypothesized that growth factors, which induce tissue fibrosis should play a role in the pathogenesis.

One growth factor which induces tissue fibrosis is Transforming growth factor beta 1 (TGF-β1). TGF-β1 is a pleiotropic cytokine that belongs to the TGF-superfamily. TGF-β1 is secreted by a large number of cells. This cytokine contributes to the proliferation and differentiation of cells, embryonic development, wound healing and angiogenesis (Sporn *et al.*, 1990; Lawrence, 1996; Alevizopoulos and Mermod, 1997). Additionally, it is influenced by or influences the pathogenesis of many diseases (Blobe *et al.*, 2000). Data from human medicine show variable blood concentrations, compared to healthy controls, in patients with cancer, immunological, fibrotic or sclerotic diseases (Colitz *et al.*, 2000; Prud'homme, 2007; Hills and Squires, 2009; Lopez-Novoa and Nieto, 2009; Shariat *et al.*, 2011). In veterinary medicine, elevated TGF-β1 concentrations were found in dogs with liver fibrosis and lung fibrosis (Neumann *et al.*, 2008; Krafft *et al.*, 2011).

Aim of the underlying prospective study was measurement of TGF-β1 in serum of diabetic dogs and its comparison with healthy controls and dogs with different fibrotic diseases. Further relation of TGF-β1 and diabetic cataracts as one mayor complication of diabetes mellitus in dogs should be investigated. For that reason we measured expression of TGF-β1 receptor in the epithelia of the anterior lens capsule.

Materials and Methods

Animals

Twenty healthy dogs were used as controls. All these dogs were clinical healthy and showed no abnormalities on clinical pathology, ultrasonography or radiology. These dogs were summarized as group 1. Group 2 consisted of 12 dogs with diabetes mellitus. Seven patients underwent surgery for removal of the lens material in a specialized veterinary clinic. Further diseases were excluded in this group, using clinical pathology and diagnostic imagine.

Finally, levels of TGF-β1 were measured in 12 dogs with various fibrotic diseases. Six had liver fibrosis, three had kidney fibrosis and three had lung fibrosis. All diagnoses were confirmed by histopathology.

*****Corresponding Author:** Stephan Neumann. Institute of Veterinary Medicine, University of Goettingen, Burckhardtweg 2, D-37077 Goettingen, Germany. Email: *sneuman@gwdg.de*

These dogs were summarized as group 3. All procedures of this study conform to the German "Animal welfare law" and were carried out under the supervision of the Commissioner for "animal welfare", University of Goettingen.

Sample collection

For measurement of serum TGF-β1 levels in dogs from all groups, blood was drawn from the cephalic vein. Blood samples were collected with a wide-gauge (20-gauge) needle. To obtain serum, the blood was placed in a standard serum tube and was allowed to clot at room temperature for 30 minutes. After overnight incubation at 2–8°C the blood was centrifuged for 15 minutes at 1000 x g. The supernatant was aliquoted and stored at –80°C until further investigation. Samples of the anterior lens capsule were obtained during cataract surgery from the capsulorrhexis site.

TGF-β1 measurement

Serum concentrations of TGF-β1 were determined by use of a quantitative sandwich immunoassay (Quantikine Human TGF-β1 ELISA; catalog number DB100B; R&D Systems, Minneapolis, Minnesota, USA). According to the manufacturer's instructions, the test was previously tested and validated on canine blood, on the basis of a 94% identical amino acid sequence. The assay was performed according to the manufacturer's protocol. In brief, serum was activated by 1 N HCl, incubated at room temperature and neutralized by 1.2 N NaOH/0.5 M HEPES. Prior to the assay, activated samples were diluted with calibrator diluent. Assay diluent was then applied to each well of the microplate, followed by either a standard for the standard curve, a control or the activated sample. After 2 hours' incubation at room temperature the plate was washed; TGF-β1 conjugate was added and the plate incubated for another 2 hours. Following washing, protected from light the sample was applied to the wells and the plates incubated for 30 minutes. Finally, the visualization was stopped and the optical density was measured using a TECAN GENios Pro (TECAN Austria GmbH, Groedig, Austria) at a wavelength of 450 nm and a wavelength correction of 570 nm. Each measurement was carried out in triplicate and readings were averaged for the analyses. A standard curve was created for each measurement, based on the results for the diluted standards. The concentration of each probe was calculated according to the standard curve. Owing to the initial dilution of the probes prior to the assay, concentrations were multiplied by the final dilution factor.

Immunohistochemistry

Lens material was collected during surgery from all dogs with cataracts when anterior capsulorrhexis was performed. Samples of anterior lens capsule and associated lens epithelium were fixed in 5% neutral-buffered formalin and processed for routine histology.

Immunhistochemistry was performed at the paraffin-embedded tissue using the avidin-biotin-complex (ABC) method. As the primary antibody a polyclonal anti-TGF-beta receptor, type I (Millipore, Cat. ABF17) was established on canine placenta and inflamed skin and eye samples. Best results were seen with the Dako EnVison+ System-HRP (DAB), for use with rabbit primary antibodies.

Statistics

For statistical analysis we used the software R (Version 2.8, www.r-project.org). The age dependence of TGF-β1 was calculated using the Spearmans correlation test. The distributions of data were calculated using the Kolmogorov-Smirnov Test. To assess concentration differences between the diseased dogs and healthy controls, the Mann-Whitney U-Test was applied. Significance was defined at $p < 0.05$.

Results and Discussion

The control group was composed of eight male and 12 female dogs from different breeds; they were aged between five months and ten years.

The group of dogs with diabetes mellitus consisted of 12 dogs of different breeds aged between three and 12 years. Finally the dogs with confirmed organ fibrosis comprised seven male and five female dogs. These dogs were of different breeds and aged between six and 13 years.

All dogs in the study had measurable serum concentrations of TGF-β1. The serum concentrations in the group of clinical healthy dogs (group 1) were between 30856 pg/mL and 40576 pg/mL, with a median of 37585 pg/mL. In the group of dogs with diabetes mellitus (group 2) serum concentrations of TGF-β1 between 37240 and 106674 pg/mL could be measured, with a median of 61919 pg/mL. Finally, the dogs with fibrosis in different organs (group 3) had TGF-β1 concentrations between 32625 and 91178 pg/mL, with a median of 53634 pg/mL.

There is no age dependence of TGF-β1. Comparing all three groups, highly significant differences between the healthy controls and both other groups ($p < 0.001$) could be found. The difference between group 2 (dogs with diabetes mellitus) and dogs with fibrotic diseases was not significant ($p > 0.05$) (Fig. 1).

The expression of TGF-β1 receptors in the anterior capsular epithelium was investigated in seven dogs. In four dogs no expression of TGF-β1 receptors could be found on immunohistochemistry (Fig. 2). Three dogs expressed TGF-β1 receptors with different intensity (Fig. 3). There was no correlation between the TGF-β1 serum concentration and the expression of TGF-β1 receptor on lens capsule.

In humans, elevated serum TGF-β1 were found in diabetic patients (Jakuš et al., 2012; Mou et al., 2016). As far as we know no study about serum TGF-β1in diabetic dogs exist.

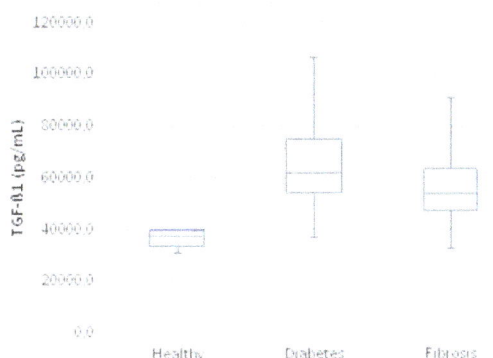

Fig. 1. Box-plot of TGF-β1 serum concentrations in all investigated groups (Healthy controls; Diabetes mellitus; Fibrotic diseases).

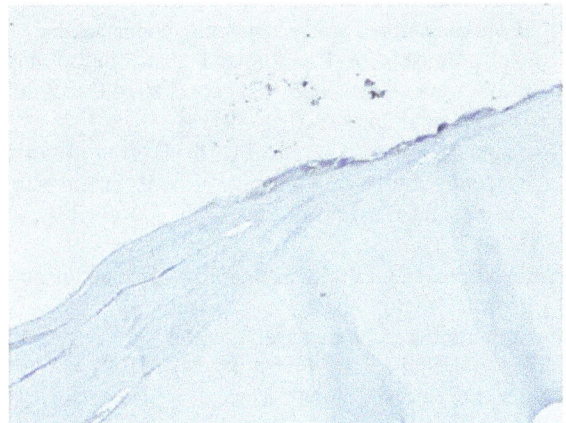

Fig. 2. No expression of the TGF-β1 receptor in the lens capsule.

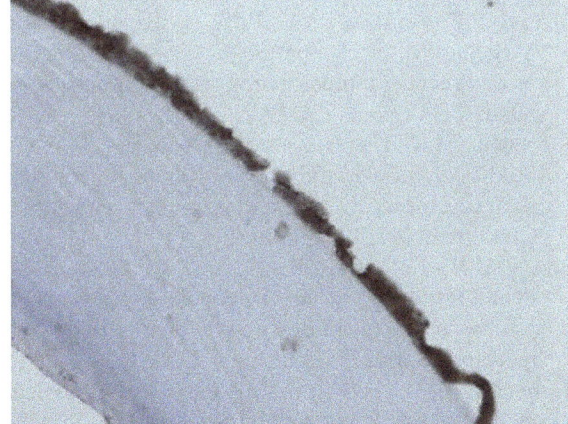

Fig. 3. Severe expression of the TGF-β1 receptor in the lens capsule.

The results of our study show that TGF-β1 serum concentrations in dogs with diabetes mellitus are comparable to those of dogs with fibrotic diseases and are significantly increased compared to healthy dogs. On that way we can confirm the results of human

patients for dogs. Because elevation of serum TGF-β1 is associated with fibrosis of different organs in dogs (Neumann *et al.*, 2008; Krafft *et al.*, 2011), we can assume that the elevation of serum TGF-β1 in diabetic dogs also induces fibrosis. The mechanism about fibrosis in diabetic patients is probably induced by hyperglycemia. Different hypothesis exist how hyperglycemia induce fibrosis. For example via polyol pathway (Greene *et al.*, 1987), via glycation of proteins (Brownlee *et al.*, 1988) or via oxidative stress (Hunt *et al.*, 1990). Further studies are necessary proofing the exact mechanism of fibrosis in diabetic dogs and its consequences.

In this study, we investigated secondly the association of TGF-β1 with canine cataracts formation. Different publications in human medicine have assumed a role of TGF-β1 in the pathogenesis of cataracts (DeIongh *et al.*, 2001; Lovicu *et al.*, 2002). For that purpose the expression of TGF-β1 receptors in lens epithelial cells was measured. However, we could not identify the receptors in all cases. A possible explanation for this finding could be an inconsistent expression of the receptor on the cell membrane during the course of the disease. This has also been reported by other researchers (Roulot *et al.*, 1999). Tissue fibrosis, as the final morphological step of organ rebuilding, is an inconsistent mechanism with periods of elevated collagen production and periods with lower production (McGee, 1977). Therefore, it is possible that TGF-β1 receptor expression is also inconsistent, resulting in the absence of receptors in some cases.

In summary the results of this study show increased serum TGF-β1 in diabetic dogs, which may can induce different complications associated with diabetes mellitus and may make dogs to a model for diabetes mellitus in humans.

Conflict of interest

The Authors declare that there are no conflict of interests.

References

Alevizopoulos, A. and Mermod, N. 1997. Transforming growth factor-beta: the breaking open of a black box. Bioessays 19, 581-591.

Blobe, G.C., Schiemann, W.P. and Lodish, H.F. 2000. Role of transforming growth factor beta in human disease. N. Engl. J. Med. 342, 1350-1358.

Brownlee, M., Cerami, A. and Vlassara, H. 1988. Advanced glycosylation end products in tissue and the biochemical basis of diabetic complications. N. Engl. J. Med. 318(20), 1315-1321.

Colitz, C.M.H., Malarkey, D., Dykstra, M.J., McGahan, M.C. and Davidson, M.G. 2000. Histologic and immunohistochemical characterization of lens capsular plaques in dogs with cataracts. Am. J. Vet. Res. 61, 139-143.

DeIongh, R., Gordon-Thomson, C., Chamberlain, C.G., Hales, A.M. and McAvoy, J.W. 2001. TGFβ Receptor Expression in Lens: Implications for Differentiation and Cataractogenesis. Exp. Eye Res. 72, 649-659.

Gangwani, R.A., Lian, J.X., Mc Ghee, S.M., Wong, D. and Li, K.K. 2016. Diabetic retinopathy screening: global and local perspective. Hong Kong Med. J. 22(5), 486-495.

Gardiner, T.A., Stitt, A.W., Anderson, H.R. and Archer, D.B. 1994. Selective loss of vascular smooth muscle cells in the retinal microcirculation of diabetic dogs. Br. J. Ophthalmol. 78(1), 54-60.

Gilbert, R.E. 2013. Endothelial loss and repair in the vascular complications of diabetes: pathogenetic mechanisms and therapeutic implications. Circ. J. 77(4), 849-856.

Greene, D.A., Lattimer, S.A. and Sima, A.A. 1987. Sorbitol, phosphoinositides, and sodium-potassium-ATPase in the pathogenesis of diabetic complications. N. Engl. J. Med. 316(10), 599-606.

Hills, C.E. and Squires, P.E. 2009. TGF-beta1-induced epithelial-to-mesenchymal transition and therapeutic intervention in diabetic nephropathy. Am. J. Nephrol. 31, 68-74.

Hunt, J.V., Smith, C.C. and Wolff, S.P. 1990. Autoxidative glycosylation and possible involvement of peroxides and free radicals in LDL modification by glucose. Diabetes 39(11), 1420-1424.

Jakuš, V., Sapák, M. and Kostolanská, J. 2012. Circulating TGF-β1, glycation, and oxidation in children with diabetes mellitus type 1. Exp. Diabetes Res. 2012: 510902. doi: 10.1155/2012/510902.

Juster-Switlyk, K. and Smith, A.G. 2016. Updates in diabetic peripheral neuropathy. F1000Res. doi: 10.12688/f1000research.7898.1.

Krafft, E., Heikkila, H.P. and Jespers, P. 2011. Serum and bronchoalveolar lavage fluid endothelin-1 concentrations as diagnostic biomarkers of canine idiopathic pulmonary fibrosis. J. Vet. Intern. Med. 25, 990-996.

Lawrence, D.A. 1996. Transforming growth factor-beta: a general review. Europ. Cytokine Network 7, 363-374.

Leung, W.K., Gao, L., Siu, P.M. and Lai, C.W. 2016. Diabetic nephropathy and endothelial dysfunction: Current and future therapies, and emerging of vascular imaging for preclinical renal-kinetic study. Life Sci. 166, 121-130.

Lopez-Novoa, J.M. and Nieto, M.A. 2009. Inflammation and EMT: an alliance towards organ fibrosis and cancer progression. EMBO Mol. Med. 1, 303-314.

Lovicu, F.J., Schulz, M.W., Hales, A.M., Vincent, L.N., Overbeek, P.A., Chamberlain, C.G. and McAvoy, J.W. 2002. TGFβ induces morphological and molecular changes similar to human anterior subcapsular cataract. Brit. J. Ophthalmol. 86, 220-226.

McGee, J.D. 1977. Collagen deposition in liver disease. Annual Rheumat. Dis. 36, 29-36.

Mou, X., Zhou, D.Y., Zhou, D.Y., Ma, J.R., Liu, Y.H., Chen, H.P., Hu, Y.B., Shou, C.M., Chen, J.W., Liu, W.H. and Ma, G.L. 2016. Serum TGF-β1 as a Biomarker for Type 2 Diabetic Nephropathy: A Meta-Analysis of Randomized Controlled Trials. PLoS One. 2016 Feb 22; 11(2):e0149513. doi: 10.1371/journal.pone.0149513.

Neumann, S., Kaup, F.J. and Beardi, B. 2008. Plasma concentration of transforming growth factor-beta1 and hepatic fibrosis in dogs. Can. J. Vet. Res. 72, 428-431.

Prud'homme, G.J. 2007. Pathobiology of transforming growth factor beta in cancer, fibrosis and immunologic disease, and therapeutic considerations. Lab. Invest. 87, 1077-1091.

Roulot, D., Sevcsik, A.M., Coste, T., Strosberg, A.D. and Marullo, S. 1999. Role of transforming growth factor β type II receptor in hepatic fibrosis: Studies of human chronic hepatitis C and experimental fibrosis in rats. Hepatol. 29, 1730-1738.

Shariat, S.F., Semjonow, A., Lilja, H., Savage, C. and Vickers, A.J. 2011. Bjartell A. Tumor markers in prostate cancer I: blood-based markers. Acta Oncol. 50, 61-75.

Siperstein, M.D., Unger, R.H. and Madison, L.L. 1968. Studies of muscle capillary basement membranes in normal subjects diabetic, and prediabetic patients. J. Clin. Invest. 47, 1973-1999.

Sporn, M.B., Roberts, A.B., Born, G.V., Cuatrecasas, P. and Herken, H. 1990. Handbook of experimental pharmacology: Peptide growth factors and their receptors. Springer Berlin, New York.

Tsilibary, E.C. 2003. Microvascular basement membranes in diabetes mellitus. J. Pathol. 200, 537-546.

14

Lateral patellar luxation in nine small breed dogs

F. Di Dona[1,*], G. Della Valle[1], C. Balestriere[1], B. Lamagna[1], L. Meomartino[2], G. Napoleone[1], F. Lamagna[1] and G. Fatone[1]

[1]*Department of Veterinary Medicine and Animal Productions, University of Napoli "Federico II", Italy*
[2]*Interdepartmental Center of Veterinary Radiology, University of Napoli "Federico II", Italy*

Abstract

The objective of this paper was to describe the clinical features, the management and the outcome of nine small breed dogs affected with lateral patella luxation referred during the period between January 2010 and December 2014. Patellar luxations were classified according to: breed, age, sex, weight, and grade of patellar luxation, as well as if unilateral or bilateral, and concurrent cranial cruciate ligament lesion. In affected dogs, surgical correction consisted in the combination of tibial tuberosity transposition and soft tissue procedure. Adjunctive condroplasty or trochleoplasty was performed as needing. The outcome was found positive after surgical management with low complication rate and complications have been easily managed with high success rate.

Keywords: Dog, Lateral, Luxation, Patellar.

Introduction

Patellar luxation (PL) is one of the most common orthopedic disease in dogs, and can affect both large and small dogs and may be seen in cats as well (Nunamaker, 1985; DeAngelis, 1996; Ness *et al.*, 1996; Linney *et al.*, 2011). Lateral patellar luxation (LPL) occurs less frequently than does medial patellar luxation (MPL) (Roush, 1993). LPL is commonly diagnosed in large or giant breed dogs, especially the St. Bernard, while it seems to be an unusual occurrence in small breed dogs (Roush, 1993; Hayes *et al.*, 1994; LaFond *et al.*, 2002; L'Eplattenier and Montavon, 2002; Harasen, 2006). In a recent study, which evaluated retrospectively 65 dogs of all breeds with LPL, medium and large breed dogs were more affected; and less than 10% (6/65) of all dogs were small breed dogs (Kalff *et al.*, 2014).

The purpose of this paper is to describe clinical presentation, radiographic findings, management and outcome of 9 small breed dogs with a diagnosis of LPL.

Materials and Methods

Medical records of small breed dogs with confirmed diagnosis of LPL admitted to the Veterinary Teaching Hospital at the University of Napoli (2010–2014) were identified. According to Kennel Club standards for weight, dogs with a physical weight less than 9 kg were considered small breed (Priester, 1972; Hayes *et al.*, 1994; Bound *et al.*, 2009). Data collection included: breed, age, sex, weight, grade of PL, as well as if unilateral or bilateral, and concurrent cranial cruciate ligament (CrCL) lesion. Grade of PL was determined by referencing the description of PL to a simplified grading system by Roush (1993). Grade I: Patella can

be manually luxated but returns to normal position when released. Grade II: Patella luxates with stifle flexion or on manual manipulation and remains luxated until stifle extension or manual replacement occurs. Grade III: Patella luxated continually, and can be manually replaced but will reluxate spontaneously when manual pressure is removed. Grade IV: Patella luxated continually and cannot be manually replaced.

Orthopedic examination consisted in gait evaluation by visual inspection, joint flexion-extension movements and range of motion evaluation, and grade of PL. Radiographic images in both medio-lateral and cranio-caudal projections were taken. All dogs were treated surgically and were evaluated at clinical follow-up.

Surgery

All surgical procedures were executed throughout a cranio-medial, parapatellar, incision to the stifle joint. The surgical techniques used in dogs with LPL were grouped in soft tissue procedures (STP) and osseous procedures (medial tibial tuberosity transposition [TTT]; femoral recession trochleoplasty or chondroplasty). The soft tissue techniques included lateral retinacular release and medial imbrication (Roush, 1993); the deep fascia was released laterally and imbricated medially in order to produce slight medial tension. The osseous procedures included TTT, femoral recession trochleoplasty (TP) or chondroplasty (CP). TTT consisted in osteotomy of the tuberosity with intact distal attachment; tibial crest was then moved medially a sufficient distance to provide straight alignment of the quadriceps mechanism and was stabilized with two Kirschner wires (0.8 to 1.5 mm; Alcyon Italia S.p.A., Italy) without using tension band

*Corresponding Author: Francesco Di Dona. Department of Veterinary Medicine and Animal Productions, University of Napoli "Federico II". Via Federico Delpino, 1 – 80138 Napoli, Italy. Email: *francesco.didona@unina.it*

fixation. Femoral recession trochleoplasty was performed when the trochlear sulcus was shallow or absent; trochlear block recession was performed through elevating an osteochondral block from the patellar groove, removing bone from the bottom of the incised block to deepen the sulcus, and then replace the osteochondral block (Priester, 1972; Bound *et al.*, 2009). In young dogs (less than 8 months) chondroplasty was performed by elevating the hyaline cartilage and removing subcondral bone beneath the cartilage flap (Roush, 1993). The adjunctive surgical technique used in dogs with concurrent CrCL injury consisted in the medial and lateral fabellae suturing (FS) (DeAngelis and Lau, 1970; Shaver *et al.*, 2014). Two unilateral-session surgeries were performed in dogs bilaterally affected.

Pre- and post-operative care
All dogs were premedicated with intramuscular administration of methadone (0.3 mg/kg; Eptadone: L. Molteni & C. S.p.A., Italy) or morphine (0.4 mg/kg; Morfina cloridrato: L. Molteni & C. S.p.A., Italy) and dexmedetomidine (5µg/kg; Dexdomitor: Vetoquinol Italia S.r.l., Italy). Intravenous administration of propofol (4-6 mg/kg; Propovet: Esteve S.p.A., Italy) was used to induce anesthesia, then maintained via gaseous mixture of oxygen and isoflurane (Isoflurane Vet: Merial Italia S.p.A., Italy). Peripheral sciatic and femoral nerve block with lidocaine (2 mg/kg; Lidocaina Cloridrato: A.T.I. S.r.l., Italy) was obtained. Perioperative antibiotic therapy included intravenous administration of cephazolin (22 mg/kg; Cefazolina Teva: Teva Italia S.r.l., Italy). Postoperative analgesia included intramuscular administration of methadone (0.3 mg/kg; Eptadone: L. Molteni & C. S.p.A., Italy) as required for up to 48h and either carprofen (2 mg/kg SID; Rimadyl: Pfizer Italia S.r.l., Italy) or firocoxib (5 mg/kg SID; Previcox: Merial Italia S.p.A., Italy) for 6 to 10 days following surgery. Dogs were dismissed from the hospital 24-48h following surgery.

Outcome and Complications
Clinical follow was performed for each dog at 7 and 14 days, then at 4 to 12 weeks following surgery, and thereafter by telephone interview. The outcome of surgical correction was classified, according to dogs' status, in: excellent (no gait abnormality), good (mild or intermittent gait abnormality), fair (moderate gait abnormality), and poor (severe gait abnormality). Frequency and type of postoperative complication associated with LPL stabilization were registered. Dogs that underwent a revision surgery were considered as having a major complication. Whereas complication did not required additional treatments were classified as minor.

Statistical analysis
All statistical analyses were performed using commercial software (Prism GraphPad Software, Inc,

USA). Descriptive statistics were calculated and data were reported as median and range. Categorical data were expressed as frequencies. Statistical power was inadequate to compare outcome measures or incidence of complications with signalment or surgical variables.

Results and Discussion
Of the one hundred thirty-seven dogs with a diagnosis of PL in the reference period, LPL was present in fourteen dogs. However only nine of them met the inclusion criteria and were classified as small breed dogs. Seven dogs were female (one neutered) and the remaining two were intact male. Dogs ranged in age from 5 to 132 months (median = 18 months). Body weight ranged from 1.3 to 8.8 kg (median = 4 kg). The following breed were registered: Poodle (n=3), Pinscher (n=2), Pekingese, Yorkshire, Cavalier King Charles Spaniel and mixed-breed. Five dogs had a diagnosis of grade III luxation and one of them was bilaterally affected. The remaining four dogs were equally affected with grade I and II luxation, whereas none of the dogs had a diagnosis of a grade IV luxation. One dog had a history of vehicular trauma, while another one experienced an acute lameness due to a CrCL injury.

Surgical correction was performed in 10 stifles and consisted in TTT and STP for all the dogs included. Two dogs received adjunctive chondroplasty because of their young age, whereas in other three dogs, the deepening of the trochlear groove was obtained through a block recession trochleoplasty. One dog was managed in a single session surgery for both LPL and CrCL injury, through medial TTT and subsequently FS.

Major complications were observed only in two dogs that experienced a lateral reluxation, and were managed with a second soft tissue procedure to improve medial tension. Two dogs had implant migration and concomitant seroma, and were considered as having a minor complication. Follow-up was performed for all dogs. Four dogs with five stifles treated were classified as having excellent outcome; three dogs as having good outcome; and two dogs as having fair outcome. These last two dogs with moderate gait abnormalities at last examination were both affected by concurrent injuries (CrCL injury; aftereffects of a pelvic trauma) (Table 1). PL is a common stifle disorder in dogs, and MPL occurs more frequently than does LPL, especially in small breed dogs (Nunamaker, 1985; Vasseur, 2003; Shaver *et al.*, 2014).

The clinical picture of the population referred to our hospital is dominated by MPL, while LPL occurred in 10.2% of the dogs. According to the literature, lateral dislocation has been observed approximately in 5% to 12% of dogs with PL, however, this was increased in large and giant breed dogs to reach 17% to 33% (Hayes *et al.*, 1994; Arthurs and Langley-Hobbs, 2006; Alam *et al.*, 2007; Shaver *et al.*, 2014).

Table 1. Distribution of lateral patellar luxation. Surgical management, complications, and outcome.

Cases	Breed	Sex	Age (months)	Weight (kg)	Grade	CrCL	Surgery	Complications	Outcome
1[*]	Poodle	F	5	2.2	3		TTT, STP, CP		excellent
2	Poodle	F[**]	36	3	3		TTT, STP, TP	Seroma; implant migration	good
3	Poodle	F	7	5.2	3		TTT, STP, CP		excellent
4	Cavalier King Charles Spaniel	M	48	7.9	1	Yes	TTT, STP, FS	Seroma; implant migration	fair
5	Mixed-breed	M	36	8.8	1		TTT, STP		excellent
6	Pekingese	F	84	6.8	2		TTT, STP		excellent
7	Pinscher	F	132	2.3	3		TTT, STP, TP	Reluxation	fair
8	Pinscher	F	12	4	2		TTT, STP		good
9	Yorkshire	F	18	1.3	3		TTT, STP, TP	Reluxation	Good

(TTT): Tibial tuberosity transposition; (STP): Soft tissue procedure; (CP): Condroplasty; (TP): Throcleoplasty; (FS): Fabellar suture.
* With bilateral patellar luxation. ** Neutered.

Most of dogs included were young at the time of examination, which is consistent with previous reports (Hayes *et al.*, 1994; Arthurs and Langley-Hobbs, 2006; Kalff *et al.*, 2014; Shaver *et al.*, 2014). The young age was frequently associated to grade III or IV of lateral luxation due to congenital reasons as a result of under-development of the trochlear groove. However, the disease may be diagnosed in older dogs, as low-grade luxations are usually asymptomatic in early stages (Kalff *et al.*, 2014).

Surgical treatment was advised for all dogs with a diagnosis of PL. TTT may be the most important component of surgical treatment for dogs with PL since quadriceps malalignment is a key feature in the development of all grades of PL (Robins, 1990). A previous study evaluated the effect of the sole TTT without trochlear groove deepening in 91 dogs with MPL, and concluded that trochlear groove deepening procedures are not always necessary, and patients that undergo these techniques should be carefully selected (Linney *et al.*, 2011). Dog included in this report received adjunctive trochlear groove deepening when a clinical and radiographic evidence of shallow groove was observed.

Complications after surgical treatment of LPL have been previously reported, however one of the major limitation was the highly variable nature of surgical correction of LPL, which made impossible to draw conclusions about the effect of specific treatments (Shaver *et al.*, 2014). The population reported here was managed with the same techniques (TTT and STP), with adjunctive procedures as needing, and our results support the effectiveness of the procedure that can result in definitive stabilization of the patella in its trochlear groove.

In the present case series, reluxation is the most important complication after surgical correction and occurred in 20% of stifle joints treated. Arthurs and Langley-Hobbs (2006) and Shaver *et al.* (2014) found respectively that 17% and 21.3% of stifle joints with LPL have reluxated, and this data is comparable with the percentage reported here. Kalff *et al.* (2014), accounting this complication in 6/65 of the dogs treated, reported the lower incidence of lateral reluxation. Minor complications included the migration of the pins and the following development of a seroma, and were easily managed through pins removal. Even though pin migration requires a minor surgical procedure for removing the Kirschner wires, it has been classified as minor complication (Kalff *et al.*, 2014).

Previous studies detected a correlation between body weight and a higher risk of complications and reluxation after corrective surgery (Arthurs and Langley-Hobbs, 2006; Gibbons *et al.*, 2006; Cashmore *et al.*, 2014). Because the dogs included are lightweight, probably stresses on stifle joints are lower, and the response to surgery may be better; furthermore the young age of affected dogs may play a central role in better recovery, due to the great tendency of tissues to have fast healing, and also for the absence of chronic degenerative joint lesions.

Shaver *et al.* (2014) stated that bilateral surgery during a single session was the only variable significantly associated with reluxation, accounting odds of reluxation 12.5 times higher than dogs that had unilateral surgery. We cannot confirm this data as most of the dogs were unilaterally affected, and the only one dog with a bilateral luxation was managed in double session surgery. Moreover, the limited number of stifles studied is a main limitation. Wangdee *et al.* (2013) evaluating the surgical management of MPL in Pomeranian dogs, established that grade II luxation had good outcome with a 100% success rate following surgery. Dogs with grade III luxation had recurrent PL in about 11% of the stifle joints treated; while dogs with grade IV luxation had higher rate of reluxation, accounting 36% of the dogs subjected to surgery, because varying degree of skeletal deformities.

Most of the dogs included in this sample had positive outcome. Whereas our hypothesis about the two dogs that experienced fair outcome is that it may be more linked to the concurrent CrCL and pelvic injuries than to the PL.

The knowledge about LPL in the dog is still limited. The present report suggests that small breed dogs seems to be affected as well as medium, large and giant breed dogs. It can be concluded that previous studies analyzed populations with different prevalence of each breed and data obtained cannot be compared, LPL is a growing disease in small breed dogs and that LPL in small breed dogs is underestimated.

References

Alam, M.R., Lee, J.I., Kang, H.S., Kim, I.S., Park, S.Y., Lee, K.C. and Kim, N.S. 2007. Frequency and distribution of patellar luxation in dogs. 134 cases (2000 to 2005). Vet. Comp. Orthop. Traumatol. 20, 59-64.

Arthurs, G.I. and Langley-Hobbs, S.J. 2006. Complications associated with corrective surgery for patellar luxation in 109 dogs. Vet. Surg. 35, 559-566.

Bound, N., Zakai, D., Butterworth, S.J. and Pead, M. 2009. The prevalence of canine patellar luxation in three centres. Clinical features and radiographic evidence of limb deviation. Vet. Comp. Orthop. Traumatol. 22, 32-37.

Cashmore, R.G., Havlicek, M., Perkins, N.R., James, D.R., Fearnside, S.M., Marchevsky, A.M. and Black, A.P. 2014. Major complications and risk factors associated with surgical correction of congenital medial patellar luxation in 124 dogs. Vet. Comp. Orthop. Traumatol. 27, 263-270.

DeAngelis, M. 1996. Patellar luxation in dogs. Vet. Clin. North Am. Small Anim. Pract. 1, 403-415.

DeAngelis, M. and Lau, R.E. 1970. A lateral retinacular imbrication technique for the surgical correction of anterior cruciate ligament rupture in the dog. J. Am. Vet. Med. Assoc. 157, 79-84.

Gibbons, S.E., Macias, C., Tonzing, M.A., Pinchbeck, G.L. and McKee, W.M. 2006. Patellar luxation in 70 large breed dogs. J. Small Anim. Pract. 47, 3-9.

Harasen, G. 2006. Patellar luxation: Pathogenesis and surgical correction. Can. Vet. J. 47, 1037-1039.

Hayes, A.G., Boudrieau, R.J. and Hungerford, L.L. 1994. Frequency and distribution of medial and lateral patellar luxation in dogs: 124 cases (1982-1992). J. Am. Vet. Med. Assoc. 205, 716-720.

Kalff, S., Butterworth, S.J., Miller, A., Keeley, B., Baines, S. and McKee, W.M. 2014. Lateral patellar luxation in dogs: a retrospective study of 65 dogs. Vet. Comp. Orthop. Traumatol. 27, 130-134.

LaFond, E., Breur, G.J. and Austin, C.C. 2002. Breed susceptibility for developmental orthopedic diseases in dogs. J. Am. Anim. Hosp. Assoc. 38, 467-477.

L'Eplattenier, H.F. and Montavon, P. 2002. Patellar luxation in dogs and cats: management and prevention. Comp. Cont. Edu. Pract. Vet. 24, 292-300.

Linney, W.R., Hammer, D.L. and Shott, S. 2011. Surgical treatment of medial patellar luxation without femoral trochlear groove deepening procedures in dogs: 91 cases (1998– 2009). J. Am. Vet. Med. Assoc. 238, 1168-1172.

Ness, M.G., Abercromby, R.H., May, C., Turner, B.M. and Carmichael, S. 1996. A survey of orthopaedic conditions in small animal veterinary practice in Britain. Vet. Comp. Orthop. Traumatol. 9, 43-52.

Nunamaker, D.M. 1985. Patellar luxation. In Textbook of Small Animal Orthopaedics, Eds., Newton, C.D. and Nunamaker, D.M.: Lippincott, Philadelphia, pp: 941-947.

Priester, W.A. 1972. Sex, size, and breed as risk factors in canine patellar luxation. J. Am. Vet. Med. Assoc. 4, 633-636.

Robins, G.M. 1990. The canine stifle joint. In Canine Orthopedics, Ed., Whittick, W.G.: Lea and Febiger, Philadelphia, pp: 693-760.

Roush, J.K. 1993. Canine patellar luxation. Vet. Clin. North Am. Small Anim. Pract. 23, 855-868.

Shaver, S.L., Mayhew, K.N., Sutton, J.S., Mayhew, P.D., Runge, J.J., Brown, D.C. and Kass, P.H. 2014. Complications after corrective surgery for lateral patellar luxation in dogs: 36 cases (2000–2011). J. Am. Vet. Med. Assoc. 244, 444-448.

Vasseur, P.B. 2003. Stifle joint. In Textbook of Small Animal Surgery, Ed., Slatter, D.S.: Saunders, Philadelphia, pp: 2090-2133.

Wangdee, C., Theyse, L.F.H., Techakumphu, M., Soontornvipart, K. and Hazewinkel, H.A. 2013. Evaluation of surgical treatment of medial patellar luxation in Pomeranian dogs. Vet. Comp. Orthop. Traumatol. 26, 435-439.

15

Post-surgical treatment of thyroid carcinoma in dogs with retinoic acid 9 cis improves patient outcome

V. Castillo[1,*], P. Pessina[2], P. Hall[3], M.F. Cabrera Blatter[1], D. Miceli[1], E. Soler Arias[1] and P. Vidal[1]

[1]*Cat. Clin. Méd. Peq. An. and U. Endocrinología, Escuela Medicina Veterinaria, Facultad de Ciencias Veterinarias, Universidad de Buenos Aires. Av.Chorroarín 280, C. Autónoma de Buenos Aires, Argentina*
[2]*Laboratorio de Técnicas Nucleares, Facultad de Veterinaria, Universidad de la República, Lasplaces 1550, Montevideo, Uruguay*
[3]*Cat. Cirugía and U. Cirugía, Hosp., Escuela Medicina Veterinaria, Facultad de Ciencias Veterinarias, Universidad de Buenos Aires. Av.Chorroarín 280, C. Autónoma de Buenos Aires, Argentina*

Abstract

The objective of the present study was to compare the effects of isotretinoin 9-cis (RA9-cis) as a post-surgery treatment of thyroid carcinoma to a traditional treatment (doxorubicin) and no treatment. Owners who did not want their dogs to receive treatment were placed into the control group A (GA; n=10). The remaining dogs were randomly placed into either group B (GB; n=12) and received doxorubicin at a dose of 30 mg/m^2 every three weeks, for six complete cycles or group C (GC; n=15) and treated with RA9-cis at a dose of 2 mg/kg/day for 6 months. The time of the recurrence was significantly shorter in the GA and GB compared to GC (P=0.0007; P=0.0015 respectively), while we did not detect differences between GA and GB. The hazard ratio of recurrence between GA and GB compared to GC were 7.25 and 5.60 times shorter, respectively. We did not detect any differences between the other groups. The risk ratio of recurrence was 2.0 times higher in GA compared to GC and 2.1 times higher in GB compared to GC. The type of carcinoma had an effect on time of survival with follicular carcinomas having an increased mean survival time than follicular-compact carcinomas (P<0.0001) and follicular-compact carcinomas had a longer mean survival time than compact carcinomas. The interaction among treatment and type was significant, but survival time in follicular carcinomas did not differ between treatments. In follicular-compact carcinomas the survival time of GC was greater than GB (P<0.05), but we did not detect a difference between GA and GB. In conclusion, this study shows that the use of surgery in combination with RA9-cis treatment significantly increases survival rate and decreases the time to tumor recurrence when compared to doxorubicin treated or untreated dogs. The histological type of carcinoma interacted with treatment for time to recurrence and survival time, with more undifferentiated carcinomas having a worse prognosis than differentiated carcinomas.

Keywords: Differentiated follicular carcinoma, Retinoic acid, Thyroid carcinoma, Thyroid tumour.

Introduction

The vast majority (90%) of thyroid tumours in dogs are thyroid carcinomas (TC), which is a frequent endocrine cancer in dogs (Barber, 2007). Thyroid carcinomas are classified according to their histological features and origin as: a) follicular thyroid carcinoma (FTC, arises from follicular cells); b) medullary thyroid carcinoma; and c) anaplastic (Kiupel *et al.*, 2008; Meissner and Warren, 1969; Wucherer and Wilke, 2010). Follicular thyroid carcinomas are further divided into well differentiated (dFTC) follicular, dFTC follicular compact, dFTC compact, dFTC papillary, poorly differentiated, undifferentiated, or carcinosarcoma. Follicular thyroid carcinoma is the most frequently diagnosed histological variants with follicular-compact and compact the most common forms (Campos *et al.*, 2014; Mitchell and Tjian 1989; Klein *et al.*, 1995; Worth *et al.*, 2005). The histological origin of dFTC tumours will influence its progression, local invasion, tumour recurrence after

surgery, and median survival time (Haugen, 1999). However, the dFTC functional characteristics (iodine uptake, thyroid hormones synthesis) vary by histological origin (Verschueren *et al.*, 1991).

The median survival time for dogs with untreated thyroid carcinoma is only three months (Worth *et al.*, 2005), but in freely movable non-metastatic thyroid tumours, the median survival time with surgery alone has been reported to be from 7-8 months (Page, 2001; Morris and Dobson, 2002) to over 36 months (Klein *et al.*, 1995). Campos *et al.* (2014) report that macro- or microscopic evidence of vascular invasion is a negative predictor of disease free-survival time in dogs after surgically excised TC.

In humans it is well known that therapeutic options for TC and prognosis after treatment will depend on the type of tumour, its iodine uptake, the vascular endothelial growth factor, and Ki-67 expression (Capp *et al.*, 2010; Coelho *et al.*, 2011; Klein *et al.*, 2000; Soh

---

*Corresponding Author:** Prof. Dr. Victor A. Castillo. Department of Companion Animals, Chief of Endocrinology Unit, Faculty of Veterinary Sciences, University of Buenos Aires, Buenos Aires, Argentina. E-mail: *vcastill@fvet.uba.ar*

et al., 1997; Tallini *et al.*, 1999); although, no similar studies have been conducted in dogs except for one study examining Ki-67 labeling, which was associated with local invasiveness (Campos *et al.*, 2014).

Regarding TC treatment in dogs, particularly dFCT, the first and main therapeutic procedure is surgical removal of the tumour, if removal is feasible. For dFTC removal, whether or not there is invasion of adjacent tissues must be taken into account. Recurrence of the tumour after surgery is dependent on the histological subtype of the tumour. The worst prognosis is seen with the follicular-compact or compact thyroid carcinoma (Klein *et al.*, 1995; Radinsky, 2007). After surgery ^{131}I therapy is recommended to eliminate remnant cancer tissue, but only if the tumour shows ^{99m}Tc uptake. Radiation is not effective when ^{99m}Tc uptake does not occur because poor uptake only occurs in poorly differentiated tumours or undifferentiated tumours (Worth *et al.*, 2005; Turrel *et al.*, 2006). In dFCT cases, radiation therapy has been associated with a median survival time of 28 months (Verschueren *et al.*, 1991; Turrel *et al.*, 2006). Despite the apparent success of surgery and radiation in the management of localized TC, up to 80% of canine patients have recurrences of TC or develop metastases during the course of their disease (Patnaik and Lieberman, 1991; Carver *et al.*, 1995; DeLellis, 2004; Kiupel *et al.*, 2008; Sipos *et al.*, 2008; Wucherer *et al.*, 2010). The limitation of radiotherapy is its high costs, the need of an appropriate infrastructure, and the legal regulations in each country. The use of chemotherapy for non-surgical TC or metastasis has had limited results. Doxorubicin has been the most frequently used drug, but it is only affective on differentiated TC tumours (Jeglum and Whereat, 1983; Ogilvie *et al.*, 1989). Studies using cisplatine and nevirapine have reported similar results (Fineman *et al.*, 1998; Muscella *et al.*, 2009; Dong *et al.*, 2013). On the other hand, chemotherapy after thyroidectomy has been reported to not provide a survival benefit (Nadeu *et al.*, 2011; Tuohy *et al.*, 2012).

Haugen *et al.* (2014) showed that thyroid tumours express both retinoic X receptor (RXR) and retinoic acid receptors (RAR) and their different isoforms. These authors also reported that the 9-cis form of retinoic acid (isotretinoin 9-cis, RA9-cis) inhibits thyroid tumour growth, but this action depends on the expression of the RXR or RAR isofroms. The results obtained in thyroid cell lines and few clinical studies in humans on RA9-cis treatment are promising (Coelho *et al.*, 2011 Simon *et al.*, 2002; Short *et al.*, 2004; Trojanowicz *et al.*, 2010); however, no reports of RA9-cis treatment on TCs in dogs are available. The effect of RA9-cis was also studied on cultured corticotroph cell tumour in dogs and in humans with Cushing's disease (Castillo *et al.*, 2006; Labeur *et al.*, 2009; Paez-Pereda *et al.*, 2001; Pecori *et al.*, 2012). These studies showed a reduction of the tumour growth, a reduction in the tumour size, and a reduction of the clinical signs and biochemical markers.

The objective of the present study was to compare the effects of RA9-cis as a novel post-surgery treatment of TC in dogs with the traditional treatment (doxorubicin), and a non-treatment control group. We compared treatment methods by analysing the time of recurrence of the tumour and survival time of the patient after treatment, while taking into account the TC histopathology.

Materials and Methods

Animals and treatments

This study was conducted at the School Hospital of Veterinary Medicine, Faculty of Veterinary Sciences, University of Buenos Aires, Argentina. All procedures were conducted in accordance with the regulations of the Animal Experimentation Committee (Faculty of Veterinary Sciences, University of Buenos Aires, Argentina). All dog owners gave their signed consent for the participation of their animals in this study. All dogs included in the present study were diagnosed with unilateral TC (one lobe affected) without evidence of metastases according to physical examination. The physical examination was done using ultrasonography with Doppler (vascularisation into the tumour is highly suspect of malignancy), scintigraphy in gamma camera with [99m]Tc (full body scan), and scan computed tomography of neck, thorax and abdomen (Fig. 1). According to the radiotracer concentration (uptake) in the gammagraphy study, (Verschueren *et al.*, 1991) tumours were classified as hot (high uptake compared to the contralateral lobe and the salivary glands that are inhibited), cold (low uptake with respect to the contralateral lobe and salivary glands, with normal uptake), or normal-uptake (both thyroid lobes uptake and the salivary glands uptake are equals). Dogs that presented any lymph node affected with local invasion or distal metastasis were excluded from the experiment.

Histological procedures and thyroid tumour classification

The thyroid tumour was surgically removed, fixed in formalin, paraffin-embedded, and stained with hematoxylin and eosin (HE). All HE-stained slides were reviewed by a two pathologist who were blinded to clinical reports. Thus, tumours were classified according to their histological characteristics in adenomas or carcinomas and their subtypes (Kiupel *et al.*, 2008; Wucherer and Wilke 2010). The distinction between adenoma and carcinoma was based on histological evidence of capsular invasion, vascular invasion, or metastases. Tumour staging was performed as described previously (Owen, 1980). All dogs included in the study had tumour staging S-II-$T2_{a/b}$-No-Mo (size between 2-5 cm, freely movable or fixed, no lymph node involvement, no evidence of distant metastases, or local invasion). In the present study, we only used dFTC follicular, follicular-compact, and compact tumours. This was done to analyse tumour recurrence, survival time, and their interaction with the treatments (Fig. 2). The other types were excluded by their low presentation in dogs (papillary, one case) or aggressive biological behaviour (anaplasic or poorly differentiated, one of each).

Thyroid hormones evaluation

At the moment of TC diagnosis, canine TSH and canine specific free thyroxine (fT4) were determined to evaluate the thyroid status. We measured canine TSH and fT4 using a chemiluminescent immunometric assay Immulite/Immulite 1000 Canine TSH and Immulite/Immulite 1000 fT4; Siemens Healthcare Diagnostics Products Ltd., Llanberis, Gwynedd, LL55 4EL, UK) according to manufacturer's instructions.

A dog was considered to be hypothyroid when TSH was elevated ($\geq$0.4 ng/mL) with fT4 levels within the reference range (0.6-2.5 ng/dL, subclinic hypothyroidism) or below 0.6 ng/dL (clinic hypothyroidism) as previously described (Borretti *et al.*, 2006; Castillo *et al.*, 2001; Ferm *et al.*, 2009). A dog was considered to be hyperthyroid when fT4 was above 2.5 ng/dL with TSH less than 0.06 ng/mL or undetectable by the assay (<0.03 ng/mL). Both hormones were evaluated before the thyroid lobule was removed and at 90 days and 360 days post-removal.

Groups performed

Dogs that did not receive any treatment, because of the owner's decision, were placed in a control group (group A [GA]). The rest of the dogs were randomly placed into two groups. Dogs placed in group B (GB) were treated with doxorubicin (dose 30 mg/m² every three weeks, six complete cycles) and dogs placed in group C were treated with RA9-cis (dose 2 mg/kg/day as enteric capsules according to the body weight of the dog for six months, as previously described (Castillo *et al.*, 2006).

The GA (n=10) included six females and four males with a median age of 7.5 (range 5-10) years; five dogs were mixed breeds and the remaining breeds consisted of: one Golden Retriever: one Labrador: one Rottweiler: one Beagle; and one Doberman. Tumours were freely movable in four dogs (S-II, T2a, No, Mo) and fixed in the six other dogs (S-II, T2b, No, Mo).

The GB (n=12) included six females and six males with a median (range) age of 8.5 (4-11) years; five dogs were mixed breeds and the remaining breeds consisted of: two Beagles; one Dachshund; one Poodle; one Pekinese; one Boxer; and one Labrador. In five dogs tumours were freely movable (S-II, T2a, No, Mo) and tumours were fixed in seven dogs (S-II, T2b, No, Mo).

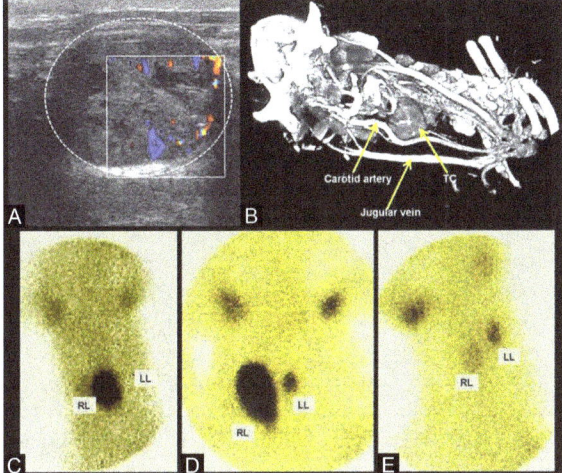

Fig. 1. Upper panel: Images of doppler ultrassonography (A), multiple slices computed tomography (B) and scintigraphy in gamma camera (C-E). Doppler ultrassonography (A) show a vascular invasion in the tumours (dotted circle show the thyroid tumour and the solid square the doppler signal). Multiple slices computed tomography (B) with extraction of the neck showing (arrow) the thyroid tumour (TC) and its relationship to the Carotid artery and Jugular vein. Bottom panel: Example of scintigraphy in dogs with follicular carcinoma and hyperthyroid (C) where the Right lobe (RL) has hot uptake and the left lobe (LL) has cold uptake; a follicular-compact carcinoma in an euthyroid dog (D) with normal uptake in both thyroid lobes, if well the size of the RL is bigger than the LL; compact carcinoma in a hypothyroid dog (E) where RL is cold (very low uptake); Add the tumour type and thyroid condition.

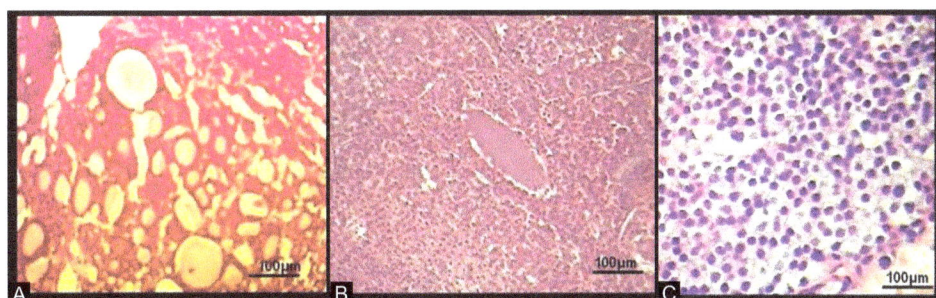

Fig. 2. Histology analysis of 3 different dFTC: A) follicular (dog was hyperthyroid); B) follicular-compact (dog was euthyroid); and C) compact (dog was hypothyroid). Bar=100 μm. Staining haematoxylin and eosin.

The GC (n= 15) included nine females and six males with a median age of 8 (6-12) years; ten dogs were mixed breeds and the remaining dog breeds consisted of: two Boxers; one Dalmatian; one Doberman; and one Labrador. Seven tumours were freely movable (S-II, T2a, No, Mo), and the remaining eight were fixed tumours (S-II, T2b, No, Mo).

The follow-up of the cases was 540 days (1.5 years) after surgery. The first 180 days the patients received the corresponding treatment. The remaining 360 days of the follow-up no treatment was given.

All hypothyroid dogs were treated with levothyroxine (10 to 20 µg/kg twice a day), which continued after surgery.

Statistical analysis

The evaluation of recurrence and survival were analysed by the Long-Rank (Mantel-Cox) test, in which each step represents the recurrence or death of the individual cases. A p-value <0.05 was considered significant for all analyses. To calculate the risk of recurrence and the time of survival (expressed as relative risk (RR) and hazard ratio (HR), a contingent table was made to analyse differences among groups by Fisher test with a P<0.05. The statistical software used was STATA 14 (StataCorp 4905 Lakeway Dr. College Station, TX 77845, USA). To analyse the effect of the type of tumour, the genmod procedure with the Poisson distribution was used (Statistical Analysis System version 9.0, SAS Institute, NC, USA) and the model included the effect of treatment, type of tumour (follicular, follicular-solid and solid carcinomas) and their interaction. Values are expressed as mean ± SEM with significance at P<0.05.

Results

Thyroid status

Before thyroid lobectomy, 32.4% (12/37) of dogs were hypothyroid. Five of these dogs had follicular-compact tumours and the remaining seven dogs had compact carcinomas. We detected hyperthyroidism in 10.8% (4/37) of dogs with follicular carcinoma well differentiated. The remaining 56.8% (21/37) of cases were euthyroid. Eight of these dogs had histological type follicular tumours, 12 had follicular-compact tumours and one had a compact carcinoma (Table 1).

Thyroid status by group was: GA 3/10 (30%) hypothyroid; 2/10 (20%) hyperthyroid; 5/10 (50%) euthyroid; GB 4/12 (33.3%) hypothyroid; 1/12 (8.3%) hyperthyroid; 7/12 (58.3%) euthyroid, and GC 5/15 (33.3%) hypothyroid; 1/15 (6.7%) hyperthyroid; 9/15 (60%) euthyroid (Fig. 3). After we removed the carcinomatous thyroid lobe from dogs with hyperthyroidism, both TSH and fT4 returned to their references range for the remainder of the study. We did not detect a change in TSH and fT4 was show in euthyroid dogs at 90 and 180 days (data no show).

Table 1. Thyroid status with respect to differentiate thyroid follicular carcinoma found in 37 dogs studied.

Thyroid status	Type of differentiate thyroid folliculwar carcinoma			Total
	Follicular	Follicular-compact	Compact	
Hypothyroid (32.4%)	---------	5	7	12
Hyperthyroid (10.8%)	4	--------	--------	4
Euthyroid (56.8%)	8	12	1	21

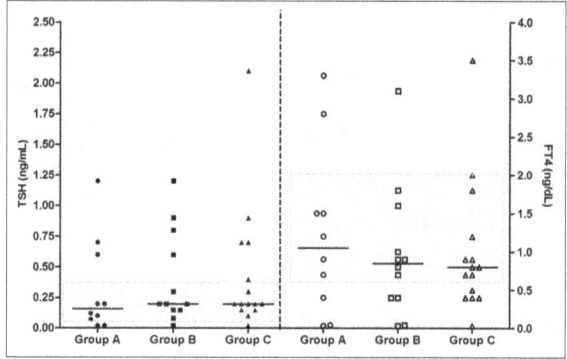

Fig. 3. Concentrations of TSH and fT4 in the control (Group A), doxorubicin (Group B), isotretinoin 9-cis (Group C) groups with follicular carcinomas. Grey areas correspond to the normal interval for the laboratory. Each dot represent one case. Horizontal lines represent the mean values.

Regardless of tumour type, thyroid carcinoma in dogs with hypothyroidism had low 99mTc uptake (cold). Conversely, follicular tumours in dogs with hyperthyroidism 99mTc uptake was enhanced (hot). In the euthyroid dogs with follicular-compact or compact tumours, the uptake of 99mTc were similar in both lobes (Fig. 1).

There were not differences between freely movable or fixed tumour with respect to the 99mTc uptake or thyroid status.

Recurrence and survival time

The time of the recurrence was significantly shorter in GA and GB compared to GC (P=0.0007 and P=0.0015 respectively; Fig. 4). The median time for tumour recurrence for 50% of GA and GB groups was 195 days (95% CI: 180-390) and 225 days (95% CI: 210-420), respectively. In contrast only 13.3% of GC presented recurrence after 360 days. At the end of the experiment, recurrence was detected in 80%, 83.3% and 40% of the GA, GB, and GC, respectively. The HRs of tumour recurrence were 7.25 (95% CI: 2.2-24.4) times shorter in GA compared to GC and 5.6 (95% CI: 1.8-17.4) times shorter in GB compared to GC. We did not detected any difference in the HR between GA and GB (HR 1.37; 95% CI: 0.5-3.7). The RR of recurrence was 2.0 times (95% CI: 1.2-4.3, P=0.017) higher in GA when compared to the GC and 2.1 times (95% CI: 1.07-4.07, P<0.05) higher in GA compared to GC. We did not detect any differences between GA and GB (RR 1.08; 95% CI: 0.78-1.5).

We also detected an increased survival time for GC compared to GA and GB (Fig. 5), but no difference between GA and GB. Median survival time was 220 days (95% CI: 180-450) for GA and 390 days (95% CI: 240-540) for GB. Because of the increased survival in GC, we were unable to obtain an accurate mean survival time for this group. At the end of the experiment, 20% of the dogs in GA, 33.3% of the dogs in GB, and 80% of the dogs in GC survived. The HR was 7.8 (95% CI: 2.0-29.7) between GA and

GB, 5.5 (95% CI: 1.5-19.6) between GB and GC, and 1.6 (95% CI: 0.5-4.4) between GA and GB.

Interaction: type of carcinoma, treatment, recurrence and survival time

The type of carcinoma affected time of recurrence. Follicular carcinomas had a greater length of time to recurrence than follicular-compact (503±15 vs. 289±13 days, P<0.0001). Follicular compact tumours had a greater length of time to recurrence than compact carcinomas (215±21 days, P<0.0001). Treatment affected recurrence time as GC had greater time of recurrence than the GB and GA (462±15 vs. 277±17 and 268±18 days, P<0.0001), while the recurrence time of the latter two groups did not differ. The interaction between treatment and type of carcinoma was significant (P<0.001). We did not detect differences between treatments in follicular carcinomas, but GC had a greater time of recurrence than GB and GA in both follicular-compact and compact carcinomas (Fig. 6A and B). In GC the time to recurrence in follicular compact carcinomas was similar to follicular carcinomas, but time to recurrence in compact carcinomas was lower to the other two types (P<0.05).Freely movable (T2a) or fixed tumours (T2b) did not show significant differences with respect to the recurrences or survival time.

Discussion

This trail shows a novel post-surgery treatment for thyroid carcinoma in dogs. We showed that dogs treated withRA9-cis had increased survival and lower risk of

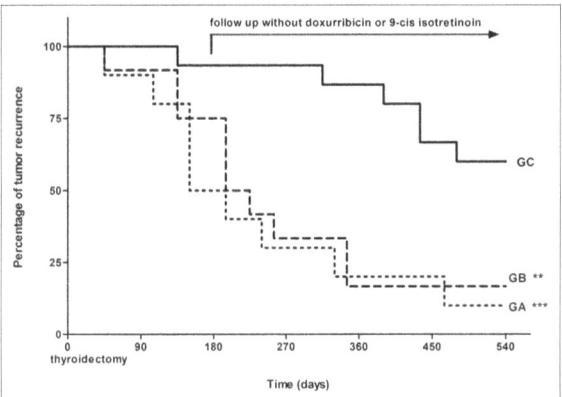

Fig. 4. Kaplan-Meier recurrence curves of thyroid tumour after surgery according to control (GA), doxorubicin (GB) and isotretinoin 9-cis (GC). Median recurrence time after surgery: GA: 195 days; GB: 225 days; GC: 360 days. ***P=0.0007 vs GC; **P=0.002 vs GC (Long-rank test).

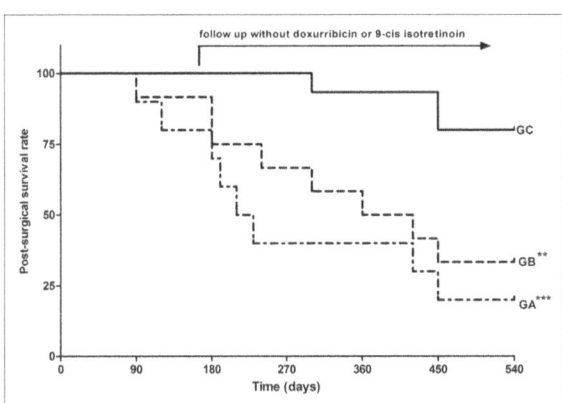

Fig. 5. Kaplan-Meier survival curves of dogs with thyroid tumour after surgery according to control (GA), doxorubicin (GB) and isotretinoin 9-cis (GC). Median survival time after surgery: GA: 220 days; GB: 390 days. In GC only 3/15 dogs had died at the end of the study (540 days). ***P=0.0004 vs GC; **P=0.006 vs GC (Long-rank test).

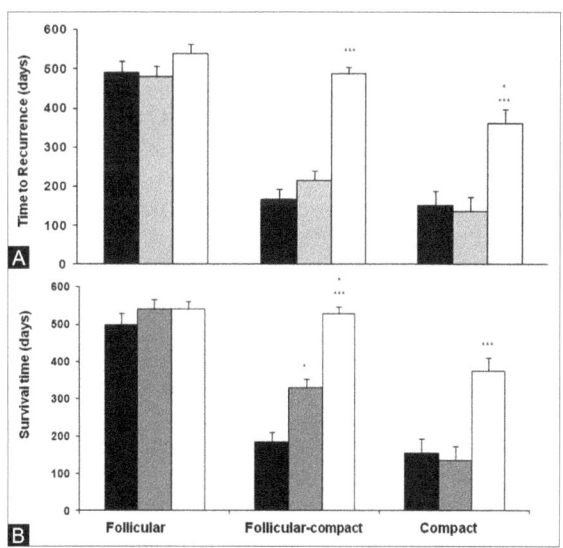

Fig. 6. Time of recurrence (A) and survival time (B) of dogs with thyroid tumour after surgery, and to the type of cancer (follicular, follicular-compact and compact). Recurrence (A): ***P<0.001 vs GA and GB in the same group; *P<0.05 Compact vs Follicular-compact of the GC and ***P<0.001 Compact vs Follicular of the GC. Survival (B): Follicular-compact: ***P<0.001 GC vs GA; *P=0.026 GC vs GB; *P<0.05 GB vs GA; Compact: ***P<0.001 GC vs GA and GB. Black bar: GA; Grey bar: GB; White bar: GC.

tumour recurrence compared to dogs that received the traditional treatment (doxorubicin) or no treatment. We also showed that the treatment effect on recurrence and survival time depended on the clinical and histological type of carcinoma.This result is supported by several previous studies (Campos *et al*., 2014, Capp *et al*., 2010; Coelho *et al*., 2011). Follicular-compact and compact carcinomas were detected more frequently than follicular carcinomas in our study, which is in agreement with previous research (Owen, 1980; Leav *et al*., 1976; Théon *et al*., 2000). Euthyroidism status was the main feature related with the follicular-compact carcinoma, whereas hypothyroidism is associated with the compact subtype and hyperthyroidism with follicular carcinoma.

As expected, all hypothyroid patients had a low uptake of ^{99m}Tc, whereas in hyperthyroid patients that uptake was higher. There are few reports regarding the relation among thyroid carcinoma functionality and/or TC histopathology. Regarding the functional characteristics, Verschueren *et al*. (1991) reported that the greater the undifferentiated thyroid carcinoma profile, the less binding sites for TSH and ^{99m}Tc uptake were found. Similarly, a greater expression of thyroglobulin and TSH-R was found in follicular cells within the carcinoma tissue where the remaining thyroid follicle architecture was found. This suggests that the functionality is associated to the degree of differentiation of the tumour (Pessina *et al*., 2014). In this study we showed that time to recurrence and survival time is affected by the histopathological subtype of the thyroid tumour (follicular, follicular-compact and compact carcinomas).

Worth *et al*. (2005) and Théon *et al*. (2000) reported that without surgery, removal, and subsequent medical treatment of TC the median survival time is three months. Although the use of chemotherapy in dogs is controversial, it improves the prognosis in non-surgical thyroid carcinoma or metastasis (Jeglum and Whereat, 1983; Ogilvie *et al*., 1989), but in dogs with TC treated with surgery and chemotherapy, the median survival time was not different from dogs treated with surgery alone (Nadeau and Kitchell, 2011). Since we did not detect a difference between GA and GB, the results from our study support these previous results.

Retinoic acid regulates tumour suppressor genes; therefore, it can inhibit tumour growth (Connolly *et al*., 2013). Retonic acid has been used successfully for the treatment of hematological cancers (acute promyelocytic leukemia), as well as a therapy and chemoprevention of solid cancers (Hansen *et al*., 2000; Lengfelder *et al*., 2005). Although there are few studies, the results of RA9-cis treatment on TC in humans are promising (Short *et al*., 2004; Simon *et al*., 2002; Trojanowicz *et al*., 2010). In tumour cells culture lines and human TC, retinoic acid acts as anti-proliferative

and redifferentiation agent of this disease (Coelho *et al*., 2005; Coelho *et al*., 2011; Oh *et al*., 2011; Trojanowicz *et al*., 2009). Although there has been investigated *in vitro* models for different tumours in dogs (de Mello Souza *et al*., 2010; Miyajima *et al*., 2006; Ohashi *et al*., 2006), there is only one report of using RA9-cis to treat Cushing's disease in dogs (Castillo *et al*., 2006). Our results clearly show that tumour recurrence is lower and survival time is longer in dogs treated with RA9-cis after surgery compared with dogs that were treated with doxorubicin. Retinoic acid was shown to be less effective in dogs with compact carcinoma. These dogs had faster tumour recurrence and shorter survival time than those with other subtypes of dFTC. The reason for this difference is attributable to compact tumours being less differentiated than the other tumour types. Therefore, they have a more aggressive behavior and are more prone recurrence (Campos *et al*., 2014). However, in dogs with the same tumour type, RA9-cis improved the time to recurrence than in those that were treated with doxorubicin and those that did not receive treatment post-surgery. Although this data is preliminary due to the low number of cases, the results of treatment with RA9-cis are promising in TC patients, mainly in those with follicular or follicular-carcinoma. Moreover, it should be noted that we did not detect any adverse effects (hepatotoxicity) related to RA9-cis treatment. This was also observed in one previous study (Ortemberg *et al*., 2007), and suggests that the drug is not only effective but also safe.

The most interesting finding of this study was the post-surgical survival rate of dogs treated with RA9-cis and the interaction with the type of cancer. While in doxorubicin and control dogs, time to recurrence and survival time were shorter in follicular-compact carcinomas than in follicular carcinomas. In RA9-cis treated dogs we did not detect any differences between these two types of carcinomas. A similar profile was found in the comparison of follicular-compact and compact carcinomas; although, compact carcinomas presented a lower time of recurrence and survival time in RA9-cis treated dogs. The therapy response with RA9-cis in both follicular-compact and compact carcinomas (e.g. more undifferentiated cells when compared with follicular carcinomas) are consistent with the function of the retinoic receptors. Therapy with RA for thyroid cancer requires intact receptor pathways in the thyroid tumour tissues and the expression of certain isoforms mainly RARβ and RXRγ (Haguen *et al*., 2004; Simon *et al*., 2002). We have recently shown (Pessina: personal communication), that follicular cells of both follicular-compact and compact carcinomas expressed RARα and RXR in similar magnitude as healthy thyroid glands.

In conclusion, this study shows that the use of surgery in combination with RA9-cis treatment significantly increase survival rate and time to tumour recurrence when compared to doxorubicin treated or untreated dogs. Moreover, it also demonstrates that treatment effect on recurrence and survival time depended on the histological type of the thyroid cancer.

Acknowledgments

We are grateful to Drs. Ana Meikle, Cecilia Ricart, and Nélida Gómez for the helpful support and critical reading of the manuscript. This work was supported by a grant from University of Buenos Aires-UBACyT, Argentina and University of the Republic, Laboratory of Nuclear Techniques, Uruguay.

Conflict of interest

The Author(s) declare(s) that there is no conflict of interest

---

References

Barber, L.G. Thyroid tumors in dogs and cats. 2007. Vet. Clin. North Am. Small Anim. Pract. 37, 756-773.

Boretti, F.S. and Reusch, C.E. 2006. Diagnostic specificity of canine thyrotropin in the diagnosis of Hypothyroidism in dogs. EJCAP. 16, 185-189.

Campos, M., Ducatelle, R., Rutteman, G., Kooistra, H.S., Duchateau, L., de Rooster, H., Peremans, K. and Daminet, S. 2014. Clinical, pathologic, and immunohistochemical prognostic factors in dogs with thyroid carcinoma. J. Vet. Intern. Med. 28, 1805-1813.

Carver, J.R., Kapatkin, A. and Patnaik, A.K. 1995. A comparison of medullary thyroid carcinoma and thyroid adenocarcinoma in dogs: a retrospective study of 38 cases. Vet. Surg. 24, 315-319.

Castillo, V., Giacomini, D., Páez-Pereda, M., Stalla, J., Labeur, M., Theodoropoulou, M., Holsboer, F., Grossman, A., Stalla, G. and Arzt, E. 2006. Retinoic Acid as a Novel Medical Therapy for Cushing's Disease in Dogs. Endocrinology 147, 4438-4444.

Castillo, V., Rodriguez, M.S., Lalia, J. 2001. Estimulación con TRH y evaluación de la respuesta de la TSH en perros. Su importancia en el diagnóstico de enfermedad tiroidea subclínica (hipotiroidismo subclínico y tiroiditis autoinmune eutiroidea). Rev. Cient-Fac. Cien. V. 11, 23-27.

Coelho, S.M., Vaisman, M. and Carvalho, D.P. 2005. Tumour re-differentiation effect of retinoic acid: a novel therapeutic approach for advanced thyroid cancer. Curr. Pharm. Des. 11, 2525-2531.

Coelho, S.M., Vaisman, F., Buescu, A., Mello, R.C., Carvalho, D.P. and Vaisman, M. 2011. Follow-up of patients treated with retinoic acid for the control of radioiodine non-responsive advanced thyroid carcinoma. Braz. J. Med. Biol. Res. 44, 73-77.

Connolly, R.M., Nguyen, N.K. and Sukumar, S. 2013. Molecular pathways: current role and future directions of the retinoic acid pathway in cancer prevention and treatment. Clin. Cancer Res. 19, 1651-1659.

De Lellis, R.A. 2004. International Agency for Research on Cancer. World Health Organization, International Academy of Pathology, International Association for the Study of Lung Cancer. Pathology and genetics of tumours of endocrine organs. Lyon: IARC Press, pp: 320.

de Mello Souza, C.H., Valli, V.E., Selting, K.A., Kiupel, M. and Kitchell, B.E. 2010. Immunohistochemical detection of retinoid receptors in tumors from 30 dogs diagnosed with cutaneous lymphoma. J. Vet. Intern. Med. 24, 1112-1127.

Dong, J.J., Zhou, Y., Liu, Y.T., Zhang, Z.W., Zhou, X.J., Wang, H.J. and Liao, L. 2013. In vitro evaluation of the therapeutic potential of nevirapine in treatment of human thyroid anaplastic carcinoma. Mol. Cell Endocrinol. 370, 113-118.

Ferm, K., Björnerfeldt, S., Karlssony, A., Andersson, G., Nachreinerz, R. and Hedhammar, A. 2009. Prevalence of diagnostic characteristics indicating canine autoimmune lymphocytic thyroiditis in giant schnauzer and hovawart dogs. J. Small Anim. Pract. 50, 176-179.

Fineman, L.S., Hamilton, T.A., de Gortari, A. and Bonney, P. 1998. Cisplatin chemotherapy for treatment of thyroid carcinoma in dogs: 13 cases. J. Am. Anim. Hops. Assoc. 34, 109-112.

Hansen, L.A., Sigman, C.C., Andreola, F., Ross, S.A., Kelloffm, G.J. and De Luca, L.M. 2000. Retinoids in chemoprevention and differentiation therapy. Carcinogenesis 21, 1271-1279.

Haugen, B.R., Larson, L.L., Pugazhenthi, U., Hays, W.R., Klopper, J.P., Kramer, C.A. and Sharma, V. 2004. Retinoic acid and retinoid X receptors are differentially expressed in thyroid cancer and thyroid carcinoma cell lines and predict response to treatment with retinoids. J. Clin. Endocrinol. Metab. 89, 272-280.

Jeglum, K.A. and Whereat, A. 1983. Chemotherapy of canine thyroid carcinoma. Comp. Cont. Educ. Pract. 5, 96-98.

Kebebew, E., Peng, M., Treseler, P.A., Clark, O.H., Duh, Q.Y., Ginzinger, D. and Miner, R. 2004. Id1 gene expression is up-regulated in hyperplastic and neoplastic thyroid tissue and regulates growth and differentiation in thyroid cancer cells. J. Clin. Endocrinol. Metab. 89, 6105-6111.

Kiupel, M., Capen, C., Miller, M. and Smedley, R. 2008. Histological classification of the endocrine system of domestic animals. In: Schulman FY, ed. WHO international histological classification of tumors of domestic animals. Washington: Armed Forces Institute of Pathology.

Klein, M.K., Powers, B.E., Withrow, S.J., Curtis, C.R., Straw, R.C., Ogilvie, G.K., Dickinson, K.L., Cooper, M.F. and Baier, M. 1995. Treatment of thyroid carcinoma in dogs by surgical resection alone: 20 cases (1981-1989). J. Am. Vet. Med. Assoc. 206, 1007-1009.

Labeur, M., Paez-Pereda, M., Arzt, E. and Stalla, G.K. 2009. Potential of retinoic acid derivatives for the treatment of corticotroph pituitary adenomas. Rev. Endocr. Metab. Disord. 10, 103-109.

Leav, I., Schiller, A.L., Rijnberk, A., Legg, M.A. and der Kinderen, P.J. 1976. Adenomas and carcinomas of the canine and feline thyroid. Am. J. Pathol. 83, 61-93.

Mayer, M.N. and MacDonald, V.S. 2007. External beam radiation therapy for thyroid cancer in the dog. Can. Vet. J. 48, 761-763.

Meissner, W.A. and Warren, S. 1969. Tumors of the thyroid gland. Atlas of Tumor Pathology,

Second series. Fascicle 4. Washington DC, Armed Forces Institute of Pathology.

Mitchell, M., Hurov, L.I. and Troy, G.C. 1979. Canine thyroid carcinomas: clinical occurrence, staging by means of scintiscans and therapy of 15 cases. Vet. Surg. 8, 112-118.

Miyajima, N., Watanabe, M., Ohashi, E., Mochizuki, M., Nishimura, R., Ogawa, H., Sugano, S. and Sasaki, N. 2006. Relationship between retinoic acid receptor alpha gene expression and growth-inhibitory effect of all-trans retinoic acid on canine tumor cells. J. Vet. Intern. Med. 20, 348-354.

Muscella, A., Urso, L., Calabriso, N., Vetrugno, C., Fanizzi, F.P., Storelli, C. and Marsigliante, S. 2009. Functions of epidermal growth factor receptor in cisplatin response of thyroid cells. Biochem. Pharmacol. 77, 979-992.

Nadeau, M.E. and Kitchell, B.E. 2011. Evaluation of the use of chemotherapy and other prognostic variables for surgically excised canine thyroid carcinoma with and without metastasis. Can. Vet. J. 52, 994-998.

Oh, S.W., Moon, S.H., Park Do, J., Cho, B.Y., Jung, K.C., Lee, D.S. and Chung, J.K. 2011. Combined therapy with ^{131}I and retinoic acid in Korean patients with radioiodine-refractory papillary thyroid cancer. EJNMMI. 38, 1798-1805.

Ohashi, E., Miyajima, N., Nakagawa, T., Takahashi, T., Kagechika, H., Mochizuki, M., Nishimura, R. and Sasaki, N. 2006. Retinoids induce growth inhibition and apoptosis in mast cell tumor cell lines. J. Vet. Med. Sci. 68, 797-802.

Ogilvie, G.K., Reynolds, H.A., Richardson, R.C., Withrow, S.J., Norris, A.M., Henderson, R.A., Klausner, J.S., Fowler, J.D. and McCaw, D. 1989. Phase II evaluation of doxorubicin for the treatment of various canine neoplasms. J. Am. Vet. Med. Assoc. 195, 1580-1583.

Ortemberg, L., Loiza, M., Martiarena, B., Cabrera Blatter, M.F., Ghersevich, M.C. and Castillo, V. 2007. Retinoic acid as a therapy for Cushing's

disease in dogs: evaluation of liver enzymes during treatment. Slov. Vet. Res. 44, 73-81.

Owen, N. 1980. TNM classification of tumours in domestic animals World Health Organization, Geneva, pp: 51-52.

Page, R.L. 2001. Tumors of the endrocrine system. In: Withrow SJ, MacEwen EG (eds). Small Animal Clinical Oncology. 3rd ed. W B Saunders, Philadelphia, USA, pp: 423-433.

Páez-Pereda, M., Kovalovsky, D., Hopfner, U., Theodoropoulou, M., Pagotto, U., Uhl, E., Losa, M., Stalla, J., Grübler, Y., Missale, C., Arzt, E. and Stalla, G.K. 2001. Retinoica cid prevents experimental Cushing síndrome. J. Clin. Invest. 108, 1123-1131.

Patnaik, A.K. and Lieberman, P.H. 1991. Gross, histologic, cytochemical, and immunocytochemical study of medullary thyroid carcinoma in sixteen dogs. Vet. Pathol. 28, 223-233.

Pecori, G., Ambrogio, A.G., Andrioli, M., Saguin, F., Karamouzis, I., Corsello, S.M., Scaroni, C., Arvat, E., Pontecorvi, A. and Cavagnini, F. 2012. Potential role for retinoic acid in patients with cushing's disease. J. Clin. Endocrinol. Metab. 10, 3577-3583.

Pessina, P., Castillo, V., Sartore, I., Borrego, J. and Meikle, A. 2014. Semiquantitative immunohistochemical marker staining and localization in canine thyroid carcinoma and normal thyroid gland. Vet. Comp. Oncol. Aug 1. doi: 10.1111/vco.12111.

Radlinsky, M.G. 2007. Thyroid surgery in dogs and cats. Vet. Clin. North Am. Small Anim. Pract. 37, 789-798.

Short, C.S., Suovuori, A., Cook, G., Viviany, G. and Harmer, C. 2004. A phase II study using retinoids as redifferentiation agents to increase iodine uptake in metastatic thyroid cancer. Clin. Oncol. 16, 569-574.

Simon, D., Körber, C., Krausch, M., Segering, J., Groth, P., Görges, R., Grünwald, F., Müller-Gärtner, H.W., Schmutzler, C., Köhrle, J., Röher, H.D. and Reiners, C. 2002. Clinical impact of retinoids in redifferentiation therapy of advanced thyroid cancer: final results of a pilot study. EJNMI 29, 775-782.

Sipos, J.A. and Mazzaferri, E.L. 2008. Differentiated thyroid carcinoma. In: Cooper DS, ed. Medical Management of Thyroid Disease, Second ed. New York: Informa Healthcare USA, Inc. pp: 237-295.

Tallini, G., Garcia-Rostan, G., Herrero, A., Zelterman, D., Viale, G., Bosari, S. and Carcangiu, M.L. 1999. Downregulation of p27KIP1 and Ki67/Mib1 labeling index support the classification of thyroid carcinoma into prognostically relevant categories. Am. J. Surg. Pathol. 23, 678-685.

Théon, A.P., Marks, S.L., Feldman, E.S. and Griffey, S.

2000. Prognostic factors and patterns of treatment failure in dogs with unresectable differentiated thyroid carcinomas treated with megavoltage irradiation. J. Am. Vet. Med. Assoc. 216, 1775-1779.

Trojanowicz, B., Sekulla, C., Lorenz, K., Köhrle, J., Finke, R., Dralle, H. and Hoang-Vu, C. 2010. Proteomic approach reveals novel targets for retinoic acid-mediated therapy of thyroid carcinoma. Mol. Cell Endocrinol. 325, 110-117.

Tuohy, J.L., Worley, D.R. and Withrow, S.J. 2012. Outcome following simultaneous bilateral thyroid lobectomy for treatment of thyroid gland carcinoma in dogs: 15 cases (1994-2010). J. Am. Vet. Med. Assoc. 24, 95-103.

Turrell, J.M., McEntee, M.C., Burke, B.P. and

Page, R.L. 2006. Sodium iodide I 131 treatment of dogs with nonresectable thyroid tumors: 39 cases (1990-2003). J. Am. Vet. Med. Assoc. 229, 542-548.

Verschueren, C.P., Selman, P.J., Mol, J.A., Vos, J.H., van Dijk, J.E., Sjollema, B.E. and de Vijlder, J.J. 1991. Circulating thyroglobulin measurements by homologous radioimmunoassay in dogs with thyroid carcinoma. Acta Endocrinol. (Copenh). 125, 291-298.

Worth, A.J., Zuber, R.M. and Hocking, M. 2005. Radioiodide (I131) therapy for the treatment of canine thyroid carcinoma. Aust. Vet. J. 83, 208-214.

Wucherer, K.L. and Wilke, V. 2010. Thyroid cancer in dogs: an update based on 638 cases (1995-2005). J. Am. Anim. Hops. Assoc. 46, 249-25.

16

Craniocervical junction abnormalities with atlantoaxial subluxation caused by ventral subluxation of C2 in a dog

Harumichi Itoh[1], Kazuhito Itamoto[1,*], Shotaro Eto[2], Tomoya Haraguchi[1], Shimpei Nishikawa[1], Kenji Tani[2], Yoshiki Itoh[3], Masato Hiyama[2], Toshie Iseri[3], Munekazu Nakaichi[3] and Yasuho Taura[2]

[1]*Department of Small Animal Clinical Science, Joint Faculty of Veterinary Medicine, Yamaguchi University, 1677-1 Yoshida, Yamaguchi City, Yamaguchi, 753-8511, Japan*
[2]*Department of Veterinary Surgery, Joint Faculty of Veterinary Medicine, Yamaguchi University, 1677-1 Yoshida, Yamaguchi City, Yamaguchi, 753-8511, Japan*
[3]*Laboratory of Veterinary Radiology Yamaguchi University, 1677-1 Yoshida, Yamaguchi City, Yamaguchi, 753-8511, Japan*

Abstract
Craniocervical junction abnormalities with atlantoaxial subluxation caused by ventral subluxation of C2 were diagnosed in a 6-month-old female Pomeranian with tetraplegia as a clinical sign. Lateral survey radiography of the neck with flexion revealed atlantoaxial subluxation with ventral subluxation of C2. Computed tomography revealed absence of dens and atlanto-occipital overlapping. Magnetic resonance imaging showed compression of the spinal cord and indentation of caudal cerebellum. The diagnosis was Chiari-like malformation, atlantoaxial subluxation with ventral displacement of C2, atlanto-occipital overlapping, and syringomyelia. The dog underwent foramen magnum decompression, dorsal laminectomy of C1, and ventral fixation of the atlantoaxial joint. Soon after the operation, voluntary movements of the legs were recovered. Finally, the dog could stand and walk without assistance. The dog had complicated malformations at the craniocervical junction but foramen magnum decompression and dorsal laminectomy for Chiari-like malformation, and ventral fixation for atlantoaxial subluxation resulted in an excellent clinical outcome.
Keywords: Atlantoaxial subluxation, Atlanto-occipital overlapping, Chiari-like malformation, Craniocervical junction abnormalities, Foramen magnum decompression.

Introduction

Atlantoaxial subluxation (AAS) is a disorder of C1-C2 causing impairment of stability; the causes of instability are associated with aplasia, hypoplasia, dorsal angulation, or non-union of the dens with the C2, and congenital absence of the transverse ligament (Thomas *et al.*, 1991). Recently, craniocervical junction abnormalities (CJA) were identified as complicated congenital malformations at the region of the caudal occiput and first two cervical vertebrae. Chiari-like malformation (CLM) appears commonly in CJA patients, and other abnormalities are atlanto-occipital overlap (AOO), dorsal constriction at C1/C2, and AAS (Dewey *et al.*, 2013).

Most cases of AAS subluxate C2 dorsally and many surgical approaches for AAS with dorsal subluxation have been reported. It have been suggested ventral stabilization may be safer than dorsal stabilization of the atlas and axis (Aikawa *et al.*, 2013) and the application of ventral pins and polymethylmethacrylate has been used successfully in the surgical treatment of congenital and traumatic AAS with dorsal subluxation of C2 (Schulz *et al.*, 1997). However, there has been no report of AAS with ventral subluxation of C2 and surgical treatment in dogs. The following case report describes AAS with ventral subluxation of C2.

Case Details

A 6-month-old female Pomeranian presented (body weight = 1.0 kg) with tetraplegia for 3 days and was referred to the Animal Medical Centre of Yamaguchi University. The neurological examination showed loss of proprioception and upper motor neuron paresis of fore- and hindlimbs. Lateral radiography of the cervical region revealed ventral subluxation of C2. Ventrodorsal radiography showed a deficit of the dens at C2. Stress radiography of the cervical region with ventral flexion revealed that the distance between the caudal margin of dorsal arch of C1 and the cranial margin of spinal process of C2 was 3.7 mm (Fig. 1) (normal range <4 mm). Sagittal MRI of the cranial cervical spine revealed severe compression of the spinal cord at C1 to C2 level and indentation of the caudal cerebellum (Fig. 2). Sagittal computed tomography (CT) revealed an occipital bony defect, and the cranial-most aspect of the dorsal arch of C1 was inserted into the intracranial region from the foramen magnum (Fig. 3).

*****Corresponding Author:** Kazuhito Itamoto. Yamaguchi University, Animal Medical Center 1677-1, Yoshida, Yamaguchi-shi, Japan. Email: *kaz2356@yamaguchi-u.ac.jp*

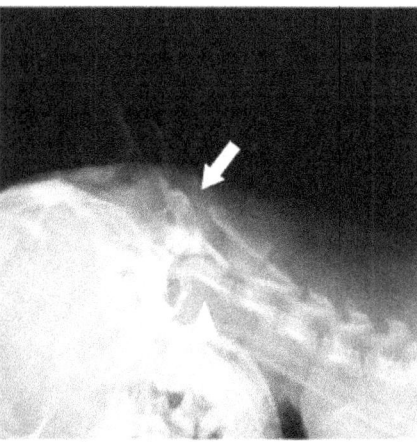

Fig. 1. Stress radiography of the cervical region with ventral flexion. The space between the dorsal lamina of the C1 and the dorsal spinous process of the C2 was 3.7mm (arrow). Ventral subluxation of C2 (arrowhead).

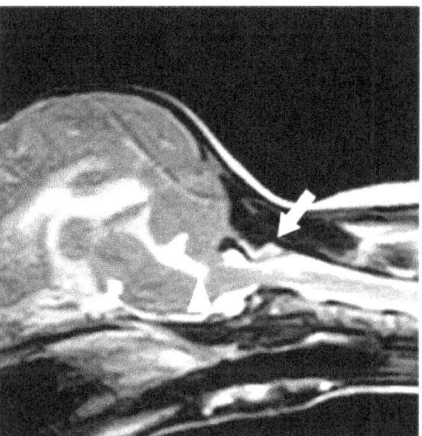

Fig. 2. Sagittal MRI image (T2-weighted) of the cranial cervical spine. Severe compression of spinal cord at C1 to C2 level (arrow) and indentation of caudal cerebellum (arrowhead).

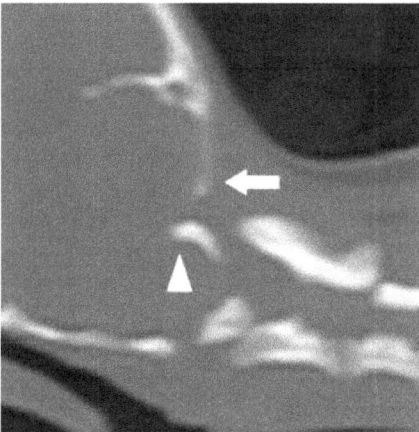

Fig. 3. Sagittal CT image of the cervical region. Occipital bony defect (arrow). Cranial-most aspect of dorsal arch of the C1 was inserted to intracranial region from foramen magnum (arrowhead).

According to these examinations, the patient was diagnosed as AAS complicated by AOO, CLM, and syringomyelia. The operative approach was divided into two phases. First, in order to treat AOO, CLM and syringomyelia, foramen magnum decompression (FMD) and dorsal laminectomy of C1 were planned to decompress the cerebellum and spinal cord. Then, in order to stabilize the atlantoaxial joint, ventral fixation of the joint was planned for the second phase. The first phase of surgery (FMD and dorsal laminectomy of C1) was performed on the 7th day after the first consultation. Anaesthesia was induced with propofol IV (7 mg kg^{-1} propofol; Intervet, Tokyo, Japan). An endotracheal tube was inserted and isoflurane (Isoflu; DS Pharma Animal Health Co, Osaka, Japan) anaesthesia was maintained at 1-2% using a low-flow, semi-closed circuit. Analgesia was performed by preoperative intara muscular administration of ketamine hydrochloride (5 mg kg^{-5} Ketalar; Daiichi Sankyo, Tokyo, Japan) and bolus administration of fentanyl (Fentanyl; Daiichi Sankyo, Tokyo, Japan). In addition, continuous rate infusion of fentanyl citrate (5 to 30 μg/kg/min) was used for intra-operative analgesia.

The patient was positioned in sternal recumbency with the neck ventroflexed. A dorsal midline incision was made extending from external occipital protuberance cranially to the second cervical vertebra caudally. The superficial dorsal cervical musculature was separated at the median raphe, exposing the underlying paired biventer cervicis muscles. The paired muscles were separated at the midline, exposing the rectus capitis dorsalis muscles. The caudal aspects of the rectus capitis dorsalis muscles were removed from the cranial half of the second cervical vertebra and the muscle bellies were split at the midline. The cranial aspects of the rectus capitis dorsalis muscles were then sharply incised from the nuchal crest, exposing the caudal portion of the occiput and the arch of the atlas.

The occiput and the dorsal aspect of the C1 vertebra were removed using a high-speed air drill with round drill. The dorsal atlanto-occipital membrane was incised and expansile duroplasty was performed by using artificial dura mater (Gore-Tex; Japan Gore, Tokyo, Japan) (Fig. 4). Closure was routine. Postoperative analgesia was performed appropriately by intramusucular administration of morphine hydrochloride (0.5 mg kg^{-1} Morphine; Takeda, Osaka, Japan). Ventral fixation of the atlantoaxial joint was performed to stabilize it on the 14th day after the first consultation. Anaesthesia and analgesia were performed as in the previous surgery. The dog was placed in dorsal recumbency with the neck hyperextended. A ventral midline skin incision was made over the cranial half of the neck.

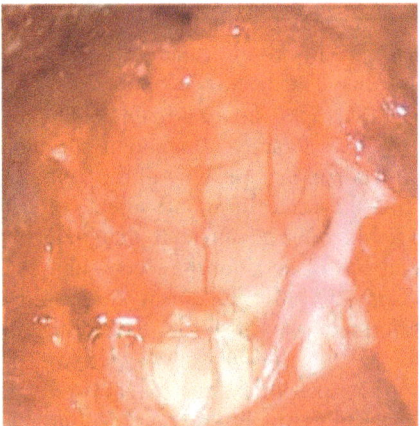

Fig. 4. The dorsal atlanto-occipital membrane were incised and expansile duroplasty by using artificial dura mater.

The sternohyoideus muscles were divided in the midline and the trachea and oesophagus were retracted toward the dog's left side. The larynx was also retracted toward the left, once the attachments of the right sternohyoideus muscle were severed close to the larynx. The thyroid gland, recurrent laryngeal nerve, right vagus, and carotid were identified and protected throughout the surgery. The longus colli muscle was elevated from the ventral surface of the axis and atlas and retracted.

Two threaded-pins (0.9 × 75 mm; IMEX, Tokyo, Japan) were placed across each of the ventral articular facets between the axis and atlas. Then, removal of cartilage of the atlantoaxial joint and autografting of cancellous bone collected from the humerus were performed to create bone union at the atlantoaxial joint. Finally, implanted pins were fixed by using bone cement (Osteobond; Zimmer, Tokyo, Japan) (Fig. 5).

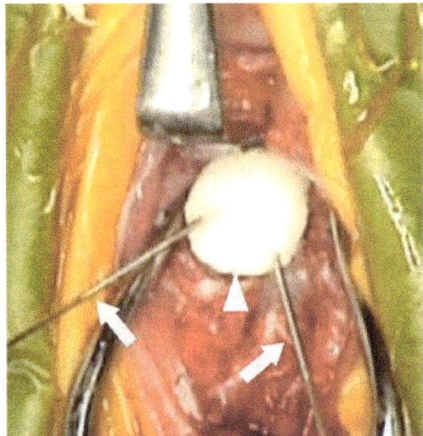

Fig. 5. Two threaded-pins are placed across each of the ventral articular facets between the axis and atlas (arrows). Implanted pins are fixed by using bone cement (arrowhead).

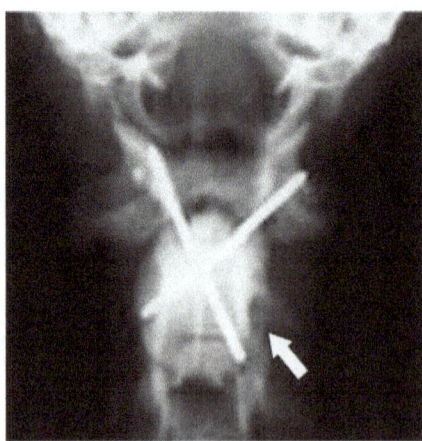

Fig. 6. 134 days after the first consultation, ventro-dorsal radiograph of the cervical region revealed no loosening of thread pins and bone cement (arrow).

The dog stood and walked by herself and left the medical centre. Ventro-dorsal radiograph of the cervical region in 134 days after the first consultation revealed no loosening of thread pins and bone cement (Fig. 6).

Discussion

In AAS, dorsal subluxation of the C2 into the vertebral canal causes direct compressive and concussive effects on the cervical spinal cord. Usually, the subluxation of C2 would occur dorsally in accordance with the direction of cervical flexion when stability is lost. However, in this case, C2 subluxated ventrally. We found no previous report about AAS with ventral subluxation of C2 in dogs.

In human cases, a form of AAS similar to this case is known as rotatory subluxation type IV (rotatory subluxation with posterior displacement of the atlas). Rotatory subluxation type IV is rare, but secondary rotatory subluxation type IV has been reported in patients with rheumatoid arthritis (Kauppi, 1994). If the erosions of the dens increase progressively in rheumatoid arthritis patients, the dens may shorten, disappear, or fracture. If the dens does not limit the posterior movement of the atlas during extension, the anterior atlas arch may glide over the whole anterior part of the axis. However, not of all AAS patients with rheumatoid arthritis and erosion of the dens shows rotatory subluxation type IV and details of mechanism about rotatory subluxation type IV have not been investigated even now.

On the other hand, we found no previous report of AAS with ventral subluxation of C2 even in dogs with rheumatoid arthritis. Anatomically, atlantoaxial joint ligaments in dogs constructed by four major ligaments. Apical, left and right alar, transverse and dorsal atlantoaxial ligaments are known commonly. A previous report concluded alar ligaments are the most important in prevending dorsal angulation (Reber *et al.*, 2013).

According to these issues, it is suggested that absence of dens allows dorsal angulation of axis by lose their functional ability of alar ligaments. In fact, some AAS patients with dorsal subluxation of C2 with deficit of the dens have been reported (Patton *et al.*, 2010; Stigen *et al.*, 2013). Therefore, the patient who has AAS with absence of dens shows higher opportunity to dorsal subluxation of C2 than normal AAS patients. Compared to these previous reports, the patient in this case report shows ventral subluxation. The exact details why this case report showed ventral subluxation are unclear. However, further investigation about this issues and follow-up to the case is necessary.

In this case, AOO was also observed. AOO can be seen in toy and small breed dogs (Cerda-Gonzalez and Dewey, 2010). A previous report described 4 cases of AOO. In this report, 3 cases had AAS (Cerda-Gonzalez *et al.*, 2009). A case report of surgical stabilization for AOO was reported. The case was performed with combined FMD with cranioplasty and stabilization of the atlanto-occipital junction (Dewey *et al.*, 2009). We also performed FMD and dorsal laminectomy of C1.

The treatment of AAS has long been performed and many treatment methods have been reported. Surgical treatment with dorsal and ventral technique has been reported. These include the dorsal Kishigami AATB technique (Pujol *et al.*, 2010), dorsal cross-pinning (Jeffery, 1996), and others. Ventral surgical treatment using transarticular lag screws/pins (Riedinger *et al.*, 2015) and screws, and polymethylmethacrylate (Platt *et al.*, 2004; Schulz *et al.*, 1997), have better clinical outcomes than dorsal surgical treatments (Aikawa *et al.*, 2013). In this case, we chose ventral fixation to treat AAS. Usually, dorsal fixation of the atlantoaxial joint needs traction on C1 in a dorsal direction when there is dorsal subluxation of C2. However, in this case, AAS was difficult to correct because of the opposite direction of subluxation. In addition, we planned FMD and dorsal laminectomy at the first operation.

In this case, AAS was concomitant with AOO, CLM, and syringomyelia. The deficit of dens, foramen magnum hypoplasia, and indentation of the caudal cerebellum were also observed. The occipital region of the skull and the first two cervical vertebrae develop together embryologically (Dewey *et al.*, 2013). Therefore, atlantoaxial instability sometimes has other concurrent abnormalities. For example, occipital dysplasia and AOO lead to CLM. Malformations of the dens and absence of the transverse ligament also lead to atlantoaxial joint instability. These malformations occur together. Recently, these complicated malformations were named "Craniocervical Junction Abnormalities" (Cerda-Gonzalez and Dewey, 2010).

Our case also had combined AAS, CLM, and AOO. Therefore, it was categorized as a CJA.

In conclusion, this was the first reported case of AAS with ventral subluxation and complicated malformations of CJA. The combination of FMD and ventral fixation of the atlanto-axial joint resulted in an excellent clinical outcome.

References

Aikawa, T., Shibata, M. and Fujita, H. 2013. Modified ventral stabilization using positively threaded profile pins and polymethylmethacrylate for atlantoaxial instability in 49 dogs. Vet. Surg. 42, 683-692.

Cerda-Gonzalez, S. and Dewey, C.W. 2010. Congenital diseases of the craniocervical junction in the dog. Vet. Clin. North Am. Small Anim.Pract. 40, 121-141.

Cerda-Gonzalez, S., Dewey, C.W., Scrivani, P.V. and Kline, K.L. 2009. Imaging features of atlanto-occipital overlapping in dogs. Vet. Radiol. Ultrasound 50, 264-268.

Dewey, C.W., Cerda-Gonzalez, S. and Scrivani, P.V. 2009. Case report --surgical stabilization of a craniocervical junction abnormality with atlanto-occipital overlapping in a dog. Compend. Contin. Educ. Vet. 31, E1-6.

Dewey, C.W., Marino, D.J. and Loughin, C.A. 2013. Craniocervical junction abnormalities in dogs. N. Z. Vet. J. 61, 202-211.

Jeffery, N.D. 1996. Dorsal cross pinning of the atlantoaxial joint: new surgical technique for atlantoaxial subluxation. J. Small. Anim. Pract. 37, 26-29.

Kauppi, M. 1994. A method for classification of the posterior atlanto-axial subluxation. Clin. Rheumatol. 13, 492-495.

Patton, K.M., Almes, K.M. and de Lahunta, A. 2010. Absence of the dens in a 9.5-year-old rottweiler with non-progressive clinical signs. Can. Vet. J. 51, 1007-1010.

Platt, S.R., Chambers, J.N. and Cross, A. 2004. A modified ventral fixation for surgical management of atlantoaxial subluxation in 19 dogs. Vet. Surg. 33, 349-354.

Pujol, E., Bouvy, B., Omana, M., Fortuny, M., Riera, L. and Pujol, P. 2010. Use of the Kishigami Atlantoaxial Tension Band in eight toy breed dogs with atlantoaxial subluxation. Vet. Surg. 39, 35-42.

Reber, K., Burki, A., Vizcaino Reves, N., Stoffel, M., Gendron, K., Ferguson, S.J. and Forterre, F. 2013. Biomechanical evaluation of the stabilizing function of the atlantoaxial ligaments under shear loading: a canine cadaveric study. Vet. Surg. 42, 918-923.

Riedinger, B., Burki, A., Stahl, C., Howard, J. and Forterre, F. 2015. Biomechanical Evaluation of the Stabilizing Function of Three Atlantoaxial Implants Under Shear Loading: A Canine Cadaveric Study. Vet. Surg. 44, 957-963.

Schulz, K.S., Waldron, D.R. and Fahie, M. 1997. Application of ventral pins and polymethylmethacrylate for the management of atlantoaxial instability: results in nine dogs. Vet. Surg. 26, 317-325.

Stigen, O., Aleksandersen, M., Sorby, R. and Jorgensen, H.J. 2013. Acute non-ambulatory tetraparesis with absence of the dens in two large breed dogs: case reports with a radiographic study of relatives. Acta. Vet. Scand. 55, 31.

Thomas, W.B., Sorjonen, D.C. and Simpson, S.T. 1991. Surgical management of atlantoaxial subluxation in 23 dogs. Vet. Surg. 20, 409-412.

17

Effects of topical flurbiprofen sodium, diclofenac sodium, ketorolac tromethamine and benzalkonium chloride on corneal sensitivity in normal dogs

Raquel de Araújo Cantarella[1], Juliana Kravetz de Oliveira[1], Daniel M. Dorbandt[2,3] and Fabiano Montiani-Ferreira[1,*]

[1]*Universidade Federal do Paraná (UFPR), Departamento de Medicina Veterinária, Rua dos Funcionários, 1540, Bairro Juvevê, 80035-050, Curitiba – PR, Brazil*
[2]*Department of Veterinary Clinical Medicine, College of Veterinary Medicine, University of Illinois at Urbana-Champaign, 1008, West Hazelwood Drive, Urbana, Illinois 61802, USA*
[3]*Central Hospital for Veterinary Medicine, North Haven, Connecticut 06473, USA*

Abstract

To evaluate corneal sensitivity by using the Cochet-Bonnet® esthesiometer in normal canine eyes at different time points following instillation of three different topical non-steroidal anti-inflammatory drugs (flurbiprofen sodium 0.03%, diclofenac sodium 0.1% and ketorolac tromethamine 0.5%) and benzalkonium chloride 0.01%. Six healthy mixed breed dogs from the same litter were used in two different stages. First, one drop of flurbiprofen sodium 0.03% and diclofenac sodium 0.1% in each eye; second, one drop of ketorolac tromethamine 0.5% and benzalkonium chloride 0.01% in each eye. Baseline esthesiometry was obtained before eye drop application and every 15 minutes thereafter until a total of 105 minutes of evaluation time. A one-week interval was allowed between the two treatment phases. Statistical analysis was used to compare means according to time of evaluation and drug used. Diclofenac sodium 0.1% decreased corneal sensitivity at 75 and 90 minutes (P > 0.015) with possible interference on neuronal nociceptive activity and analgesic effect while ketorolac tromethamine 0.5% did not show any variation for esthesiometry means along the evaluation. Flurbiprofen sodium 0.03% resulted in increased esthesiometry values 30 minutes after instillation (P > 0.013), increasing corneal sensitivity and possibly producing a greater irritant corneal effect over its analgesic properties. Benzalkonium chloride 0.01% significantly increased corneal sensitivity at 15 minutes of evaluation (P > 0.001), most likely resulting from its irritating effect. Esthesiometry did not allow a definite conclusion over the analgesic effect of the NSAIDs tested; however it was effective in detecting fluctuations in corneal sensitivity.
Keywords: Cochet-Bonnet, Cornea, Nociceptors, NSAID.

Introduction

Corneal and bulbar conjunctival innervation is supplied by a relatively small number of primary sensorial nerves originating from the ipsilateral trigeminal ganglion (about 1.5% of the neurons from ganglion's total number) (De Felipe et al., 1999). However, the small dimension of the corneal surface with the vast branching of peripheral nerve axons results in the cornea being the most densely innerved structure of the body (De Felipe et al., 1999). Additionally, 70% of these sensorial fibers are classified as polymodal nociceptors (Belmonte et al., 2004).

Non-steroidal anti-inflammatory drugs (NSAIDS) are a group comprised of several drugs that are able control inflammation, promote analgesia and reduce hyperthermia by inhibiting cyclooxygenases activity, thereby reducing eicosanoid synthesis created through the arachinodic acid cascade (Bloom, 1996; Insel, 1996; Aragona et al., 2000). Prostaglandins are one of the primary eicosanoids released upon insult to the canine eye (Maggs, 2008). After biosynthesis, prostaglandins bind to receptors called pain facilitators (Tranquilli and Thurman, 1999; Marfurt et al. 2001), which promote variations in the resting potential of neuronal membranes. These variations in membrane resting potentials result in pain amplification (Bloom, 1996; Tasaka, 1999; Acosta et al., 2005; Tranquilli and Thurman, 1999).

NSAIDS are commonly used in ophthalmology to control pain caused by tissue injury and reduce localized inflammation and after surgical procedures (Chen et al., 1997; Aragona et al., 2000; Weaver and Terrell, 2003; Giuliano, 2004; Acosta et al., 2007; Kim et al., 2015). Topical NSAIDs such as flurbiprofen, diclofenac and ketorolac tromethamine are commonly prescribed in human and veterinary medicine due to their availability and relatively low cost. Topical NSAIDS are primarily used for inflammatory ocular conditions such as the suppression of uveitis that may be present before and after intraocular surgery

*Corresponding Author: Fabiano Montiani-Ferreira. Universidade Federal do Paraná (UFPR), Departamento de Medicina Veterinária, Rua dos Funcionários, 1540, Bairro Juvevê, 80035-050, Curitiba – PR, Brazil. Email: montiani@ufpr.br

(Giuliano, 2004; Sigle and Nasisse, 2006; Kim *et al.*, 2010; Maca *et al.*, 2010; Klein *et al.*, 2011).

Chen *et al.* (1997) showed that the application of topical NSAID ophthalmic solutions effectively reduced corneal sensitivity as well as the sensitivity of polymodal nociceptors. These findings support that analgesia and ocular comfort reported by human beings may, in part, be due to decreased PGs excitatory activity on nervous fibers (Martini *et al.*, 1984; Yamada *et al.*, 2002).

The aim of this study is to evaluate variations in the corneal sensitivity of dogs after topical application of three different NSAIDS and one preservative agent using a Cochet-Bonnet esthesiometer, which measures the corneal surface sensitivity threshold. In dogs, the accepted criteria for measurement of corneal sensitivity threshold is the degree of corneal stimulation that is required to elicit a blink reflex (Barrett *et al.*, 1991; Stiles *et al.*, 2001; Good *et al.*, 2003; Blocker *et al.*, 2007; Venturi *et al.*, 2016; Dorbandt *et al.*, 2017).

Materials and Methods

This study followed ARVO´s Statement for the Use of Animals in Ophthalmic and Vision Research and was approved by the Ethics Committee of the Agrarian Sciences Sector, Federal University of Parana.

Six nine-month-old nonbrachycephalic mixed breed dogs, all littermates, were used in the study. Three males and three females were used, and all dogs were previously evaluated, vaccinated and free from signs of systemic or ophthalmic diseases. Prior to enrollment in the study, a complete ophthalmic examination was performed including a Schirmer tear test I (STT-I) (Drogavet, Curitiba, Brazil), fluorescein stain (fluorescein sodium; Drogavet, Curitiba, Brazil), tonometry (Tono-Vet; Icare Finland, Espoo, Finland), slit-lamp biomicroscopy (Hawk Eye; Dioptrix, L'Union, France), and indirect ophthalmoscopy (Heine Omega 180 Headworn Binocular Indirect Ophthalmoscope, Dove, USA). Additionally, a complete blood count, serum biochemical analysis, and urinalysis were obtained.

A masked prospective study design was used to determine the immediate effects of three commonly available ophthalmic NSAIDS and one common ophthalmic preservative on corneal sensitivity in normal canine eyes. The ophthalmic NSAIDS evaluated were flurbiprofen sodium 0.03% (ALLERGAN; Syntex Inc., USA), diclofenac sodium 0.1% (ALLERGAN; Syntex Inc., USA) and ketorolac tromethamine 0.5% (ALLERGAN; Syntex Inc., USA). The ophthalmic preservative evaluated was benzalkonium chloride 0.01%, which is the preservative agent found in ketorolac tromethamine. Benzalkonium chloride eye drops were specially prepared in a compounding pharmacy (OPHTHALMOS, São Paulo, Brazil).

Corneal sensitivity data were acquired using a Cochet-Bonnet esthesiometer (Luneau Ophtalmologie, Chartres Cedex, France) following a previously described protocol (Barrett *et al.*, 1991; Good *et al.*, 2003). Data collection began approximately two weeks after the screening examination. The handheld esthesiometer possesses a thin, retractable, nylon monofilament that extends up to 6 cm in length. Since normal baseline corneal sensitivity threshold range of the normal dog varies from 1.0 to 3.5 cm (Stiles *et al.* 2001; Blocker *et al.*, 2007; Kobashigawa *et al.*, 2015; Venturi *et al.*, 2016), measurements started with a nylon monofilament length of 4 cm, which is a usual initial set point for corneal sensitivity evaluation in dogs (Venturi *et al.*, 2016).

The esthesiometer was gently advanced perpendicularly toward the center of corneal surface until a slight deflection of the monofilament was noted after contact. If a blink reflex was not observed on at least three attempts, the length of the monofilament was decreased 0.25 cm, and the procedure was then repeated. The length of the filament is directly proportional to corneal sensitivity such that a longer nylon monofilament length required to stimulate a blinking reflex equates to a more sensitive cornea. The experiment was conducted in two different stages, and for each stage, a repetition was made in the same group of animals.

The drug bottles were labeled as 'A', 'B,' 'C', 'D', and the investigators responsible for application of the study drug and esthesiometry measurements were masked to the drug being used. The key was maintained by the principal investigator and revealed to the study investigators at the conclusion of the study. In the first stage, one drop of flurbiprofen sodium (drug A) was administered onto the right eye, and one drop of diclofenac sodium (drug B) was administered onto the left eye of each animal. In the second stage, after a washout period of 7 days, one drop of ketorolac tromethamine (drug C) was administered onto the right eye and one drop of benzalkonium chloride was administered onto the left eye (drug D).

For each stage, the length of the nylon monofilament able to stimulate the dogs' blink reflex was recorded. Baseline esthesiometry (before the administration of any drug) was represented as time 0. Once each eye drop was applied onto the ocular surface, subsequent esthesiometry data were collected every 15 minutes after initial administration until one hour and 45 minutes after the last drop (105 minutes).

Each stage was performed with same room conditions, controlling external variables such as weather, noise, and people and animal traffic inside and outside the room. Only two study investigators were present during the data collection, one responsible for esthesionometry and the other responsible for animal restraint. The same study investigator was responsible for each function throughout the experiment. Temperature and humidity were evaluated during each stage of the investigation using a wireless thermos hygrometer (TM005X-M Meade Instruments, Irvine, CA).

Statistical analyses were performed to compare the esthesiometry data obtained in relation to time (in minutes) and each drug used. To check whether or not the distribution of the data errors followed a Gaussian distribution, a Shapiro-Wilk test was applied. The test revealed that the data did not follow a non-Gaussian distribution. Therefore the non-parametric Friedman´s test (similar to the parametric repeated measures ANOVA) was used to detect differences in treatments across multiple test attempts on the same group of animals (paired data). Descriptive and inferential statistical analysis were performed using the JMP v7 (SAS Institute, Cary, NC, EUA), statistical package for computers.

Results

In the first stage, the mean environmental conditions during the time in which the experiment was conducted was 21°C and 71% humidity. During the second stage, temperature was 18°C with 77% humidity.

Table 1 shows the esthesiometry results (medians) by each evaluation time for each drug tested. No significant difference was found comparing baseline results (time 0). An overall (considering all drugs together) significant difference for higher corneal sensitivity values within the initial 15 (P = 0.001) and 30 minutes (P = 0.03) after topical administration of all eye drops tested was observed compared to baseline values. This initial increase in corneal sensitivity was followed by a gradual and significant decrease in mean values (P≤ 0.025) compared to baseline values. Considering the results for the individual drugs, after the topical use of flurbiprofen sodium 0.03%, an increase in corneal sensitivity at 30 minutes was observed (P = 0.013) when compared with baseline values. Subsequently, a tendency towards a decrease in mean corneal sensitivity values was observed until the last evaluation time. However these lower mean corneal sensitivity values were not significantly different than baseline values. A slight increase of esthesiometry means also was observed 30 minutes after topical administration of diclofenac sodium 0.1%; however, this slight increase was not statistically significant (P=0.75).

Subsequently, however, significant decreases (P ≤ 0.034) in corneal sensitivity were observed between 75 and 90 minutes post-application of diclofenac sodium 0.1% when compared to baseline values. Nonetheless, at 105 minutes after initial topical administration of diclofenac, the difference was no longer significant. Corneal sensitivity data obtained after topical application of ketorolac tromethamine 0.5% showed no

significant differences between esthesiometry data means and baseline means at 15 minutes (P = 0.1), 30 minutes (P = 0.8) or at any other time point after topical administration. After topical application of benzalkonium chloride 0.01%, a significant increase (P = 0.001) in corneal sensitivity values compared with baseline values was observed at 15 minutes.

Discussion

It is well known that corneal sensitivity exhibits a great variability and it is influenced by several factors. For instance, corneal sensitivity is significantly reduced in brachycephalic and corneal region evaluated, with the central part being more sensitive that the peripheral cornea in dogs (Barrett et al., 1991) and cats (Blocker and Van Der Woerdt, 2001). Humans over the age of 40 have a significantly reduced corneal sensitivity (Millodot, 1972). Interestingly, the influence of age was not observed in dogs (Barrett et al., 1991) or cats (Blocker and Van Der Woerdt, 2001). These variables were controlled in the present study since a repeated measure statistical design was used with the same test-subjects (paired data), including the initial control. Data were collected in a longitudinal fashion in which change over time was assessed and time 0 is the control of each subject. This method reduces the variance of estimates of treatment-effects, allowing statistical inference to be made with fewer subjects (Gueorguieva and Krystal, 2004). Additionally, to reduce the influence of different examiners on data variability, the same study investigator was responsible for all corneal sensitivity evaluations.

Topical application of diclofenac sodium 0.1% was the only study drug that resulted in a decrease in corneal sensitivity, and this occurred at 75 and 90 minutes post-application. Paradoxically, topical application of flurbiprofen sodium 0.03% demonstrated a significant increase in corneal sensitivity 30 minutes post-application while a nonsignificant trend for an increase in corneal sensitivity occurred for all other study drugs during the initial 15 to 30 minutes. For all treatment protocols, this initial increase in corneal sensitivity was followed by a steady decrease (Table 1).The magnitude and significance of the initial increase and subsequent decrease is different between drugs, but this trend is consistently observed for each specific anti-inflammatory drug evaluated.The control of corneal pain has limited options, as topical sodium channel blockers, such as proparacaine and tetracaine, are not acceptable due to their limited duration of activity and epitheliotoxic effects (Grant and Acosta, 1994; Herring et al., 2005; Venturi et al., 2016). Topical morphine has been shown to provide acceptable analgesia without a delay of corneal epithelialization (Peyman et al., 1994; Stiles et al., 2003; Clark et al., 2011); however, the corneal analgesic effectiveness in dogs has recently come into question (Thomson et al., 2013).

Table 1. Esthesiometry values (median in cm) in relation with each time point evaluated after topical use of sodium flurbiprofen 0.03%, sodium diclofenac 0.01%, ketorolac tromethamine 0.5% and benzalkonium chloride 0.01% on corneal surface in dogs.

Drugs	Time (minutes)							
	0	15	30	45	60	75	90	105
Flurbiprofen Sodium 0.03%	0.875	1.125	1.375*	0.875	1.000	1.000	0.875	0.875
Diclofenac Sodium 0.1%	1.250	1.125	1.250	1.000	1.00	0.750*	0.750*	0.875
Ketorolac Tromethamine 0.5%	1.250	1.375	1.250	1.250	1.250	1.000	1.000	1.000
Benzalkonium Chloride 0.01%	1.000	1.5*	1.375	1.125	1.000	1.000	1.250	1.000

*Means that presented significant differences compared with the baseline esthesiometry, $P < 0.05$.

Therefore, it is paramount to identify alternative options for corneal analgesia. In humans, the use of topical NSAIDS has been shown to decrease corneal pain (Weaver and Terrell, 2003; Kim et al., 2015). To the authors' knowledge, there are no studies evaluating the antinociceptive effect of topical NSAIDS on dogs with corneal ulcers. The current study provides evidence that diclofenac decreases corneal sensitivity, and this may correlate with improved comfort when used in the presence of a corneal ulceration; however, controlled studies should be performed to evaluate its efficacy. This decrease in corneal sensitivity after topical application of diclofenac has also been reported in humans (Szerenyi et al., 1994; Seitz et al., 1996).

In contrast to the effect of diclofenac, topical application of flurbiprofen demonstrated a possible increase of nociceptor excitatory activity after 30 minutes. However, between 45 to 105 minutes after application, corneal sensitivity decreased, and nociceptor activity conceivably started to decline as well. During this period of decreasing sensitivity, mean corneal sensitivity values still remained higher than baseline. Our data support that flurbiprofen may result in a more evident irritant action than an analgesic one. The authors hypothesize that the initial increase reflects a common time pattern for the irritant action on the canine corneal surface after topical administration of all drugs tested.

The authors believe that blocking prostaglandin action in peripheral nociceptors is able to promote a decrease of neuronal excitatory activity even in non-inflamed eyes, which is supported by previous studies (Chen, et al., 1997; Aragona et al., 2000). Esthesiometry data obtained after topical application of diclofenac in the current study suggests the peak analgesic action of this drug to occur 75 to 90 minutes after topical application. After this period, however, corneal sensitivity returned to baseline values. Topical application of ketorolac did not produce significant changes in corneal sensitivity.

Data obtained after topical application of benzalkonium chloride demonstrates a significant increase in corneal sensitivity at 15 minutes compared with baseline values. Additionally, higher mean sensitivity values were obtained when compared to other study treatments during the same time point, which may represent a potentially higher corneal irritant effect. This finding was interesting, as a change in corneal sensitivity was not expected because benzalkonium chloride is a preservative devoid of anti-inflammatory properties and is instead used in ophthalmic solutions to increase drug penetration through the lipid cell membrane (Madhu et al., 1996; Malhotra and Majumdar, 2006). It is also an ingredient present in ketorolac ophthalmic solution. Importantly, benzalkonium chloride has also been shown to promote eicosanoid synthesis and, consequently, ocular irritation suggests that topical application of this preservative, even in concentrations as low as 0.0001%, decreases proliferative cellular activity and promotes apoptosis (Madhu et al., 1996; De Saint Jean et al., 1999).

Although the present study demonstrated an increase in corneal sensitivity after application of benzalkoniun chloride, the same effect was not observed with ketorolac, despite containing benzalkonium chloride as a preservative. It is possible that the anti-inflammatory action of ketorolac may reduce the irritant effect of benzalkonium chloride on corneal nociceptor fibers.

The results of flurbiprofen and diclofenac identified in the current study are somewhat different than the results obtained in a recent study (Dorbandt et al., 2017), and this may be explained, in part, by variations in study design as well as differences in ambient humidity between the two studies. The current study evaluated corneal sensitivity with decreasing increments of 0.25 cm, and this may have allowed the investigators to assess for smaller changes in corneal sensitivity. The current study also evaluated corneal sensitivity up to 105 minutes after application of the specified study drug. Specifically, for diclofenac, a decrease in corneal sensitivity was observed at 75 and 90 minutes after application (Table 1). One of the most important differences between the two studies is the ambient humidity. In the current study, ambient humidity values during data collection were 71% to 77%, and it has been shown that humidity may have profound effects on corneal esthesiometry measurements (Dorbandt et al., 2017). In the recent comparable study, ambient humidity ranged from 19% to 44%, which may explain the higher sensitivity values, as the same study found that a lower humidity results in a higher corneal sensitivity measurement (increased filament length) (Dorbandt *et al.*, 2017). With these results of humidity kept in mind, it can explain why corneal sensitivity values (filament length) obtained in the present study are lower than those obtained in previous studies (Barrett *et al.*, 1991; Good *et al.*, 2003; Dorbandt *et al.*, 2017).

Although some previous studies in humans and dogs demonstrated the analgesic action of flurbiprofen and ketorolac (Sigle and Nasisse, 2006; Maca *et al.*, 2010), the present study suggests that the ophthalmic application of these two drugs do not promote analgesic activity on corneal nociceptor activity in healthy canine eyes. Another recent study (Dorbandt *et al.*, 2017) also demonstrated a lack of analgesic activity after topical application of flurbiprofen to canine eyes. Nevertheless, Acosta *et al.* (2007) found that topical ketorolac 0.4% resulted in analgesic efficacy in healthy feline eyes and that this drug was capable of decreasing peripheral nociceptor activity. Although the study by Acosta *et al.* (2007) also uses the Cochet-Bonnet esthesiometer as mechanical stimuli, data collection was performed using the evaluation of the evoked potential of neuronal fibers. This methodology, previously developed by Chen *et al.* (1997), comprises a more quantifiable parameter for the evaluation of corneal nociceptors. In this way, the single use of a blinking reflex in the current investigation as an indirect observational parameter of corneal sensitivity promoted by Cochet-Bonnet esthesiometry may have resulted in insufficient data due to inherent variability in the blink response.

Studies in humans have found that topical application of diclofenac demonstrates comparatively higher corneal analgesic potential (Szerenyi *et al.*, 1994; Seitz *et al.*, 1996) which corroborates the results from Aragona *et al.* (2000). Studies have also demonstrated evidence for the interaction of diclofenac with β-endorphin (endogenous inhibitory neurotransmitter) and substance P (nociceptors endogenous excitatory neurotransmitter). In these studies, there was an observed increase in plasma β-endorphins (Martini *et al.*, 1984) and a decrease in levels of substance P in tears (Yamada *et al.*, 2002), which may contribute to the potential analgesic action of this drug. Thus, the authors believe that topical diclofenac effectively caused inhibition of the eicosanoid production in the arachidonic acid metabolic pathway in the canine corneas. This mechanism was then responsible for decreasing corneal nociceptor activity of polymodal nociceptors, which are present in the cornea and are responsive to prostaglandins and bradykinin (Belmonte *et al.*, 2004). This decrease in corneal nociception generated a clinically-detectable degree of topical analgesia (Bloom, 1996). This assumption corroborates the findings from other authors (Szerenyi *et al.*, 1994;

Seitz *et al.*, 1996; Chen *et al.*, 1997; Aragona *et al.*, 2000; Yamada *et al.*, 2002; Acosta *et al.*, 2005, 2007). A limitation of the current study is that the low number of individuals evaluated may have a profound effect on significance (Type II statistical error), and it is possible that a significant increase would have been achieved with higher study numbers. Topical administration of all eye drops tested (considered together) show a significant increase in corneal sensitivity values within the initial 15-30 minutes. However, when evaluated individually only flurbiprofen (at 30 minutes) and benzalkonium chloride (at 15 minutes) demonstrated an increase in corneal sensitivity. For diclofenac, although not statistically significant, a trend exists towards an increase in corneal sensitivity values 30 minutes after topical application. Another limitation is that the only preservative evaluated was benzalkonium chloride. Given the result of benzalkonium chloride application alone, the initial increase in corneal sensitivity noted between 15 and 30 minutes may suggest an irritant action caused by different preservative agents present in each of these ophthalmic solutions: thimerosal 0.005% for flurbiprofen; boric acid for diclofenac; benzalkonium chloride 0.01% for ketorolac. For ketorolac, the trend towards an increase in sensitivity after the administration was an expected result given the significant increase in corneal sensitivity after benzalkonium chloride alone was observed. The fact that benzalkonium chloride did not show a significant difference when used in combination with ketorolac may be due to the slightly higher variation of the corneal sensitivity means observed at baseline. This overall effect also might be responsible by the burning sensation reported by several human patients that use these drugs topically (Chen *et al.*, 1997; Aragona *et al.*, 2000; Acosta *et al.*, 2005). However, new investigations are necessary to prove the mechanism of action for these agents on the corneal surface. Although the subjectivity of the blink reflex by observational evaluation may have interfered directly in obtaining esthesiometry results, both baseline and experimental values were always evaluated by the same observer, thus minimizing the possibility of subjectivity on variable measurement.

The results of the current study demonstrate that corneal sensitivity of normal, nonbrachycephalic dogs is decreased by topical diclofenac sodium 0.1% at 75 and 90 minutes after application. However, the topical administration of flurbiprofen sodium 0.03% and benzalkonium chloride 0.01% result in an immediate increase in corneal sensitivity between 15 and 30 minutes after application while ketorolac tromethamine 0.5% has no effect. The results of topical diclofenac demonstrated in the current study mimics those found in humans in that diclofenac was the only topical NSAID observed to cause an immediate, but transient, decrease in corneal sensitivity. More studies with controlled variables, including the use of new methodologies of corneal nociceptor electrophysiological activity, are necessary to obtain trustworthy data regarding analgesic efficacy of anti-inflammatories tested in this study.

Conflict of interest

The authors declare that they have no competing interests.

References

Acosta, M.C., Luna, C., Graff, G., Mesenguer, V.M., Viana, F., Gallar, J. and Belmont, C. 2007 Comparative effects of the nonsteroidal anti-inflammatory drug nepafenac on corneal sensory nerve fibers responding to chemical irritation. Invest. Ophthal. Vis. Sci. 48, 182-188.

Acosta, M.C., Berenguer-Ruiz, L., García-Gálvez, A., Perea-Tortosa, D., Gallar, J. and Belmont, C. 2005. Changes in mechanical, chemical, and thermal sensitivity of the cornea after topical application of nonsteroidal anti-inflammatory drugs. Invest. Ophthal. Vis. Sci. 46, 282-286.

Aragona, P., Tripodi, G., Spinella, R., Laganá, E. and Ferreri, G. 2000. The effects of the topical administration of non-steroidal anti-inflammatory drugs on corneal epithelium and corneal sensitivity in normal subjects. Eye 14, 206-210.

Barrett, P.M., Scagliotti, R.H., Merideth, R.E., Jackson, P. and Alarcon, F. 1991. Absolute corneal sensitivity and corneal trigeminal nerve anatomy in normal dogs. Prog. Vet. Comp. Ophthalmol. 1, 245-254.

Belmonte, C., Acosta, M.C. and Gallar, J. 2004. Neural basis of sensation in intact and injured corneas. Exp. Eye Res. 78, 513-525.

Blocker, T., Hoffman, A., Schaeffer, D.J. and Wallin, J.A. 2007. Corneal sensitivity and aqueous tear production in dogs undergoing evisceration with intraocular prosthesis placement. Vet. Ophthalmol. 10, 147-154.

Blocker, T. and Van Der Woerdt, A. 2001. A comparison of corneal sensitivity between brachycephalic and Domestic Short-haired cats. Vet. Ophthalmol. 4, 127-130.

Bloom, F.E. 1996. Neurotransmission and the central nervous system. In Goodman & Gilman's The Pharmacological Basis of Therapeutics. 9th edition. Eds Hardman, J.G., Limbird, L.E. Molinoff, P.B., Ruddon, R.W. and Gilman, A.G. New York. McGraw-Hill, pp: 267-294.

Chen, X., Gallar, J. and Belmont, C. 1997. Reduction by anti-inflammatory drugs of the response of corneal sensory nerve fibers to chemical irritation. Invest. Ophthal. Vis. Sci. 38, 1944-1953.

Clark, J.S., Bentley, E. and Smith, L.J. 2011. Evaluation of topical nalbuphine or oral tramadol as analgesics for corneal pain in dogs: a pilot study. Vet. Ophthalmol. 14, 358-364.

De Felipe, C., González, G.G., Gallar, J. and Belmonte, C. 1999. Quantification and immunocytochemical characteristics of trigeminal ganglion neurons projecting to the cornea: effect of corneal wounding. Eur. J. Pain 3, 32-39.

De Saint Jean, M., Brignole, F., Bringuier, A.F., Bauchet, A., Feldmann, G. and Baudouin, C. 1999. Effects of benzalkonium chloride on growth and survival of Chang conjunctival cells. Invest. Ophthal. Vis. Sci. 40, 619-630.

Dorbandt, D.M., Labelle, A.L., Mitchell, M.A. and Hamor, R.E. 2017. The effects of topical diclofenac, topical flurbiprofen, and humidity on corneal sensitivity in normal dogs. Vet. Ophthalmol. 20, 160-170.

Giuliano, E.A. 2004. Nonsteroidal anti-inflammatory drugs in veterinary ophthalmology. Vet. Clin. North Am. Small Anim. Pract. 34, 707-723.

Good, K.L., Maggs, D.J., Hollingsworth, S.R., Scagliotti, R.H. and Nelson, R.W. 2003. Corneal sensitivity in dogs with diabetes mellitus. Am. J. Vet. Res. 64, 7-11.

Grant, R.L. and Acosta, D. 1994. Comparative toxicity of tetracaine, proparacaine and cocaine evaluated with primary cultures of rabbit corneal epithelial cells. Exp. Eye Res. 58, 469-478.

Gueorguieva, R. and Krystal, J.H. 2004. Move over ANOVA: progress in analyzing repeated-measures data and its reflection in papers published in the Archives of General Psychiatry. Arch. Gen. Psychiatry 61, 310-317.

Herring, I.P., Bobofchak, M.A., Landry, M.P. and Ward, D.L. 2005. Duration of effect and effect of multiple doses of topical ophthalmic 0.5% proparacaine hydrochloride in clinically normal dogs. Am. J. Vet. Res. 66, 77-80.

Insel, P.A. 1996. Analgesic-antipyretic and anti-inflammatory agents and drugs employed in the treatment of goat. In Goodman & Gilman's The Pharmacological Basis of Therapeutics. 9th edition. Eds Hardman, J.G., Limbird, L.E. Molinoff, P.B., Ruddon, R.W. and Gilman, A.G. New York. McGraw-Hill, pp: 617-658.

Kim, S.J., Flach, A.J. and Jampol, L.M. 2010. Nonsteroidal anti-inflammatory drugs in ophthalmology. Surv. Ophthalmol. 55, 108-133.

Kim, S.K., Hong, J.P., Nam, S.M., Stulting, R.D. and Seo, K.Y. 2015. Analgesic effect of preoperative topical nonsteroidal antiinflammatory drugs on postoperative pain after laser-assisted subepithelial keratectomy. J. Cataract Refract. Surg. 41, 749-755.

Klein, H.E., Krohne, S.G., Moore, G.E. and Stiles, J. 2011. Postoperative complications and visual outcomes of phacoemulsification in 103 dogs (179 eyes): 2006–2008. Vet. Ophthalmol. 14, 114-120.

Kobashigawa, K.K., Lima, T.B., Padua, I.R.M., Barros Sobrinho, A.A.F., Marinho, F.A., Ortêncio, K.P. and Laus, J.L. 2015. Ophthalmic parameters in adult Shih Tzu dogs. Ciência Rural 45, 1280-1285.

Maca, S.M., Amon, M., Findl, O., Kahraman, G. and Barisani-Asenbauer, T. 2010. Efficacy and tolerability of preservative-free and preserved diclofenac and preserved ketorolac eyedrops after cataract surgery. Am. J. Ophthalmol. 149, 777-784.

Madhu, C., Rix, P.J., Shackleton, M.J., Nguyen, T.G. and Tang-Liu, D.D. 1996. Effect of benzalkonium chloride/EDTA on the ocular bioavailability of ketorolac tromethamine following ocular instillation to normal and de-epithelialized corneas of rabbits. J. Pharm. Sci. 85, 415-418.

Maggs, J.D. 2008. Ocular pharmacology and therapeutics. In Slatter's Fundalmentals of Veterinary Ophthalmology. 5th edition. Eds, Maggs, D., Miller, P. and Ofri, R. Elsevier Inc., pp: 33-61.

Malhotra, M. and Majumdar, D.K. 2006. Aqueous, oil, and ointment formulations of ketorolac: efficacy against prostaglandin E2-induced ocular inflammation and safety: a technical note. AAPS PharmSciTech. 7(4), 96.

Marfurt, C.F., Murphy, C.J. and Florczak, J.L. 2001. Morphology and neurochemistry of canine corneal innervation. Invest. Ophthal. Vis. Sci. 42, 2242-2251.

Martini, A., Bondiolotti, G.P., Sacerdote, P., Pierro, L., Picotti, G.B., Panerai, A.E., Restelli, L., Zancaner, F. and Monza, G. 1984. Diclofenac increases beta-endorphin plasma concentrations. J. Int. Med. Res. 12, 92-95.

Millodot, M. 1972. Diurnal variation of corneal sensitivity. Br. J. Ophthalmol. 56, 844-847.

Peyman, G.A., Rahimy, M.H. and Fernandes, M.L. 1994. Effects of morphine on corneal sensitivity and epithelial wound healing: implications for topical ophthalmic analgesia. Br. J. Ophthalmol. 78, 138-141.

Seitz, B., Sorken, K., LaBree, L.D., Garbus, J.J. and McDonnell, P.J. 1996. Corneal sensitivity and burning sensation: comparing topical ketorolac and diclofenac. Arch. Ophthalmol. 114, 921-924.

Sigle, K.J. and Nasisse, M.P. 2006. Long-term complications after phacoemulsification for cataract removal in dogs: 172 cases (1995–2002). J. Am. Vet. Med. Assoc. 228, 74-79.

Stiles, J., Honda, C.N., Krohne, S.G. and Kazacos, E.A. 2003. Effect of topical administration of 1% morphine sulfate solution on signs of pain and corneal wound healing in dogs. Am. J. Vet. Res. 16, 813-818.

Stiles, J., Krohne, S., Rankin, A. and Chang, M. 2001. The efficacy of 0.5% proparacaine stored at room temperature. Vet. Ophthalmol. 4, 205-207.

Szerenyi, K., Sorken, K., Garbus, J.J., Lee, M. and McDonnell, P.J. 1994. Decrease in normal human corneal sensitivity with topical diclofenac sodium. Am. J. Ophthalmol. 118, 312-315.

Tasaka, A.C. 1999. Antinflamatórios não-esteroidais. In Farmacologia Aplicada à Medicina Veterinária. 2ª edição. Eds, Spinosa, H.S., Gorniak, S.L., Bernardi, M.M. Guanabara Koogan: Rio de Janeiro, pp: 212-226.

Thomson, S.M., Oliver, J.A., Gould, D.J., Mendl, M. and Leece, E.A. 2013. Preliminary investigations into the analgesic effect of topical ocular 1% morphine solution in dogs and cats. Vet. Anaesth. Analg. 40, 632-640.

Tranquilli, W.J. and Thurman, J.C. 1999. Perioperative pain and its management. In Essentials of Small Animal Anesthesia & Analgesia. Eds, Thurman, J.C., Tranquilli, W.J., Benson, G.J. 1st edition. Lippincott Williams & Wilkins. Baltimore, pp: 28-60.

Venturi, F., Blocker, T., Dees, D.D., Madsen, R. and Brinkis, J. 2016. Corneal anesthetic effect and ocular tolerance of 3.5% lidocaine gel in comparison with 0.5% aqueous proparacaine and 0.5% viscous tetracaine in normal canines. Vet. Ophthalmol. doi: 10.1111/vop.12440.

Weaver, C.S. and Terrell, K.M. 2003. Evidence-based emergency medicine. Update: do ophthalmic nonsteroidal anti-inflammatory drugs reduce the pain associated with simple corneal abrasion without delaying healing? Ann. Emerg. Med. 14, 134-140.

Yamada, M., Ogata, M., Kawai, M., Mochizuki, H. and Mashima, Y. 2002. Topical diclofenac sodium decreases the substance P content of tears. Arch. Ophthalmol. 120, 51-54.

18

Primary leiomyosarcoma of the jugular vein in a dog

Alessio Pierini[1,*], Filippo Cinti[1], Diana Binanti[2] and Guido Pisani[1]

[1]Centro Veterinario Luni Mare, Ortonovo (SP), 19034, Italy
[2]AbLab, Laboratorio di Analisi Veterinarie, Sarzana (SP), 19038, Italy

Abstract

A four-year-old, male, Labrador retriever was referred for removal of a spindle cell sarcoma involving the right jugular vein. A post-contrast CT scan showed a seven-centimeter subcutaneous mass originated from the right external jugular vein, which was partially obstructed and showing contrast stasis, suggested a primary intravascular tumor of the jugular vein. The mass was resected, and histological evaluation was consistent with grade II intravenous spindle cell sarcoma of the jugular vein. Immunohistochemical positivity for vimentin, desmin, and αSMA antibody and negativity for S-100 protein confirmed venous leiomyosarcoma. The dog received five doses of intravenous doxorubicin, and there was no recurrence of the tumor 30 months post treatment. In dogs, primary intravascular sarcomas are rare and primary venous leiomyosarcoma has not been described. A venous tumor may be considered as a differential diagnosis in dogs with ventral neck swelling.

Keywords: Dog, Doxorubicin, Intravascular sarcoma, Jugular vein, Leiomyosarcoma.

Introduction

Primary intravascular sarcoma is rare in dogs and only intra-arterial tumors have been reported (Anderson et al., 1988; Callanan et al., 2000; Mellanby et al., 2003; Ranck et al., 2008; Cohen et al., 2010; Lee et al., 2011; Stieger-Vanegas et al., 2016). In people, primary intravascular sarcomas also are rare and almost all intravenous sarcomas were classified as leiomyosarcomas (Burke and Virmani, 1993). In humans, a high metastatic rate has been reported for intravenous leiomyosarcoma (Tilkorn et al., 2010).

Leiomyosarcoma is rare in companion animals. In the dog, it is most common in the alimentary tract, spleen, and liver and is considered to have a moderate to high metastatic tendency (Kapatkin et al., 1992).

To authors' knowledge, primary venous leiomyosarcoma has not been described in dogs. This report describes clinical, tomographic and pathological features, treatment and outcome of a primary leiomyosarcoma of the jugular vein in a dog.

Case history

A four-year-old, 39.3 kg, male Labrador retriever was referred for removal of a spindle cell tumor involving the right jugular vein. The dog had been examined initially at a primary care clinic because of a neck swelling that had increased in size over 2 weeks. Cytological evaluation of aspirate collected by fine needle biopsy revealed spindle cell sarcoma. Excisional biopsy was attempted at the primary care clinic but abandoned because of severe hemorrhage. Computed tomography (CT) showed a 7.2 cm x 5.7 cm x 5.2 cm mass at the thoracic inlet in the right caudoventral neck

area (Fig. 1). The mass originated from the right external jugular vein, which was dilated cranially and joined the tumor in an S-configuration. Post-contrast CT showed partial obstruction of the right external jugular vein and contrast stasis. The right internal jugular vein, carotid artery, retropharyngeal and cervical lymph nodes, and thyroid gland were normal as were the thoracic and abdominal findings. The CT results were consistent with a primary intravascular venous tumor or extravascular tumor with secondary involvement of the right external jugular vein and venous thrombosis.

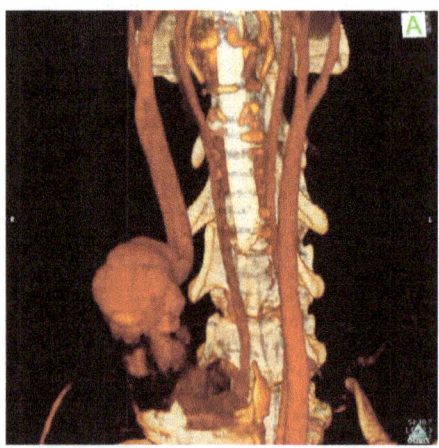

Fig. 1. 3D volume-rendered CT image of the ventral cervical region highlighting the vascular structures of the neck. The mass involving the right external jugular vein is clearly visible as well as the associated distention of the jugular vein and its S-configuration, proximal to the mass.

*Corresponding Author: Dr. Alessio Pierini. Present address: Veterinary Teaching Hospital, Department of Veterinary Sciences, University of Pisa, San Piero a Grado, Pisa, 56122, Italy. Email: pierini.alessio2004@libero.it

Physical examination of the dog at the referral clinic showed a longitudinal, 10-cm, surgical wound in the caudal third of the ventral neck region. A 7-cm, firm, painless, subcutaneous mass that extended cranially from the thoracic inlet could be palpated in the region of the wound. There was no apparent vascular obstruction or venous stasis. The cervical lymph nodes were unremarkable, and results of a complete blood cell count and serum biochemical analysis were within the reference intervals.

The dog was premedicated with dexmedetomidine (5 µg/kg IM Dexdomitor, Pfizer Italia srl, Milan, Italy) and butorphanol (0.1 mg/kg IM Dolorex, Intervet Italia srl, Latina, Italy) and a catheter was placed in the lateral saphenous vein. The dog was pre-oxygenated via a face mask, and anesthesia was induced with propofol (2 mg/kg IV Rapinovet, Intervet Italia srl, Latina, Italy) and maintained with oxygen and isoflurane after endotracheal intubation. The dog was placed in dorsal recumbency with the head extended and the ventral aspect of the neck was prepared for aseptic surgery. The surgical wound was resected, and a clean margin was maintained around the entire periphery of the tumor during its removal. The right external jugular vein was isolated, exposed with blunt dissection, and ligated (2.0 poliglyconate) cranial and caudal to the mass, which was then resected and submitted for histologic examination (Fig. 2).

The excised tissue was fixed in 10% buffered formalin, processed routinely, and embedded in paraffin wax for histologic and immunohistochemical examination. Sections were stained with hematoxylin and eosin. A streptavidin/peroxidase complex method (Vectastain Kit, Vector Laboratories Inc., Burlingame, CA, USA) was used for immunohistochemical staining. The primary antibodies used included rabbit polyclonal desmin antibody (polyclonal, Santa Cruz), mouse monoclonal vimentin antibody (clone 3B4, Dako), α-smooth muscle actin antibody (αSMA, clone 1A4, Scytek), and S-100 protein antibody (clone 4C4.9, Scytek). The expression of Ki67, a cellular marker for proliferation and prognostic indicator, was evaluated by incubating tissue sections with primary Ki67 antibody (MIB-1 mAb, DAKO, Carpinteria, CA). The tumor was encapsulated and pedunculated, and histologic evaluation showed a neoplasm composed of spindle cells arranged in interlacing bundles with a herringbone pattern and no interstitial collagen matrix (Fig. 3).

There were occasional, thin-walled, blood vessels. Neoplastic cells had indistinct borders, an intermediate nuclear-to-cytoplasmic ratio, and a moderate amount of lightly eosinophilic cytoplasm. Nuclei were round to oval, often cigar-shaped, or blunt-ended, with finely granular chromatin and one central magenta nucleolus. Mitotic figures ranged from 0-4 per high-power field (11 mitotic figures per 10 HPF), and there was

moderate anisocytosis and anisokaryosis with kariomegaly and occasional bizarre cells. Moderate multifocal foci of necrosis were evident (<50%). Histologic findings were consistent with intravenous spindle cell sarcoma of the jugular vein, most likely of smooth muscle origin (leiomyosarcoma). Based on the grading system for soft tissue sarcoma using histotype, mitotic index, and necrosis, the neoplasm was classified as grade II sarcoma (Dennis *et al.*, 2011).

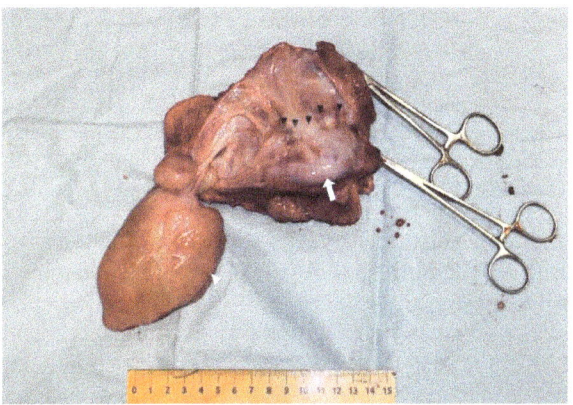

Fig. 2. The resected right external jugular vein has been opened longitudinally revealing the tunica intima (white arrow) and the leiomyosarcoma. The tumour has been turned over to show its pedunculated shape (white arrowhead) and the suture on the internal side of the jugular vein (black arrowheads) from the initial surgery.

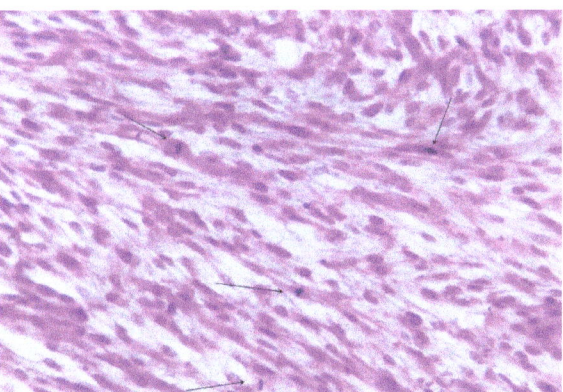

Fig. 3. The neoplasm was composed of spindle cells arranged in interlacing bundles and in a herringbone pattern. The cells have indistinct cell borders, a moderate amount of lightly eosinophilic cytoplasm, and oval or cigar-shaped nuclei. Several mitoses are evident (arrows) (H&E stain; bar = 100 µm).

Immunohistochemical staining with vimentin, desmin, and αSMA antibodies was positive in all sections (Fig. 4). Neoplastic cells were uniformly negative for S-100 protein, typically expressed in peripheral nerve sheath tumour, confirming the diagnosis of leiomyosarcoma. Ki67 positive cells were uniformly distributed in the neoplasm, and the Ki67 index was 30-40%, which was considered high.

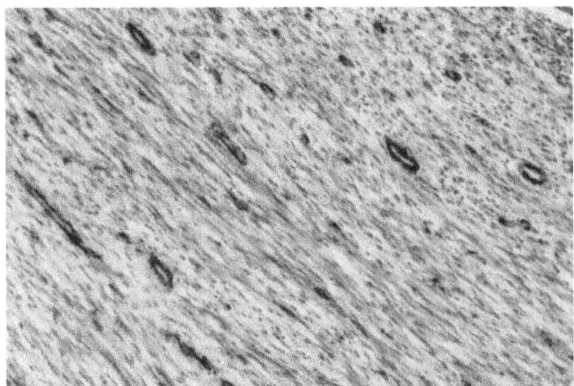

Fig. 4. Neoplastic cells showed moderate to strong αSMA immunelabeling. Small blood vessels within the tumour were strongly positive. Immunohistochemistry (IHC), diaminobenzidine, hematoxylin counterstain.

The dog was discharged the next day and healed without complications. At a follow-up examination 2 weeks postoperatively, the results of echocardiography were normal and the dog was treated with doxorubicin (30 mg/m² IV Doxorubicina, Teva Italia srl, Milan, Italy), administered over 20 minutes, once every 3 weeks for a total of five treatments. No chemotherapy side effects occurred.

The results of echocardiography 1 month after the last treatment were normal. The dog was examined clinically every three months, and there was no recurrence of the tumor at 30 months after the initial diagnosis.

Discussion

Primary intravascular sarcoma is rare in dogs and to our knowledge, only intra-arterial tumors have been reported and diagnosed histologically as aortic chondrosarcoma in 3 cases, pulmonary artery chondrosarcoma in 1 case, aortic angiosarcoma in 1 case, pulmonary artery poorly differentiated hemangiosarcoma in 1 case and pulmonary artery leiomyosarcoma in 1 case (Anderson *et al.*, 1988; Callanan *et al.*, 2000; Mellanby *et al.*, 2003; Ranck *et al.*, 2008; Cohen *et al.*, 2010; Lee *et al.*, 2011; Stieger-Vanegas *et al.*, 2016).

In people, primary intravascular sarcomas also are rare and may occur in great vessels of both the arterial and venous systems (Burke and Virmani, 1993). They are classified histologically as undifferentiated intimal sarcomas and differentiated sarcomas. Most of the latter are leiomyosarcomas and angiosarcomas (Burke and Virmani, 1993; Afzal *et al.*, 2015) and almost all intravenous sarcomas were classified as leiomyosarcomas (Burke and Virmani, 1993).

Leiomyosarcoma is rare in companion animals. In the dog, it is most common in the alimentary tract, spleen, and liver and is considered to have a moderate to high metastatic tendency (Kapatkin *et al.*, 1992). Pulmonary metastases were found in an adult dog euthanized

because of endoluminal arterial leiomyosarcoma (Callanan *et al.*, 2000). Of 12 people with venous leiomyosarcoma, 5 had high-grade leiomyosarcoma, 2 had distant metastases at the time of diagnosis, and 6 had distant metastases at the end of the study. All had pulmonary metastases, and the 3-year survival rate was 57% (Tilkorn *et al.*, 2010).

Based on a soft tissue grading system, the intravascular leiomyosarcoma described in this report was classified as grade II. It had an intermediate mitotic index and high Ki67 expression (Dennis *et al.*, 2011) suggesting malignant behavior (Ettinger *et al.*, 2006).

Because of the high risk of metastasis, adjuvant chemotherapy using a doxorubicin-based protocol was started; this is considered the best adjuvant treatment of dogs with high-grade soft tissue sarcoma (Ogilvie *et al.*, 1989) even though the efficacy of chemotherapy is not clear.

Edema in the head and neck region due to venous thrombosis or stasis did not occur in this dog, but was observed in 6 of 12 people with venous leiomyosarcoma (Tilkorn *et al.*, 2010). Despite the large size of the mass, the venous drainage of the head and neck could be afforded by the left external jugular vein and the internal jugular veins. Similarly, no local edema occurred after external jugular vein autografts were used to treat intrahepatic portosystemic shunts in dogs (Kyles *et al.*, 2001).

The diagnosis of leiomyosarcoma was based on histologic features (herringbone pattern, cigar-shaped nuclei), immunohistochemical expression of vimentin, desmin, and αSMA, and lack of expression of S100 (Frost *et al.*, 2003). An immunohistochemical panel that was recently introduced to better classify perivascular wall tumors was not used because frozen sections are required (Avallone *et al.*, 2007). Moreover, histological pattern was not characteristic of this group of tumours. Venous tumor may be considered as a differential diagnosis in dogs with ventral neck swelling.

Acknowledgements

The authors would like to thank Deborah Francione and Sara Rossi for their contributions.

References

Afzal, A.M., Alsahhar, J., Podduturi, V. and Schussler, J.M. 2015. Undifferentiated Intimal Sarcoma of the Inferior Vena Cava with Extension to the Right Atrium and Renal Vasculature. Case Rep. Cardiol. 1-4. doi:10.1155/2015/812374.

Anderson, W.I., Carberry, C.A., King, J.M., Trotter, E.J. and de Lahunta, A. 1988. Primary aortic chondrosarcoma in a dog. Vet. Pathol. 25(2), 180-181.

Avallone, G., Helmbold, P., Caniatti, M., Stefanello, D., Nayak, R.C. and Roccabianca, P. 2007. The spectrum of canine cutaneous perivascular wall tumors: morphologic, phenotypic and clinical characterization. Vet. Pathol. 44(5), 607-620.

Burke, A.P. and Virmani, R. 1993. Sarcomas of the great vessels. A clinicopathologic study. Cancer 71(5), 1761-1773.

Callanan, J.J., McCarthy, G.M. and McAllister, H. 2000. Primary pulmonary artery leiomyosarcoma in an adult dog. Vet. Pathol. 37(6), 663–666.

Cohen, J.A., Bulmer, B.J., Patton, K.M. and Sisson, D.D. 2010. Aortic dissection associated with an obstructive aortic chondrosarcoma in a dog. J. Vet. Cardiol. 12(3), 203-210.

Dennis, M.M., McSporran, K.D., Bacon, N.J., Schulman, F.Y., Foster, R.A. and Powers, B.E. 2011. Prognostic factors for cutaneous and subcutaneous soft tissue sarcomas in dogs. Vet. Pathol. 48, 73-84.

Ettinger, S.N., Scase, T.J., Oberthaler, K.T., Craft, D.M., McKnight, J.A., Leibman, N.F., Charney, S.C. and Bergman, P.J. 2006. Association of argyrophilic nucleolar organizing regions, Ki-67, and proliferating cell nuclear antigen scores with histologic grade and survival in dogs with soft tissue sarcomas: 60 cases (1996-2002). J. Am. Vet. Med. Assoc. 228(7), 1053-1062.

Frost, D., Lasota, J. and Miettinen, M. 2003. Gastrointestinal stromal tumors and leiomyomas in the dog: a histopathologic, immunohistochemical, and molecular genetic study of 50 cases. Vet. Pathol. 40, 42-54.

Kapatkin, A.S., Mullen, H.S., Matthiesen, D.T. and Patnaik, A.K. 1992. Leiomyosarcoma in dogs: 44 cases (1983-1988). J. Am. Vet. Med. Assoc. 201, 1077-1079.

Kyles, A.E., Gregory, C.R., Jackson, J., Ilkiw, J.E., Pascoe, P.J., Adin, C., Samii, V.F. and Herrgesell, E. 2001. Evaluation of a portocaval venograft and ameroid ring for the occlusion of intrahepatic portocaval shunts in dogs. Vet. Surg. 30, 161-169.

Lee, B., Lee, S., Lee, H., Kim, H., Kim, D.Y. and Choi, J. 2011. Abdominal aortic chondrosarcoma in a dog. J. Vet. Med. Sci. 73(11), 1473-1476.

Mellanby, R., Holloway, A., Woodger, N., Baines, E., Ristic, J. and Herrtage, M.E. 2003. Primary chondrosarcoma in the pulmonary artery of a dog. Vet. Rad. Ultrasound. 44, 315-321.

Ogilvie, G.K., Reynolds, H.A., Richardson, R.C., Withrow, S.J., Norris, A.M., Henderson, R.A., Klausner, J.S., Fowler, J.D. and McCaw, D. 1989. Phase II evaluation of doxorubicin for treatment of various canine neoplasms. J. Am. Vet. Med. Assoc. 195, 1580-1583.

Ranck, R.S., Linder, K.E., Haber, M.D. and Meuten, D.J. 2008. Primary intimal aortic angiosarcoma in a dog. Vet. Pathol. 45(3), 361-364.

Stieger-Vanegas, S.M., Bottorff, B., Sisson, D. and Löhr, C.V. 2016. Imaging diagnosis-multimodality findings in an adult dog with primary sarcoma of the pulmonary artery and myocardial metastases. Vet. Rad. Ultrasound. 57(4), 34-41.

Tilkorn, D.J., Hauser, J., Ring, A., Goertz, O., Stricker, I., Steinau, H.U. and Kuhnen, C. 2010. Leiomyosarcoma of intravascular origin--a rare tumor entity: clinical pathological study of twelve cases. World J. Surg. Oncol. 8(1), 103.

19

Survey of spatial distribution of vector-borne disease in neighborhood dogs in southern Brazil

Caroline Constantino[1], Edson Ferraz Evaristo de Paula[2], Ana Pérola Drulla Brandão[3], Fernando Ferreira[3], Rafael Felipe da Costa Vieira[1] and Alexander Welker Biondo[1,2]*

[1]*Department of Veterinary Medicine, Federal University of Paraná, Curitiba, PR, 80035-050, Brazil*
[2]*Animal Protection Section, City Secretary of Environment, Curitiba, PR, 80020-290, Brazil*
3*Department of Preventive Veterinary Medicine, University of São Paulo, São Paulo, SP, 05508-270, Brazil*

Abstract

Neighborhood dogs may act as reservoirs and disseminators of vector-borne diseases in urban areas. Accordingly, the aim of this study was to ascertain the health status and the vector-borne pathogens infecting dogs living in public areas with high levels of human movement in the city of Curitiba, southern Brazil. Blood samples from 21 neighborhood dogs that were found in nine of 22 bus stations and two public parks were subjected to a complete blood cell (CBC) count, serum biochemical profiling, a commercial rapid ELISA test and a commercial real-time PCR panel of vector-borne diseases. The CBC count and serum biochemical profiling were within the normal range for dogs and only 1/21 (4.7%) of the dogs was seroreactive for *Borrelia burgdorferi* sensu stricto. The commercial real-time PCR panel showed that 7/21 (33.3%) of the dogs had *Mycoplasma haemocanis* infection, 9/21 (42.8%) had 'Candidatus Mycoplasma haematoparvum' and 4/21 (19.0%) had both. No statistical association between infected by the agents found here and abnormalities in physical examinations, laboratory tests or ectoparasite presence was found ($p > 0.05$). In conclusion, neighborhood dogs showed low prevalence of vector-borne diseases and satisfactory wellbeing, and dogs can be used as sentinels for disease exposure.
Keywords: *Borrelia burgdorferi*, Community dogs, Hemoplasmas, Sentinel animals, Tick-borne diseases.

Introduction

Dogs have been indicated as potential public health sentinels because of their close interaction with humans, particularly their owners, while presenting associations with common infectious agents and vectors (Backer *et al.*, 2001; Schmidt, 2009; Schurer *et al.*, 2012).

Whereas true sentinels should reveal diseases without harboring them, dogs may become reservoirs for certain diseases such as visceral leishmaniasis (Dantas-Torres, 2009).

Moreover, dogs may act as potential sources of dissemination of invertebrate vectors and transmission of their zoonoses (Schmidt, 2009).

Although neighborhood dogs have been defined for more than two decades as semi-restricted or free-range animals with semi-dependence on one or more families for food and shelter (WHO/WSPA, 1990), their health status and role in maintaining and spreading zoonotic diseases has yet to be fully established.

In addition, dogs that lack healthcare such as regular vaccination, deworming, and ectoparasite control may have greater susceptibility to diseases and/or environmental bioaccumulation as well as negatively impact animal welfare (Salb *et al.*, 2008).

Owned dogs in southern Brazil have been shown to have higher exposure to tick-borne pathogens in urban areas than in rural settings (Vieira *et al.*, 2013b).

Moreover, dogs may serve as a potential source for transmission of canine vector-borne diseases (CVBDs) with zoonotic risk (Diniz *et al.*, 2007; Otranto *et al.*, 2009a, 2009b; Vieira *et al.*, 2013a; Eremeeva and Dasch, 2015). Within this scenario, neighborhood dogs can be expected to be at higher risk of infection because of their urban roaming and vector exposure. The city of Curitiba, the capital of the state of Paraná, is currently the eighth biggest city and the ninth biggest metropolitan area in Brazil, with approximately 3.5 million habitants (IBGE, 2014).

Although commonly found in low-income neighborhoods of urban areas, neighborhood dogs may find sufficient food and shelter in bus stations because of the infrastructure and high levels of human movement. Since the city of Curitiba has no subway, 1.1 million daily users rely on ground transportation interconnected by 22 main bus stations. Accordingly, the aim of the present study was to survey CVBDs in neighborhood dogs found in public areas with high daily levels of human movement (bus stations and public parks) in the city of Curitiba, southern Brazil.

*Corresponding Author: Alexander Welker Biondo. Departamento de Medicina Veterinária, Universidade Federal do Paraná, 1540, 80035 050, Curitiba, Paraná, Brazil. Email: abiondo@ufpr.br

Materials and Methods

The present study was approved by the Ethics Committee for Animal Experimentation and Animal Welfare of the Federal University of Paraná, state of Paraná, southern Brazil (protocol number 027/2015).

Cross-sectional study and sampling

All 22 bus stations and two public parks in the city of Curitiba (25°25'40" S and 49°16'23" W), in southern Brazil, were included in this study (Fig. 1).

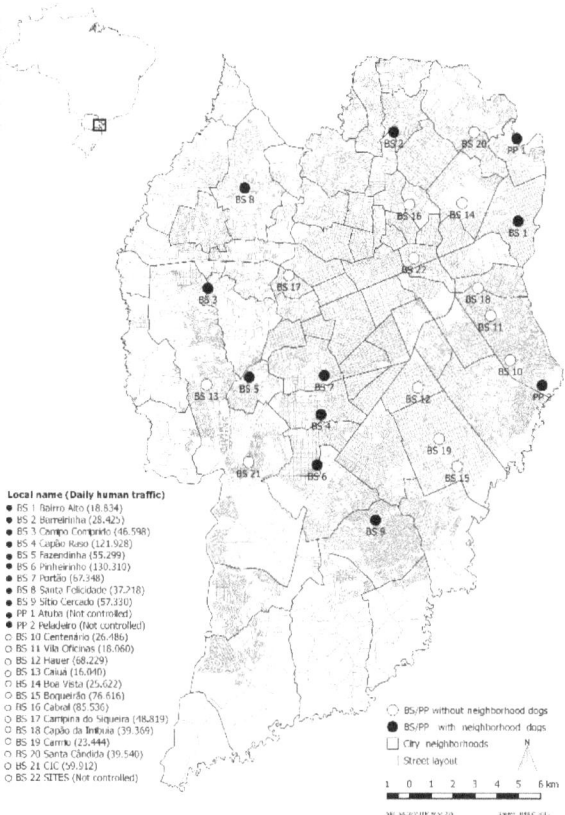

Local name (Daily human traffic)
- BS 1 Bairro Alto (18,834)
- BS 2 Boneirinha (28,425)
- BS 3 Campo Comprido (46,598)
- BS 4 Capão Raso (121,928)
- BS 5 Fazendinha (55,299)
- BS 6 Pinheirinho (130,310)
- BS 7 Portão (67,348)
- BS 8 Santa Felicidade (37,218)
- BS 9 Sítio Cercado (57,330)
- PP 1 Atuba (Not controlled)
- PP 2 Peladeiro (Not controlled)
- BS 10 Centenário (26,486)
- BS 11 Vila Oficinas (18,060)
- BS 12 Hauer (68,229)
- BS 13 Caiuá (16,040)
- HS 14 Boa Vista (25,622)
- BS 15 Boqueirão (76,616)
- BS 16 Cabral (85,536)
- BS 17 Campina do Siqueira (48,319)
- BS 18 Capão da Imbuia (39,369)
- BS 19 Carmo (23,444)
- BS 20 Santa Cândida (39,540)
- BS 21 CIC (59,912)
- BS 22 SITES (Not controlled)

○ BS/PP without neighborhood dogs
● BS/PP with neighborhood dogs
☐ City neighborhoods
Street layout

1 0 1 2 3 4 5 6 km

Fig. 1. Map of Brazil showing the locations of the state of Paraná and city of Curitiba. Enlarged map shows locations and daily human movements of the bus stations (BS) and public parks (PP) included in the study, distinguishing those at which neighborhood dogs were sampled. City of Curitiba, state of Paraná, Brazil, 2016.

At the time of the survey, the city of Curitiba had an estimated population of 1,864,416 inhabitants distributed over an area of 435,036 km^2, located at 934.6 meters above sea level. This city has humid subtropical climate, with rainfall of 1,434 mm/year and average winter and summer temperatures of 10 °C and 22 °C respectively (IBGE, 2014).

The dog inclusion criteria were applied in accordance with the World Health Organization (WHO) definition of neighborhood dogs (WHO/WSPA, 1990), as follows: semi-restricted or entirely free to wander and establish food and shelter dependency with users and

workers at the bus stations and parks. A total of 21 neighborhood dogs, 19 from 9/22 bus stations (40.9% of the bus stations) and two from each public park, were found between February and April of 2014 (Fig. 1). The dogs were all of mixed breed and aged ≥ 1 year; 8/21 (38.1%) were females and 13/21 (61.9%) were males. They were physically restrained and underwent physical examination. Since over 1.0 million people daily use the ground transportation of Curitiba, researchers were allowed by the City Secretary of Transportation to perform capture, physical restrain and dog samplings on site only between February and April (mild Autumn). Blood samples were collected by means of venipuncture of the jugular vein using commercial sterile vacuum tubes with and without EDTA. Thereafter, complete blood cell (CBC) counts and biochemical profiling were performed, and the remaining aliquots were stored at -20 °C for further molecular and serological analysis.

Laboratory tests

CBC counts and biochemical profiling were performed on all samples. CBC counts were performed in a commercial automated hematological analyzer (CC-550, Celm Ltd, São Paulo, Brazil). Blood smears were made from fresh blood samples; they were dried and stained using a commercial staining agent (Diff-Quick; Panótico Rápido LB, Laborclin, São Paulo, Brazil), and differential leukocyte counts and cell morphology analysis were performed under an optical microscope. Alanine aminotransferase (ALT) and alkaline phosphatase (ALP) activity levels and creatinine concentrations were determined by means of the kinetic method, urea concentrations by means of the enzymatic method and total protein and fractions by means of the colorimetric method, using a commercial semiautomatic analyzer (Bio-2000lL, Bioplus, São Paulo, Brazil).

Serum samples were tested for *Dirofilaria immitis*, *Ehrlichia* spp. (*E. canis*, *E. chaffeensis* and *E. ewingii*), *Borrelia burgdorferi* sensu stricto (s.s.) and *Anaplasma* spp. (*A. phagocytophilum* and *A. platys*) using a commercial rapid ELISA test (SNAP® 4Dx® Plus, IDEXX Laboratories Inc., Westbrook, ME, USA), in accordance with the manufacturer's instructions.

Whole EDTA-blood samples were tested for *Babesia* spp., *Anaplasma* spp., *Ehrlichia* spp., *Rickettsia* spp., *Hepatozoon* spp., *Leishmania* spp., *Neorickettsia risticii*, *Bartonella* spp., *Mycoplasma haemocanis* and 'Candidatus Mycoplasma haematoparvum', using a commercial real-time PCR panel of vector-borne diseases (IDEXX Laboratories, Westbrook, ME, USA). DNA was extracted from the blood samples using standard protocols on a commercial platform (Corbett XTractor-Gene, Qiagen, Valencia, CA, USA). A housekeeping gene (18S rRNA) was used to determine DNA content and quality. The primers for both the housekeeping gene and the PCR test were based on IDEXX's proprietary real-time PCR oligonucleotides (IDEXX Laboratories). Real-time PCR was performed using default-cycling conditions in commercial apparatus (Roche LC480 in the 384-well plate configuration, Roche Applied Science, Indianapolis, IN, USA).

Statistical analysis

The data were stored in electronic spreadsheets (Microsoft Excel® 2010) and subsequently analyzed using the SPSS (2008) statistical software (version 17.0). Descriptive analyses with frequency distributions were performed and in order to verify bivariate associations, nonparametric Fisher's exact tests were conducted, at the 5% significance level. In addition, to measure the relationship between daily human movement and the number of neighborhood dogs in the study locations, the Pearson correlation coefficient was calculated.

Results and Discussion

All 21 neighborhood dogs were considered to be clinically healthy and had CBC counts and biochemical profiles within the normal range for the species. Only 1/21 (4.8%) of the dogs was seroreactive for *Borrelia burgdorferi* s.s. according to the commercial rapid ELISA test. The commercial real-time PCR panel revealed that 7/21 (33.3%) of the dogs were positive for *M. haemocanis*, 9/21 (42.8%) for '*Ca.* M. haematoparvum' and 4/21 (19%) for both (Table 1). All 21 neighborhood dogs tested negative for the remaining CVBDs according to both real-time PCR and the rapid ELISA test.

No significant association was found between gender ($p = 0.337$) or presence of ectoparasites ($p = 0.638$) and infection by *M. haemocanis*, or between gender ($p = 0.642$) or presence of ectoparasites ($p = 0.642$) and infection by '*Ca.* M. haematoparvum'. The number of neighborhood dogs did not show any correlation with the daily human movement at the bus stations (*Pearson correlation coefficient* = 0.347, $p = 0.123$).

In this cross-sectional study, neighborhood dogs were screened for CVBDs by means of serological and molecular methods. Despite the WHO definition published 25 years ago, this was the first study to survey health status and CVBDs in neighborhood dogs, to the best of the authors' knowledge. Since these dogs may have spent their time continuously roaming outdoors, their exposure to vectors and pathogens was expected to be relatively higher than that of owned dogs (Azzag *et al.*, 2015). Surprisingly, despite lacking traditional ownership, these dogs were found to be healthy on clinical examination, with CBC counts and biochemical profiles within the normal range, and they mostly tested negative for CVBD. In Brazil, previous studies have shown that the prevalence of CVBDs in dogs in urban areas has varied from absence to 91.2%

(Lasta *et al.*, 2013; Spolidorio *et al.*, 2013; Vieira *et al.*, 2013b). Although the neighborhood dogs of the present study had comparatively lower CVBD prevalence (Vieira *et al.*, 2013b; Azzag *et al.*, 2015), the wide differences in CVBD prevalence may be explained by the populations studied, lifestyles, environmental occurrence of vectors and diseases, diagnostic tests used and vector competence of ticks from the *Rhipicephalus sanguineus* group (Balakrishnan *et al.*, 2014; Maia *et al.*, 2015; Moraes-Filho *et al.*, 2015).

As observed here, infection by CVBDs may occur in the absence of clinical signs (Joppert *et al.*, 2001; Maggi *et al.*, 2014; Azzag *et al.*, 2015) or hematological changes (Novacco *et al.*, 2010; Balakrishnan *et al.*, 2014; Moraes-Filho *et al.*, 2015). A previous study on owned dogs did not show any significant associations between hemoplasma infection and anemia, ectoparasite infestation, gender and clinical status (Tennant *et al.*, 2011), thus corroborating the findings from the neighborhood dogs of the present study.

Although neighborhood dogs with outdoor lives in urban areas may be at higher risk of exposure to tick-borne pathogens (Cardoso *et al.*, 2012; Vieira *et al.*, 2013b; Maia *et al.*, 2015), only 1/7 (14.3%) of the dogs infected by *M. haemocanis* and 1/9 (11.1%) by '*Ca.* M. haematoparvum' were infested by ticks. No association was found between the presence of ectoparasites and positivity for at least one species of *Mycoplasma* ($p = 0.397$). Although *Mycoplasma* spp. infection has previously been reported in dogs (Ramos *et al.*, 2010; Valle *et al.*, 2014; Vieira *et al.*, 2015) and has been correlated with exposure to ticks and fleas in Brazil (Valle *et al.*, 2014), our findings corroborate other reports from Brazil, Greece and Africa, which did not find any association between hemoplasma infection and ticks (Barker *et al.*, 2010; Tennant *et al.*, 2011; Vieira *et al.*, 2015). Since the clinical examinations were limited to the time of sampling, it is possible that these dogs may have acquired and eliminated ticks before this time.

Despite the low prevalence of *M. haemocanis* and '*Ca.* M. haematoparvum' hemoplasmas in the neighborhood dogs, these pathogens have previously been reported infecting humans (Kallick, 2010; Maggi *et al.*, 2013a, 2013b). Since neighborhood dogs may play a role as environmental CVBD reservoirs and/or disseminators, zoonotic potential should always be considered, particularly because of these animals' close contact with users at bus stations every day. Thus, these animals should be continuously monitored as environmental sentinels for hemoplasmas and other CVBDs. Although seropositivity has been already reported in dogs, human beings and horses in Brazil, no molecular evidence of *B. burgdorferi* infection has been found to date (Joppert *et al.*, 2001; Labarthe *et al.*, 2003; Spolidorio *et al.*, 2010; Montandon *et al.*, 2014).

Table 1. Location and results of molecular and serological tests performed on blood samples from 21 neighborhood dogs in the city of Curitiba, state of Paraná, Brazil, 2016.

| Neighborhood dog | | Commercial real-time PCR panel of vector-borne diseases | | | | Commercial rapid ELISA test | |
| | | *M. haemocanis* | | '*Ca.* M. haematoparvum' | | *Borrelia burgdorferi* | |
Location	Number	Positive (%)	Negative (%)	Positive (%)	Negative (%)	Positive (%)	Negative (%)
BS 1	1	0/1 (0)	1/1 (100)	1/1 (100)	0/1 (0)	0/1 (0)	1/1 (100)
BS 2	5	1/5 (20)	4/5 (80)	1/5 (20)	4/5 (80)	0/5 (0)	5/5 (100)
BS 3	1	0/1 (0)	1/1 (100)	0/1 (0)	1/1 (100)	0/1 (0)	1/1 (100)
BS 4	1	1/1 (100)	0/1 (0)	1/1 (100)	0/1 (0)	0/1 (0)	1/1 (100)
BS 5	2	1/2 (50)	1/2 (50)	2/2 (100)	0/2 (0)	0/2 (0)	2/2 (100)
BS 6	5	2/5 (40)	3/5 (60)	1/5 (20)	4/5 (80)	0/5 (0)	5/5 (100)
BS 7	2	0/2 (0)	2/2 (100)	2/2 (100)	0/2 (0)	1/2 (50)	1/2 (50)
BS 8	1	0/1 (0)	1/1 (100)	0/1 (0)	1/1 (100)	0/1 (0)	1/1 (50)
BS 9	1	1/1 (100)	0/1 (0)	0/1 (0)	1/1 (100)	0/1 (0)	1/1 (50)
PP 1	1	0/1 (0)	1/1 (100)	0/1 (0)	1/1 (100)	0/1 (0)	1/1 (50)
PP 2	1	1/1 (100)	0/1 (0)	1/1 (100)	0/1 (0)	0/1 (0)	1/1 (50)
Total	21	7/21 (33.3)	14/21 (66.6)	9/21 (42.8)	12/21 (57.1)	1/21 (4.8)	20/21 (95.2)

(BS): Bus station; (PP): Public park.

Thus, the finding of a neighborhood dog that was seropositive for *B. burgdorferi* in the present study may have potentially been a false positive. This result may have been due to the high sensitivity (94.1%) and good specificity (96.2%) for specific antibodies to the C6 synthetic peptide to *B. burgdorferi* s.s. presented by the commercial rapid ELISA test used here.

Alternatively, our findings may have been the consequence of a low tick infection rate (Spolidorio *et al.*, 2010) or a conceivably different *B. burgdorferi* strain or a similar species in Brazil (Joppert *et al.*, 2001; Montandon *et al.*, 2014). Nonetheless, further studies should be conducted in order to fully establish the potential association between antibody presence and the zoonotic Brazilian Baggio-Yoshinari syndrome.

Since direct transfer of infected ticks between dogs and human beings is considered to be a minor transmission factor (Goossens *et al.*, 2001), dogs may not be important pathogen disseminators. As previously shown, dogs may be suitable sentinels for evaluating the environmental risk of human exposure to *B. burgdorferi* (Duncan *et al.*, 2005). Moreover, since dogs may be more exposed to ticks, particularly in endemic areas, monitoring of anti-*B. burgdorferi* antibodies in neighborhood dogs may indicate an environmental risk of human exposure.

Despite relatively low number of individuals, the neighborhood dogs in the present study were randomly distributed throughout the city (Fig. 1). In addition, a high degree of result repetition was observed since all the dogs were considered to have adequate health status and were within the normal ranges for the CBC count and biochemical profile for the species, with low prevalence of CVBD.

No previous survey has been found to date on tested pathogens (*Dirofilaria immitis*, *Ehrlichia canis*, *E. chaffeensis*, *E. ewingii*, *Borrelia burgdorferi* sensu stricto, *Anaplasma phagocytophilum*, *A. platys*, *Babesia* spp., *Rickettsia* spp., *Hepatozoon* spp., *Leishmania* spp., *Neorickettsia risticii*, *Bartonella* spp., *Mycoplasma haemocanis* and '*Candidatus* Mycoplasma haematoparvum') in human samples at the city of Curitiba or surrounding areas. Anti-*Ehrlichia* spp. antibodies in human samples were reported in a rural settlement of northern Paraná state, however without molecular evidence of infection (Vieira *et al.*, 2015). Also within the Paraná state, the first detection of antibodies against *B. burgdorferi* sensu latu was reported in human beings living in the same rural area (Gonçalves *et al.*, 2013).

Finally, the adequate clinical and laboratory health status observed among these neighborhood dogs may imply that these dogs in the city of Curitiba were living under good animal sanitary and welfare conditions, particularly since some of the bus stations have a human movement of over than 100,000 daily users (Fig. 1). Furthermore, since these neighborhood dogs were receiving water, food and shelter at the bus stations, their individual CBC counts and clinical biochemical profiles together may indicate that they were in a situation of animal welfare in an overall non-harmful environment. The low prevalence of CVBD among these neighborhood dogs may show that was a low environmental risk and consequently a low risk of dissemination, particularly in the bus stations. Moreover, clinically healthy dogs with CBC counts and biochemical profiles within the normal range may represent a state of low environmental toxicity and satisfactory animal welfare. In conclusion, neighborhood dogs should be continuously monitored and may act as sentinels for environmental risk such as vector-borne diseases in public areas with highly human movement.

Acknowledgements
We thank Aline Gizzi, Cynthia Silva, Camila Martins and the staff of the Animal Service of city of Curitiba for their in-field assistance. We thank the Araucaria Support Foundation for Scientific and Technological Development of the State of Paraná for the full financial support (grant number 292/13) for this research and the Coordination Office for Improvement of Higher-Education Personnel for the master's fellowship.

Conflict of Interest
The authors declare that no competing interests exist.

References
Azzag, N., Petit, E., Gandoin, C., Bouillin, C., Ghalmi, F., Haddad, N. and Boulouis, H.J. 2015. Prevalence of select vector-borne pathogens in stray andclient-owned dogs from Algiers. Comp. Immunol. Microbiol. Infect. Dis. 38, 1-7.

Backer, L.C., Grindem, C.B., Corbett, W.T., Cullins, L. and Hunter, J.L. 2001. Pet dogs as sentinels for environmental contamination. Sci. Total Environ. 274, 161-169.

Balakrishnan, N., Musulin, S., Varanat, M., Bradley, J.M. and Breitschwerdt, E.B. 2014. Serological and molecular prevalence of selected canine vector borne pathogens in blood donor candidates, clinically healthy volunteers, and stray dogs in North Carolina. Parasit. Vectors 7, 116-125.

Barker, E.N, Tasker, S., Day, M.J., Warman, S.M., Woolley, K., Birtles, R., Georges, K.C., Ezeokoli, C.D., Newaj-Fyzul, A., Campbell, M.D., Sparagano, O.A., Cleaveland, S. and Helps, C.R. 2010. Development and use of real-time PCR to detect and quantify *Mycoplasma haemocanis* and "*Candidatus* Mycoplasma haematoparvum" in dogs. Vet. Microbiol. 140, 167-170.

Cardoso, L., Mendão, C. and de Carvalho, L.M. 2012. Prevalence of *Dirofilaria immitis, Ehrlichia canis, Borrelia burgdorferi* sensu lato, *Anaplasma* spp. and *Leishmania infantum* in apparently healthy and CVBD-suspect dogs in Portugal-a national serological study. Parasit. Vectors 5, 62-71.

Dantas-Torres, F. 2009. Canine leishmaniosis in South America. Parasit. Vectors 2, S1.

Diniz, P.P., Schwartz, D.S., de Morais, H.A. and Breitschwerdt, E.B. 2007. Surveillance for zoonotic vector-borne infections using sick dogs from southeastern Brazil. Vector Borne Zoonotic Dis. 7, 689-697.

Duncan, A.W., Correa, M.T., Levine, J.F. and Breitschwerdt, E.B. 2005. The dog as a sentinel for human infection: prevalence of *Borrelia burgdorferi* C6 antibodies in dogs from southeastern and mid-Atlantic States. Vector Borne Zoonotic Dis. 5, 101-109.

Eremeeva, M.E. and Dasch, G.A. 2015. Challenges posed by tick-borne rickettsiae: eco-epidemiology and public health implications. Front. Public Health 3, 55-72.

Gonçalves, D.D., Benitez, A., Lopes-Mori, F.M.R., Alves, L.A., Freire, R.L., Navarro, I.T., Santana, M.A.Z., Santos, L.R.A., Carreira, T., Vieira, M. L. and Freitas, J.C.D. 2013. Zoonoses in humans from small rural properties in Jataizinho, Parana, Brazil. Brazilian J. Microbiol. 44, 125-131.

Goossens, H.A., Van Den Bogaard, A.E. and Nohlmans, M.K. 2001. Dogs as sentinels for human Lyme borreliosis in The Netherlands. J. Clin. Microbiol. 39, 844-848.

IBGE. 2014. Instituto Brasileiro de Geografia e Estatística. Estimativas da População dos Municípios Brasileiros com Data de Referência em 1º de Julho de 2014 http://www.ibge.gov.br/home/presidencia/noticias/pdf/analise_estimativas_2014.pdf (Accessed on 05 may 2015).

Joppert, A.M., Hagiwara, M.K. and Yoshinari, N.H. 2001. *Borrelia burgdorferi* antibodies in dogs from Cotia county, São Paulo State, Brazil. Rev. Inst. Med. Trop. São Paulo 43, 251-255.

Kallick, C.A. 2010. Specific bacterial inclusions in bone marrow cells indicate systematic lupus erythematosus, and treatment for lupus. U.S. Patent 7, 820, 405.

Labarthe, N., Pereira, M.C., Barbarini, O., McKee, W., Coimbra, C.A. and Hoskins, J. 2003. Serologic prevalence of *Dirofilaria immitis, Ehrlichia canis*, and *Borrelia burgdorferi* infections in Brazil. Vet. Ther. 4, 67-75.

Lasta, C.S., Santos, A.P., Messick, J.B., Oliveira, S.T., Biondo, A.W., Vieira, R.F., Dalmolin, M.L. and González, F.H. 2013. Molecular detection of *Ehrlichia canis* and *Anaplasma platys* in dogs in Southern Brazil. Rev. Bras. Parasitol. Vet. 22, 360-366.

Maggi, R.G., Birkenheuer, A.J., Hegarty, B.C., Bradley, J.M., Levy, M.G. and Breitschwerdt, E.B. 2014. Comparison of serological and molecular panels for diagnosis of vector-borne diseases in dogs. Parasit. Vectors 7, 127-136.

Maggi, R.G., Compton, S.M., Trull, C.L., Mascarelli, P.E., Mozayeni, B.R. and Breitschwerdt, E.B. 2013b. Infection with Hemotropic *Mycoplasma* Species in Patients with or without Extensive Arthropod or Animal Contact. J. Clin. Microbiol. 51, 3237-3241.

Maggi, R.G., Mascarelli, P.E., Havenga, L.N., Naidoo, V. and Breitschwerdt, E.B. 2013a. Co-infection with *Anaplasma platys*, *Bartonella henselae* and *Candidatus* Mycoplasma haematoparvum in a veterinarian. Parasit. Vectors 6, 103-113.

Maia, C., Almeida, B., Coimbra, M., Fernandes, M.C., Cristóvão, J.M., Ramos, C., Martins, Â., Martinho, F., Silva, P., Neves, N., Nunes, M., Vieira, M.L., Cardoso, L. and Campino, L. 2015. Bacterial and protozoal agents of canine vector-borne diseases in the blood of domestic and stray dogs from southern Portugal. Parasit. Vectors 23, 138-145.

Montandon, C.E., Yoshinari, N.H., Milagres, B.S., Mazioli, R., Gomes, G.G., Moreira, H.N., Padilha, A.F., Wanderley, G.G., Mantovani, E., Galvão, M.A., Langoni, H. and Mafra, C. 2014. Evidence of *Borrelia* in wild and domestic mammals from the state of Minas Gerais, Brazil. Rev. Bras. Parasitol. Vet. 23, 287-290.

Moraes-Filho, J., Krawczak, F.S., Costa, F.B., Soares, J.F. and Labruna, M.B. 2015. Comparative Evaluation of the Vector Competence of Four South American Populations of the *Rhipicephalus sanguineus* Group for the Bacterium *Ehrlichia canis*, the Agent of Canine Monocytic Ehrlichiosis. PLoS One 10, 1-16.

Novacco, M., Meli, M.L., Gentilini, F., Marsilio, F., Ceci, C., Pennisi, M.G., Lombardo, G., Lloret, A., Santos, L., Carrapiço, T., Willi, B., Wolf, G., Lutz, H. and Hofmann-Lehmann, R. 2010. Prevalence and geographical distribution of canine hemotropic mycoplasma infections in Mediterranean countries and analysis of risk factors for infection. Vet. Microbiol. 142, 276-284.

Otranto, D., Dantas-Torres, F. and Breitschwerdt, E.B. 2009a. Managing canine vector-borne diseases of zoonotic concern: part one. Trends Parasitol. 25, 157-163.

Otranto, D., Dantas-Torres, F. and Breitschwerdt, E.B. 2009b. Managing canine vector-borne diseases of zoonotic concern: part two. Trends Parasitol. 25, 228-235.

Ramos, R., Ramos, C., Araújo, F., Oliveira, R., Souza, I., Pimentel, D., Galindo, M., Santana, M., Rosas, E., Faustino, M. and Alves, L. 2010. Molecular survey and genetic characterization of tick-borne pathogens in dogs in metropolitan Recife (northeastern Brazil). Parasitol. Res. 107, 1115-1120.

Salb, A.L., Barkema, H.W., Elkin, B.T., Thompson, R.C., Whiteside, D.P., Black, S.R., Dubey, J.P. and Kutz, S.J. 2008. Dogs as sources and sentinels of parasites in humans and wildlife, northern Canada. Emerg. Infect. Dis. 14, 60-63.

Schmidt, P.L. 2009. Companion animals as sentinels for public health. Vet. Clin. North Am. Small Anim. Pract. 39, 241-250.

Schurer, J.M., Hill, J.E., Fernando, C. and Jenkins, E.J. 2012. Sentinel surveillance for zoonotic parasites in companion animals in indigenous communities of Saskatchewan. Am. J. Trop. Med. Hyg. 87, 495-498.

Spolidorio, M.G., Labruna, M.B., Machado, R.Z., Moraes-Filho, J., Zago, A.M., Donatele, D.M., Pinheiro, S.R. Silveira, I., Caliari, K.M. and Yoshinari, N.H. 2010. Survey for tick-borne zoonoses in the State of Espirito Santo, Southeastern Brazil. Am. J. Trop. Med. Hyg. 83, 201-206.

Spolidorio, M.G., Minervino, A.H., Valadas, S.Y., Soares, H.S., Neves, K.A., Labruna, M.B., Ribeiro, M.F. and Gennari, S.M. 2013. Serosurvey for tick-borne diseases in dogs from the Eastern Amazon, Brazil. Rev. Bras. Parasitol. Vet. 22, 214-219.

SPSS Inc. Released 2008. SPSS Statistics for Windows, Version 17.0. Chicago: SPSS Inc.

Tennant, K.V., Barker, E.N., Polizopoulou, Z., Helps, C.R. and Tasker, S. 2011. Real-time quantitative polymerase chain reaction detection of haemoplasmas in healthy and unhealthy dogs from Central Macedonia, Greece. J. Small Anim. Pract. 52, 645-649.

Valle, S.F., Messick, J.B., dos Santos, A.P., Kreutz, L.C., Duda, N.C., Machado, G., Corbellini, L.G., Biondo, A.W. and González, F.H. 2014. Identification, occurrence and clinical findings of canine hemoplasmas in southern Brazil. Comp. Immunol. Microbiol. Infect. Dis. 37, 259-265.

Vieira, R.F., Vieira, T.S., Nascimento, D.A., Martins, T.F., Krawczak, F.S., Labruna, M.B., Chandrashekar, R., Marcondes, M., Biondo, A.W. and Vidotto, O. 2013a. Serological survey of *Ehrlichia* species in dogs, horses and humans: zoonotic scenery in a rural settlement from southern

Brazil. Rev. Inst. Med. Trop. São Paulo 55, 335-340.

Vieira, R.F., Vidotto, O., Vieira, T.S., Guimarães, A.M., Santos, A.P., Nascimento, N.C., Santos, N.J., Martins, T.F., Labruna, M.B., Marcondes, M., Biondo, W.B. and Messick, J.B. 2015. Molecular investigation of hemotropic mycoplasmas in human beings, dogs and horses in a rural settlement in southern Brazil. Rev. Inst. Med. Trop. São Paulo 57, 353-357.

Vieira, T.S., Vieira, R.F., Nascimento, D.A., Tamekuni, K., Toledo, R.S., Chandrashekar, R., Marcondes, M., Biondo, A.W. and Vidotto, O. 2013b. Serosurvey of tick-borne pathogens in dogs from urban and rural areas from Parana State, Brazil. Rev. Bras. Parasitol. Vet. 22, 104-109.

WHO/WSPA. 1990. World Health Organization/ World Society for the Protection of Animals. Guidelines for dog population management. World Health Organization, Geneva.

20

Metastatic intraocular hemangiopericytoma in a dog

Jonathan D. Pucket[1,*], Rachel A. Allbaugh[2], Mary L. Higginbotham[3], Amy J. Rankin[3] and Leandro Teixeira[4]

[1]Department of Veterinary Clinical Sciences, College of Veterinary Health Sciences, Oklahoma State University, Stillwater, OK 74078, USA
[2]Department of Veterinary Clinical Sciences, College of Veterinary Medicine, Iowa State University, Ames, IA 50011, USA
[3]Department of Clinical Science, College of Veterinary Medicine, Kansas State University, Manhattan, KS 66506, USA
[4]Department of Pathological Sciences, College of Veterinary Medicine, University of Wisconsin-Madison, WI 53706, USA

Abstract

A 10-year-old Labrador Retriever who had been undergoing therapy for a recurrent hemangiopericytoma of the right flank presented to the Kansas State University Ophthalmology service for evaluation of a painful left eye. Examination revealed secondary glaucoma and irreversible blindness of the affected eye and multifocal chorioretinal lesions in the fellow eye. Therapeutic and diagnostic enucleation of the left eye was performed and histopathologic examination demonstrated the presence of a presumed metastatic spindle cell sarcoma. Further immunohistochemical staining confirmed the intraocular neoplasia to be metastatic spread from the previously removed flank mass. Rapid progression in size and number of chorioretinal lesions in the right eye was noted in the post-operative period until the patient was euthanized one month after surgery. This case report is the first to document intraocular metastasis of hemangiopericytoma in a veterinary patient.

Keywords: Glaucoma, Hemangiopericytoma, Metastasis.

Introduction

Malignant tumors can originate throughout the body, yet despite the well vascularized nature of the uveal tract metastasis to the ocular tissues is not a common occurrence. Lymphoma is the most common of those tumors which have been noted to spread to the eye (Hendrix, 2013). Less commonly documented intraocular metastatic neoplasms include melanoma, hemangiosarcoma, malignant histiocytosis, adenocarcinoma, osteosarcoma, transitional cell carcinoma, and others (Szymanski, 1972; Schmidt, 1981; Render et al., 1982; Szymanski et al., 1984; Habin and Elsa, 1995; Esson et al., 2007; Naranjo et al., 2007; Mowat et al., 2012).

Patients with metastatic ocular neoplasia may present with systemic signs attributable to the disease or may only have observable ophthalmic signs. Although possibly asymmetric in presentation, metastatic neoplasia is more likely to affect both eyes than primary tumors (Hendrix, 2013).

This case report is the first to describe metastatic spread of hemangiopericytoma to both eyes of a dog.

Case Details

A 10 year old, male neutered Labrador Retriever was referred to the ophthalmology service at Kansas State University's College of Veterinary Medicine due to left sided ocular discomfort, diffuse corneal edema, and possible vision loss. The patient was undergoing radiation therapy for a recurrent subcutaneous right flank mass, diagnosed as a hemangiopericytoma.

The original mass was removed from the right hip 18 months prior to presentation and on histopathology presented as a poorly delineated and infiltrative neoplastic tissue, partially effacing the superficial and deep dermis and composed of spindled to round cells with small amounts of pale or eosinophilic cytoplasm, indistinct cell borders and bland vesicular nuclei, arranged in streams and bundles forming variably ectatic or compressed, thin walled branching vascular channels.

Despite multiple surgical resections and complete excision according to histopathologic evaluation, the mass continued to recur subcutaneously in the right flank region. Based on the recurrence of the mass in the face of multiple resections, radiation therapy following excision and skin grafting was performed. Routine examination 4 months after radiation therapy showed a new subcutaneous mass in the right flank and multiple pulmonary nodules visible on computerized tomography (CT) scan. Two weeks after diagnosis of the pulmonary nodules the ocular signs became evident.

*Corresponding Author: Jonathan D. Pucket. Department of Veterinary Clinical Sciences, College of Veterinary Health Sciences, Oklahoma State University, Stillwater, OK 74078, USA. Email: jonathanpucket@gmail.com

Ophthalmic examination revealed slight blepharospasm and epiphora of the left eye (OS) along with an elevated third eyelid. No pain or significant adnexal abnormalities were noted in the right eye (OD) except for a single distichia dorsally. Menace response and dazzle reflexes were present OD but were both absent OS. Direct pupillary light response was present OD and absent OS. A consensual pupillary light response was not noted in either eye. Severe conjunctival hyperemia and moderate episcleral injection were noted OS. Fluorescein staining was negative in both eyes for epithelial defects. Intraocular pressures measured by rebound tonometry (TonoVet®; Jorgensen Labs, Loveland, CO) were 6 and 60 mmHg OD and OS respectively.

On biomicroscopic examination (Kowa SL-15; Kowa Company, Tokyo, Japan) the cornea of the OS had moderate diffuse corneal edema making it difficult to visualize intraocular structures in detail, however, a dyscoric and relatively miotic pupil were detectable as well as a diffusely swollen and reddened iris profile. Extensive posterior synechia and iris swelling contributed to the dyscoria OS and structures posterior to the pupil could not be visualized. Examination of the cornea and anterior segment of the OD was unremarkable. Nuclear sclerosis was present OD as well as a ventromedial pinpoint anterior cortical incipient cataract and mild anterior vitreal syneresis. Upon indirect ophthalmoscopic examination (Vantage Plus Wireless, Keeler Instrument Inc, Bromall, PA) of the OD, multifocal lesions in the tapetal fundus were noted and photodocumented (RetCam Shuttle; Clarity Medical Systems, Pleasanton, CA) (Fig. 1A and 1B).

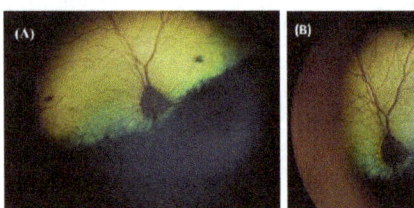

Fig. 1. Presence of chorioretinal lesions in the tapetal fundus OD noted on initial presentation. Images represent central view **(A)** and a view angled to highlight the largest chorioretinal lesion **(B)**. Multifocal pink lesions are noted throughout the tapetal fundus arising from the termination of retinal vessels representing metastatic spread of the hemangiopericytoma. Images obtained with the RetCam Shuttle.

The largest lesion was raised, pale pink in color, one optic nerve head in diameter and located dorsomedial to the optic disc arising at the termination of a retinal vessel. Other smaller lesions appeared multifocally throughout the tapetal fundus as pinpoint reddish-pink colored lesions near the termination of retinal vessels, some of which could not be differentiated from retinal

hemorrhages. Based on the clinical evidence, secondary glaucoma of the OS was diagnosed as well as suspected chorioretinal metastatic disease lesions OD.

Enucleation of the painful globe OS was recommended in order to provide comfort as well as diagnostic benefit through histopathology. Preoperative blood work was obtained and no significant abnormalities were noted. On physical examination, the patient was bright, alert and responsive as well as mildly overweight. No significant abnormalities were detected on thoracic auscultation or complete physical examination other than mild dental calculus, bilateral coxofemoral pain, and a 2 x 3 x 2 cm right flank subcutaneous mass. Fine needle aspirates of the subcutaneous mass performed five weeks prior revealed a spindle cell population with features of malignancy suggestive of a sarcoma. The left globe was removed using a transconjunctival approach and the patient recovered uneventfully. After removal, the globe was immersion fixed in 10% neutral buffered formalin and submitted to the Comparative Ocular Pathology Laboratory of Wisconsin for histopathologic evaluation.

Histopathology revealed a population of neoplastic spindle cells arranged in streams and bundles carpeting the surfaces of the iris and ciliary body, infiltrating and expanding the tapetal choroid and multifocally invading the choroidal vessels (Fig. 2A and 2B). The cells presented indistinct cell borders, small amounts of eosinophilic cytoplasm and oval to elongated nuclei with usually a large and central magenta nucleolus. Mitotic figures were common averaging 6 per high power field and cellular pleomorphism was marked with multiple karyomegalic cells. Neoplastic cells were also found to extend within scleral blood vessels (Fig. 2C). Notable secondary ocular lesions were posterior synechia, retinal detachment and secondary glaucoma, characterized by loss of ganglion cells and gliosis of the optic nerve head. The pattern of distribution of the neoplastic cells within the globe, with cells carpeting ocular surfaces and multifocally infiltrating the uveal tissue along with the presence of neoplastic cells in blood vessels was strongly suggestive of a metastatic disease. Sections of the previously excised flank hemangiopericytoma and the left globe were selected for immunohistochemistry to determine if the intraocular mass was metastatic or a separate neoplastic process. Sections were stained using the following antibodies: Skeletal muscle actin (mouse anti-sarcomeric actin, clone alpha-Sr-1, 1:150 dilution, Dako, Carpinteria, CA), Vimentin (mouse anti-vimentin, clone V9, 1:200, Dako), Alpha-smooth muscle actin (mouse anti–alpha smooth muscle actin, clone 1A4, 1:1000, Dako), S-100 (rabbit anti–S100 protein, 1:2500, Dako), CD31 (mouse anti-CD31, 1:40, Dako) and CD34 (mouse anti-CD34, 1:50, Dako).

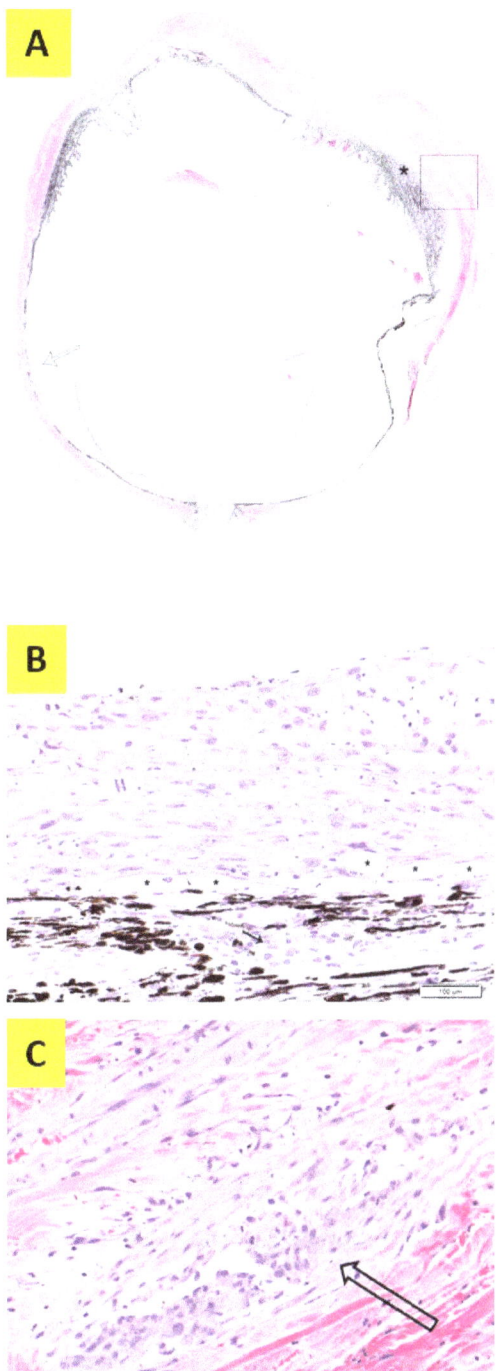

Fig. 2. (A): Metastatic spindle cell sarcoma. Subgross photograph. Note the carpet of neoplastic cells in the choroid (arrow) and in the ciliary body (*). Hematoxylin and eosin (H&E). **(B):** Tumor in the choroid. Higher magnification of the neoplastic cells near the arrow in Fig. 2A. Cells infiltrate the tapetum (*) and surround choroidal vessels (arrow). (H&E) (Bar = 100 μm). **(C):** Tumor in the scleral vessels. Higher magnification of the square in Fig. 2A. Cells surround and infiltrate scleral vessels (arrow). (H&E). (Bar = 100 μm).

The results of the immunohistochemical staining showed perfect alignment in staining patterns in that the two separate masses were vimentin, alpha-smooth muscle actin and CD34 positive, while negative for skeletal muscle actin, S-100 and CD31 (Fig. 3). Together with the microscopic features of the flank mass (fusiform cells forming irregular vascular channels with a staghorn pattern) the immunohistochemical staining pattern confirmed the diagnosis of hemangioperycitoma and a metastatic spread of the right flank neoplasm to the eye in this case (Avallone et al., 2007).

The patient returned two weeks after surgery for routine enucleation site suture removal. Upon exam of the OD fluorescein staining was negative, the intraocular pressure was 5 mmHg, the direct pupillary light reflex was positive and a menace response was present. Despite the lower intraocular pressure, there was no evidence of blepharospasm, epiphora, conjunctival hyperemia, miosis, or aqueous flare on her exam.

No changes in the lenticular opacities were observed, however, fundic examination revealed that the chorioretinal lesions had progressed significantly in size and number throughout the tapetal fundus (Fig. 4). Perilesional retinal detachments were identified around the larger pink colored lesions. Despite disease progression, the patient remained comfortable and visual. Prophylactic topical anti-inflammatory and topical anti-glaucoma therapy were discussed with the owner given the previous progression OD and previous sequelae OS but were declined. Five days after suture removal the patient presented for acute blepharospasm and epiphora of the OD. Fluorescein staining was negative and the intraocular pressure was 6 mmHg. A small fibrin clot was noted on the anterior surface of the lens capsule axially along with a trace amount of aqueous flare. No significant progression of the chorioretinal lesions was detected. The patient was started on 1% topical ophthalmic prednisolone acetate suspension (Falcon Pharmaceuticals, Hünenberg, Switzerland) every 8 hours as well as 2.2 mg/kg of oral carprofen (Rimadyl; Pfizer Inc, New York, NY) every twelve hours. In addition, despite a low but seemingly normal intraocular pressure, topical 2% dorzolamide (Dorzolamide HCL 2% ophthalmic solution; Hi-Tech Pharmacal Co, Amityville, NY) solution was instituted every 8 hours OD given previous progression to secondary glaucoma OS. A recheck was scheduled for 1 week. Three days later the patient presented on emergency for difficulty urinating and a gallop rhythm was asculted on physical exam. Radiographs showed multiple small cystic and urethral calculi, slight enlargement of the previously noted pulmonary nodules, and right sided cardiac enlargement.

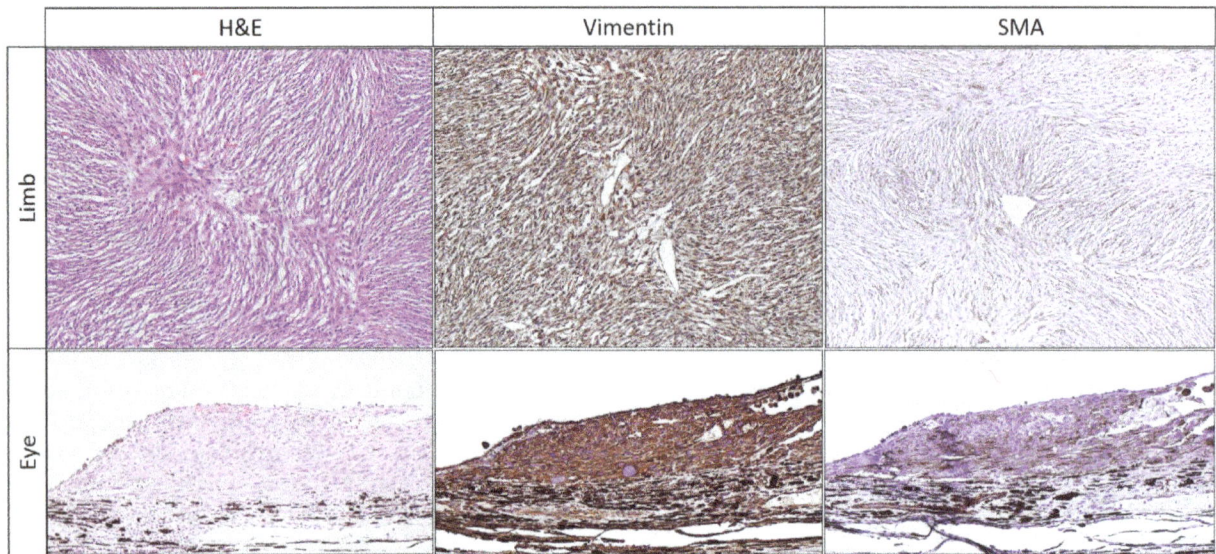

	H&E	Vimentin	SMA
Limb			
Eye			

Fig. 3. Immunohistochemical staining of both the original right flank/limb hemangiopericytoma and the left eye metastasis. Both tissues show positive staining for vimentin and alpha-smooth muscle actin (SMA).

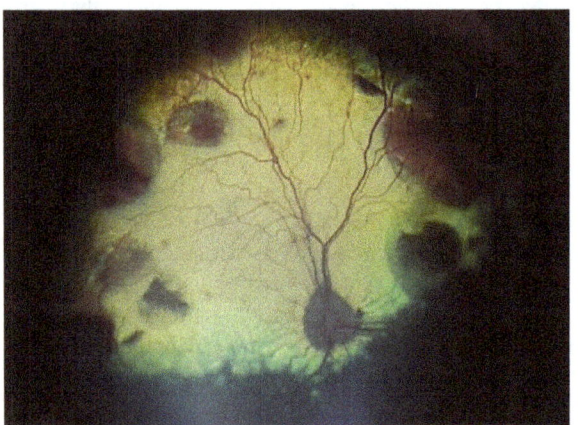

Fig. 4. Image of right tapetal fundus two weeks after initial presentation. The presence of numerous large pink/red colored lesions throughout tapetal fundus present near retinal vessel terminations showing significant progression of chorioretinal lesions. Perilesional retinal elevations are seen around each foci of metastasis and appear as halos of reduced reflectivity. Image obtained with the RetCam Shuttle.

On echocardiogram, a 5x3 cm heteroechoic mass was noted arising from the right atrium and extending into the auricle with moderate pericardial effusion but no cardiac tamponade. Due to the extensive nature and poor prognosis, the patient had a urethral catheter placed and was discharged for palliative care by the owner and referring veterinarian. One week later the patient was euthanized. A postmortem examination was not performed and no tissues were available for evaluation.

Discussion

Perivascular wall tumor is a term used to describe the grouping of soft tissue sarcomas which have origins in the structural and supportive cells of blood vessels (Avallone *et al.*, 2007).

Hemangiopericytoma refers to a sub-category of perivascular wall tumors and is a rare vascular tumor that is thought to arise from mesenchymal cells which coat capillaries and post capillary venules, known as pericytes of Zimmerman. This type of tumor was first described by Stout and Murray (1942).

Since the initial manuscript there have been numerous reports documenting this tumor in humans and various veterinary species (Mulligan, 1955; Enzinger and Smith, 1976; Richardson *et al.*, 1983; Boniuk *et al.*, 1985; Fossum *et al.*, 1988; Graves *et al.*, 1988; Mitarai *et al.*, 1998; Beltran *et al.*, 2001; McCaw *et al.*, 2001; Serena *et al.*, 2006; Silva *et al.*, 2014).

Most commonly, hemangiopericytoma is reported in dogs, of which it accounts for around 3-4% of all cutaneous neoplasia (Graves *et al.*, 1988). The tumors are reported to be well circumscribed initially with a pseudocapsule covering the mass (Henderson and Farrow, 1978; Sujatha *et al.*, 1994) and attached to deeper structures with freely movable skin over the surface (Caniatti *et al.*, 2001). If the pseudocapsule is breached during surgery or incomplete excision is noted, extensive local regrowth and metastasis can be seen (Shimura *et al.*, 2001).

Proper diagnosis of hemangiopericytomas can be challenging from a histopathologic standpoint and recent investigations show that many previous cases diagnosed as such may actually represent one of a spectrum of perivascular wall tumors (Avallone *et al.*, 2007; Palmieri *et al.*, 2013). The originally described microscopic pattern of a hemangiopericytoma consisted of concentric layers of spindle cells arranged around a central vessel which was devoid of erythrocytes, known as a "fingerprint, staghorn, or onion skin pattern" (Perez et al., 1996). This pattern is often lacking and non-specific as it can even be found in other types of vascularized soft-tissue neoplasms (Pantekoek and Schiefer, 1975).

Definitive diagnosis requires immunohistochemical staining or electron microscopy to differentiate hemangiopericytoma from other soft tissue sarcomas (Avallone et al., 2007; Palmieri et al., 2013). Previous reports have tried to elucidate the immunoreactivity patterns to aide differentiation. Hemangiopericytoma cells stain positive for vimentin and CD 34, owing to their mesenchymal and endothelial cell derivation respectively (Perez et al., 1996; Middleton et al., 1998). Staining for S-100 and CD 31 are negative, proving the neoplasms are not of peripheral nerve, melanocyte, granular cell, macrophage, or monocyte origin (Middleton et al., 1998). Staining for muscle actins can be variable depending on their location and if describing human or canine hemangiopericytoma. While canine hemangiopericytomas express muscle actins, human hemangiopericytomas are lacking this trait. This means that the human neoplasia counterpart either loses the expression during differentiation, or the cell of origin is not a true pericyte (Porter et al., 1991; Perez et al., 1996).

In dogs, the expression or not of α-smooth muscle actin depends on whether the tumor formed from capillary or arteriolar and venular pericytes (Herman and D'amore, 1985; Schürch et al., 1987). Alpha-smooth muscle actin is expressed in hemangiopericytomas that arise from arteriolar or venular pericytes and non-smooth muscle actin isoforms are derived from those of capillary origin (Herman and D'amore, 1985). This explains the variable staining noted in hemangiopericytomas with regard to α-smooth muscle actin. In our case, both the original flank mass and the intraocular metastasis lesions were in perfect alignment with regard to reported hemangiopericytoma immunohistochemical staining patterns, confirming the diagnosis.

Hemangiopericytomas tend to develop on distal extremities of older dogs and have a slow growth rate (Mulligan, 1955; Graves et al., 1988; Mazzei et al., 2002).

In humans, common locations for development of hemangiopericytoma are the thigh and pelvic retroperitoneal regions (Enzinger and Smith, 1976; Lee et al., 2003). Average age at the time masses are observed in dogs is around 10 years, with a range of 2-14 years (Graves et al., 1988; Caniatti et al., 2001; Namazi et al., 2014).

The frequency of metastasis is presumed to be low based on available cases, but local recurrence is high due to the infiltrative nature of the mass (Yost and Jones, 1958; Handharyani et al., 1999). Recurrence

rates after excision approximate 40% even if all grossly visible tumor has been removed (Graves et al., 1988). A statistically significant difference has not been shown between simple excision, excision with orthovoltage radiation, and excision with subsequent photodynamic therapy (Graves et al., 1988; McCaw et al., 2001).

Seven previous canine cases have been recognized to have metastasized, and of those the lungs and lymph nodes were sites of spread (Handharyani et al., 1999; Silva et al., 2014). In humans, the rate of metastasis has been reported to be as high as 50%, with spread to the lungs, liver, and bones occurring most frequently (Johnson, 1976). The reason for the low rate of metastasis in dogs as compared to humans has not been determined.

In humans, hemangiopericytoma is very rarely found in or around the eye with the majority of cases being retrobulbar in origin (Henderson and Farrow, 1978; Karcioglu et al., 1997; Lee et al., 2003; Manjandavida et al., 2013). Other reported locations include the lacrimal sac, optic nerve, conjunctiva, and eyelids (Boniuk et al., 1985; Grossniklaus et al., 1986; Sujatha et al., 1994; Charles et al., 1998; Parmar and Rose, 2003; Schwent et al., 2007). There have been only 5 cases of intraocular hemangiopericytoma reported to date (Papale et al., 1983; Gieser et al., 1988; Brown et al., 1991; Toth et al., 1996; Shimura et al., 2001). Of these most were considered primary lesions, however, metastatic spread from another primary location was not completely ruled out.

In veterinary patients, the reported incidence of ocular hemangiopericytoma is also low with only 2 reported cases. The first was a presumed orbital hemangiopericytoma in a seven year old mixed-breed dog presenting with progressive unilateral exophthalmos (Beltran et al., 2001). The tumor was diagnosed by histopathologic evaluation after removal, however immunohistochemical staining was not performed to differentiate from peripheral nerve sheath tumors or other soft tissue sarcomas. The other ocular hemangiopericytoma was documented in an eyelid of a fourteen year old Arabian horse (Serena et al., 2006). The mass had been present for two years but then rapidly increased in size, prompting exam and removal. The diagnosis was confirmed through immunohistochemical staining of excised tissue. One year after removal, no recurrence of the mass or spread was noted.

To the authors' knowledge, the case reported here is the first to document presumed intraocular metastatic spread of a perivascular wall tumor in a veterinary patient.

Unlike previously reported ocular manifestations, the hemangiopericytoma in our case progressed rapidly. The findings of a right sided heart mass and the suspected pulmonary metastatic lesions during the course of diagnosis and therapy are interesting but the significance is not known as diagnostic samples were never obtained.

In addition, a post mortem examination was not performed and so any attempt to correlate these to the primary hemangiopericytoma would be unfounded and only the ocular metastasis lesions were confirmed. Intraocular metastasis may represent a late stage of progression with hemangiopericytoma or could signal a more aggressive tumor as evidenced by the very short survival time of this patient after recognized intraocular spread.

Conflict of Interest

The Authors declare no conflict of interest.

References

Avallone, G., Helmbold, P., Caniatti, M., Stefanello, D., Nayak, R. and Roccabianca, P. 2007. The spectrum of canine cutaneous perivascular wall tumors: morphologic, phenotypic and clinical characterization. Vet. Pathol. 44, 607-620.

Beltran, W.A., Colle, M., Boulouha, L., Daude-Lagrave, A., Moissonnier, P. and Clerc, B. 2001. A case of orbital hemangiopericytoma in a dog. Vet. Ophthalmol. 4, 255-259.

Boniuk, M., Messmer, E. and Font, R. 1985. Hemangiopericytoma of the meninges of the optic nerve. A clinicopathologic report including electron microscopic observations. Ophthalmol. 92, 1780-1787.

Brown, H., Brodsky, M., Hembree, K. and Mrak, R. 1991. Supraciliary hemangiopericytoma. Ophthalmol. 98, 378-382.

Caniatti, M., Ghisleni, G., Ceruti, R., Roccabianca, P. and Scanziani, E. 2001. Cytological features of canine haemangiopericytoma in fine needle aspiration biopsy. Vet. Rec. 149, 242-244.

Charles, N., Palu, R. and Jagirdar, J. 1998. Hemangiopericytoma of the lacrimal sac. Arch. Ophthalmol. 116, 1677-1680.

Enzinger, F. and Smith, B 1976. Hemangiopericytoma. An analysis of 106 cases. Hum. Pathol. 7, 61-82.

Esson, D., Fahrer, C., Zarfoss, M. and Dubielzig, R. 2007. Suspected uveal metastasis of a nail bed melanoma in a dog. Vet. Ophthalmol. 10, 262-266.

Fossum, T., Couto, C., DeHoff, W. and Smeak, D. 1988. Treatment of hemangiopericytoma in a dog using surgical excision, radiation, and a thoracic pedicle skin graft. J. Am. Vet. Med. Assoc. 193, 1440-1442.

Gieser, S., Hufnagel, T., Jaros, P., MacRae, D. and Khodadoust, A. 1988. Hemangiopericytoma of the ciliary body. Arch. Ophthalmol. 106, 1269-1272.

Graves, G., Bjorling, D. and Mahaffey, E. 1988. Canine hemangiopericytoma: 23 cases (1967-1984). J. Am. Vet. Med. Assoc. 192, 99-102.

Grossniklaus, H., Green, W., Wolff, S. and Iliff, N. 1986. Hemangiopericytoma of the conjunctiva. Two cases. Ophthalmol. 93, 265-267.

Habin, D. and Else, R. 1995. Parotid salivary gland adenocarcinoma with bilateral ocular and osseous metastases in a dog. J Small Anim Pract 36, 445-449.

Handharyani, E., Ochiai, K, Kadosawa, T., Kimura, T. and Umemura, T. 1999. Canine hemangiopericytoma: an evaluation of metastatic potential. J. Vet. Diag. Invest. 11, 474-478.

Henderson, J. and Farrow, G. 1978. Primary orbital hemangiopericytoma. An aggressive and potentially malignant neoplasm. Arch. Ophthalmol. 96, 666-673.

Hendrix, D. 2013. Diseases and surgery of the canine anterior uvea. Veterinary Ophthalmology. Gelatt, K.N., B.C. Gilger and T.J. Kern. Ames, IA, John Wiley & Sons, pp: 1146-1198.

Herman, I. and D'amore, P. 1985. Microvascular pericytes contain muscle and nonmuscle actins. J. Cell Biol. 101, 43-52.

Johnson, C. 1976. Pathology of cutaneous vascular tumors. Int. J. Dermatol. 15, 256-259.

Karcioglu, Z., Nasr, A. and Haik, B. 1997. Orbital hemangiopericytoma: clinical and morphologic features. Am. J. Ophthalmol. 124, 661-672.

Lee, Y., Wang, J. and Shyu, J. 2003. Orbital hemangiopericytoma-a case report. The Kaohsiung J. Med. Sci. 19, 33-37.

Manjandavida, F., Honavar, S., Gowrishankar, S., Mulay, K., Reddy, V. and Vemuganti, G. 2013. Optic nerve meningeal hemangiopericytoma: a clinicopathologic case report. Surv. Ophthalmol. 58, 341-347.

Mazzei, M., Millanta, F., Citi, S., Lorenzi, D. and Poli, A. 2002. Hemangiopericytoma: histological spectrum, immunohistochemical characterization and prognosis. Vet. Dermatol. 13, 15-21.

McCaw, D., Payne, J., Pope, E., West, M., Tompson, R. and Tate, D. 2001. Treatment of canine hemangiopericytomas with photodynamic therapy. Lasers Surg. Med. 29, 23-26.

Middleton, L., Duray, P. and Merino, M. 1998. The histological spectrum of hemangiopericytoma: application of immunohistochemical analysis including proliferative markers to facilitate diagnosis and predict prognosis. Hum. Pathol. 29, 636-640.

Mitarai, Y., Ishikawa, Y. and Kadota, K. 1998. Hemangiopericytoma in a calf. Res. Vet. Sci. 65, 265-267.

Mowat, F., Langohr, I., Bilyk, O., Koterbay, A., Pierce, K. and Petersen-Jones, S. 2012. Bilateral uveal metastasis of a subcutaneous fibrosarcoma in a cat. Vet. Ophthalmol. 15, 391-397.

Mulligan, R. M. 1955. Hemangiopericytoma in the dog. Am. J. Pathol. 31, 773-789.

Namazi, F., Abbaszadeh Hasiri, M., Oryan, A. and Moshiri, A. 2014. Hemangiopericytoma in a young dog: Evaluation of histopathological and immunohistochemical features. Vet. Res. Forum 5, 157-160.

Naranjo, C., Dubielzig, R. and Friedrichs, K. 2007. Canine ocular histiocytic sarcoma. Vet. Ophthalmol. 10, 179-185.

Palmieri, C., Avallone, G., Cimini, M., Roccabianca, P., Stefanello, D. and Salda, L. 2013. Use of electron microscopy to classify canine perivascular wall tumors. Vet. Pathol. 50, 226-233.

Pantekoek, J. and Schiefer, B. 1975. Metastasising canine fibrosarcoma originally diagnosed as haemangiopericytoma. J. Small Anim. Pract. 16, 259-265.

Papale, J., Frederick, A. and Albert, D. 1983. Intraocular hemangiopericytoma. Arch. Ophthalmol. 101, 1409-1411.

Parmar, D. and Rose, G. 2003. Management of lacrimal sac tumours. Eye (London) 17, 599-606.

Perez, J., Bautista, M., Rollón, E., de Lara, F., Carrasco, L. and Martin de las Mulas, J. 1996. Immunohistochemical characterization of hemangiopericytomas and other spindle cell tumors in the dog. Vet. Pathol. 33, 391-397.

Porter, P., Bigler, S., McNutt, M. and Gown, A. 1991. The immunophenotype of hemangiopericytomas and glomus tumors, with special reference to muscle protein expression: an immunohistochemical study and review of the literature. Mod. Pathol. 4, 46-52.

Render, J., Carlton, W., Vestre, W. and Hoerr, F. 1982. Osteosarcoma metastatic to the globes in a dog. Vet. Pathol. 19, 323-326.

Richardson, R., Render, J., Rudd, R., Shupe, R. and Carlton, W. 1983. Metastatic canine hemangiopericytoma. J. Am. Vet. Med. Assoc. 182, 705-706.

Schmidt, R.E. 1981. Transitional cell carcinoma metastatic to the eye of a dog. Vet. Pathol. 18, 832-834.

Schürch, W., Skalli, O., Seemayer, T. and Gabbiani, G. 1987. Intermediate filament proteins and actin isoforms as markers for soft tissue tumor differentiation and origin. I. Smooth muscle tumors. Am. J. Pathol. 128, 91.

Schwent, B., Wojno, T. and Grossniklaus, H. 2007. Hemangiopericytoma of the optic nerve sheath. Am. J. Ophthalmol. 143, 904-906.

Serena, A., Joiner, K. and Schumacher, J. 2006. Hemangiopericytoma in the eyelid of a horse. Vet. Pathol. 43, 576-578.

Shimura, M., Suzuki, K., Fuse, N., Yoshida, M., Saiki, Y., Ohtani, H. and Tamai, M. 2001. Intraocular hemangiopericytoma. A case report. Ophthalmologica 215, 378-382.

Silva, E., Romero, F., Green, K., Martins, M. and Bracarense, A. 2014. Hemangiopericytoma in a female dog with direct invasion of abdominal cavity and pulmonary metastasis. Ciênc 44, 358-361.

Stout, A. and Murray, M. 1942. Hemangiopericytoma: a vascular tumor featuring Zimmerman's pericytes. Ann. Surg. 116, 22-33.

Sujatha, S., Sampath, R., Bonshek, R. and Tullo, A. 1994. Conjunctival haemangiopericytoma. Br. J. Ophthalmol. 78, 497-499.

Szymanski, C., Boyce, R. and Wyman, M. 1984. Transitional cell carcinoma of the urethra metastatic to the eyes in a dog. J. Am. Vet. Med. Assoc. 185, 1003-1004.

Szymanski, C.M. 1972. Bilateral metastatic intraocular hemangiosarcoma in a dog. J. Am. Vet. Med. Assoc. 161, 803-805.

Toth, J., Kerenyi, A., Suveges, I. and Futo, G. 1996. Leiomyoma of the ciliary body and hemangiopericytoma of the choroid. Pathol. Oncol. Res. 2, 89-93.

Yost, D. and Jones, T. 1958. Hemangiopericytoma in the dog. Am. J. Vet. Res. 19, 159-163.

21

Laryngeal paralysis associated with a muscle pseudotumour in a young dog

Francesca Rizzo[1,*], Cecilia Benetti[1], Consuelo Ballatori[1] and Diana Binanti[2]

[1]Clinica Veterinaria Colombo, Viale Colombo 153, 55041, Lido di Camaiore (LU), Italy
[2]AbLab, Laboratorio di Analisi Veterinarie, Sarzana (SP), 19038, Italy

Abstract
An 18-month-old male entire Bloodhound dog was presented with a six-week history of progressive inspiratory dyspnoea, stridor, dysphonia and exercise intolerance. CT scan performed elsewhere had revealed the presence of an unencapsulated nodular mass (3x1x5 cm) dorsal to the larynx and first tracheal rings. Laryngoscopy demonstrated the presence of bilateral laryngeal paralysis and distorted laryngeal architecture suggestive of extraluminal compression. Histopathology results of incisional biopsies from the mass were suggestive of a benign non-neoplastic muscular lesion. Surgery was performed to manage laryngeal paralysis and attempt mass excision. A second histopathology examination confirmed an inflammatory and dysplastic lesion suggestive of a pseudotumour. All clinical signs resolved after surgery and at the 13 months follow-up the dog remains asymptomatic. To the authors' knowledge, this is the first report of a case of laryngeal paralysis caused by a muscle pseudotumour in a young dog.
Keywords: Dog, Laryngeal paralysis, Larynx, Muscle pseudotumour.

Introduction
Muscle pseudotumours are benign non-neoplastic lesions arising from the skeletal muscle (Cooper and Valentine, 2002; The Armed Forces Institute of Pathology, 2007). They have been reported in humans (Gude *et al.*, 2011; Segawa *et al.*, 2014) and occasionally in animals (Cooper and Valentine, 2002; van der Woerdt, 2008; Knight *et al.*, 2009; Loderstedt *et al.*, 2010). Aetiology of muscle pseudotumours remains unknown, although several hypotheses have been postulated. Laryngeal paralysis (LP) in dogs is the most common disease involving the larynx (MacPhail, 2014) and a frequent cause of upper respiratory obstruction and dyspnoea in large breed dogs. Acquired LP is most commonly reported in older dogs. It can be idiopathic or it may result from trauma, neuromuscular disease, iatrogenic injury or mass-related compression of the recurrent laryngeal nerve (Millard and Tobias, 2009). This paper describes clinical presentation, diagnosis, treatment and follow-up of a case of LP caused by a muscle pseudotumour in an 18-month-old Bloodhound dog.

Case Details
An 18-month-old, 47 kg, male entire, Bloodhound was presented with a six-week history of progressive inspiratory dyspnoea, stridor, dysphonia and exercise intolerance. The dog had been submitted to medical therapy by previous vets with amoxicillin-clavulanic acid (Synulox; Pfizer), cephalexin (ICFVET; ICF), carprofen (Rimadyl; Pfizer) and prednisone (Deltacortene; Bruno Farmaceutici SPA) without significant clinical improvement. Previous CT scan investigation of the neck region performed by primary veterinary surgeon had revealed the presence of a space-occupying lesion 3x1x5 cm dorso-lateral to the trachea (Fig. 1).

On presentation the dog appeared bright and alert, and in good body condition. Tachypnoea, increased inspiratory effort and stridors were evident and more pronounced when the dog was excited. Remaining clinical examination was unremarkable, as was neurological examination and thorough palpation of the region of the neck, pharynx and larynx. Haematology, full serum biochemistry profile, thyroid profile and coagulation times were all within normal range. Thoracic radiographs and abdominal ultrasound were performed to rule out the presence of additional masses and did not reveal any significant findings. Direct and indirect laryngoscopy and tracheoscopy were performed under appropriate light anaesthesia. Propofol (Proposure; Merial Italia SpA) was slowly titrated intravenously in order to maintain spontaneous breathing and allow inspection of the larynx. These investigations revealed the presence of bilateral laryngeal paralysis; diffuse laryngeal oedema was also present, which extended to the proximal section of the trachea. The rima glottidis appeared of abnormal shape due to severe dorso-lateral compression suggestive of the presence of an extraluminal space-occupying mass at the right side (Fig. 2). The trachea was otherwise normal. Three incisional biopsies of the mass were obtained via a right lateral surgical approach to the neck region just dorsal to the larynx, facilitating direct visualisation of the area involved.

*Corresponding Author: Francesca Rizzo. Clinica Veterinaria Colombo, Viale Colombo 153, 55041, Lido di Camaiore (LU), Italy. Email: *frabristol@yahoo.it*

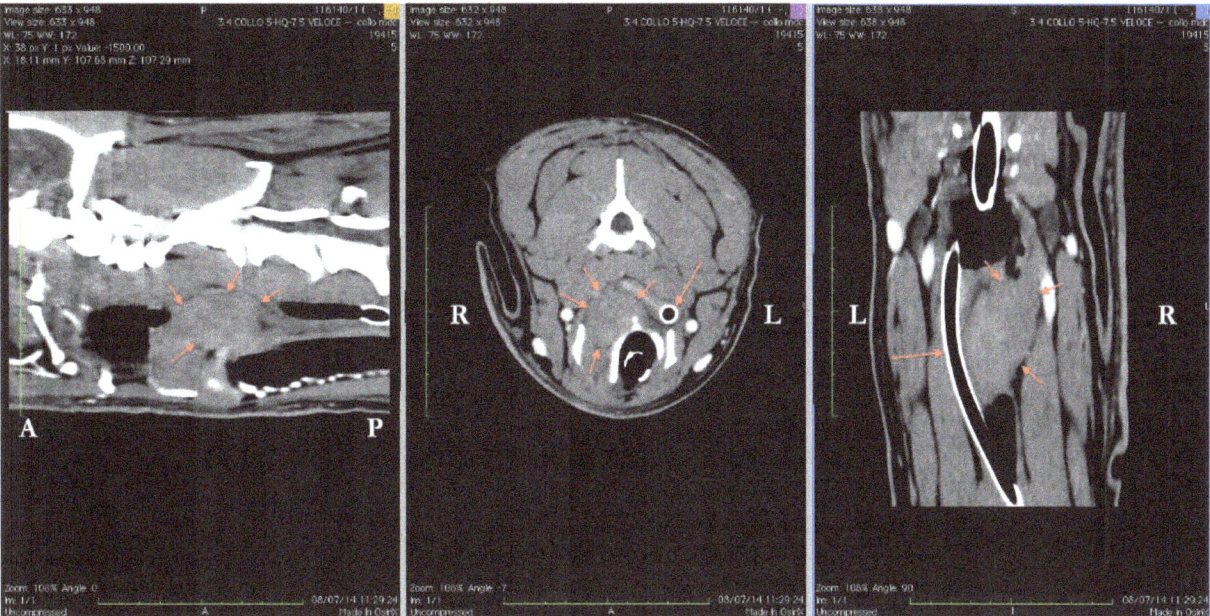

Fig. 1. CT scan images (from left to right: sagittal, transverse and dorsal plane): the mass-type lesion (short arrows) extends dorsally to the first tracheal rings and larynx, causing right lateral deviation of the proximal trachea and oesophagus; the deviation of the intraoesophageal tube appears evident (long arrows).

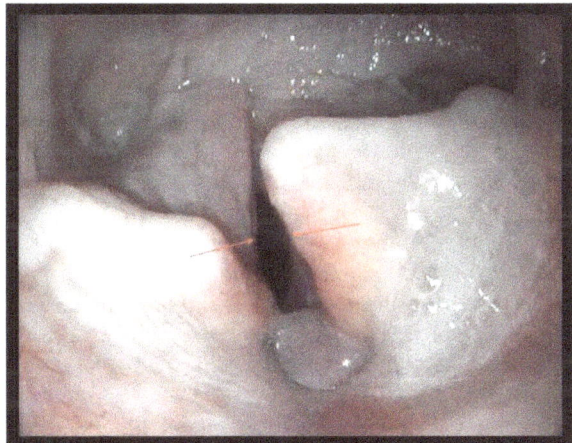

Fig. 2. Laryngoscopy image: The extraluminal mass distorts the normal laryngeal architecture causing narrowing of the glottis lumen (arrows) and bilateral laryngeal paralysis.

The abnormal tissue appeared to be muscle tissue slightly bulging, firmer and paler than the surrounding muscle on palpation. The dog recovered well from the procedure with the respiratory signs remaining unchanged.

Microscopically, the biopsy samples were represented by skeletal muscle tissue with severe degrees of dysplasia and moderate inflammation. The mass was composed of haphazardly arranged mature skeletal muscle fibers, with marked size variations, from hypertrophy to atrophy, and disarray of orientation, with some fibers in transverse section, longitudinal section, and others in oblique section.

Signs of regeneration, degeneration and necrosis of the fibres were present. Mild perimysial and endomysial fibrosis was evident. A mild multifocal inflammatory infiltrate was present and composed mainly by lymphocytes and plasma cells with scattered eosinophils and neutrophils. Findings suggestive of a neoplastic process were not evident.

Surgery was planned to manage laryngeal paralysis and perform mass removal. The patient was placed in right lateral recumbency and a unilateral cricoarytenoid lateralisation was performed (Kitshoff *et al.*, 2013). The patient was then placed in left lateral recumbency for an optimal surgical approach to the mass. A skin incision was made dorsal to the jugular vein from the caudal margin of the mandible to the first tracheal rings. Blunt and sharp dissection through the subcutaneous muscles allowed the exposition of the dorso-lateral right laryngeal region. The mass was palpable and included the right caudo-lateral portion of the thyropharyngeal and cricopharyngeal muscles. The muscle portion involved was excised via skeletisation of the laryngeal cartilages. Haemostasis was achieved by bipolar cauterisation. Muscles, subcutaneous tissues and skin were closed routinely. Recovery from surgery was uneventful and clinical signs resolved immediately. Histopathological examination of samples obtained from the mass was similar to previous results of incisional biopsy examination (Fig. 3).

The patient was re-examined 12 days after surgery for suture removal and remains asymptomatic at follow-up 13 months after surgery.

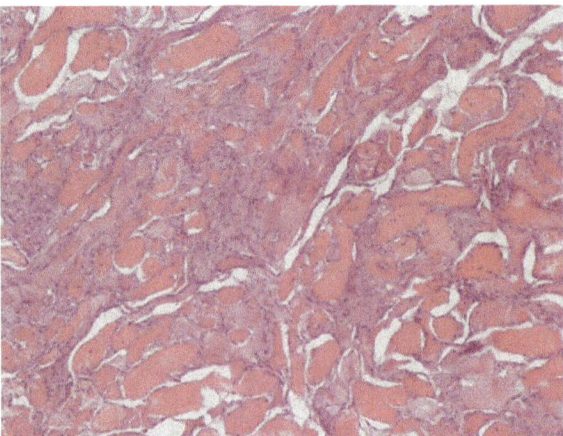

Fig. 3. Histology image: Portion of skeletal muscle with markedly distorted architecture and mild inflammatory changes. Myofibers show severe variations in size, shape and staining affinity. Disarray of orientation is evident, with fibres in transverse, longitudinal and oblique section. Degeneration, regenerative changes and fibrosis are also evident (H&E stain, 10X).

Discussion

To the authors' knowledge, this is the first report of an acquired LP in a young dog caused by the presence of a muscle pseudotumour.

The term muscle pseudotumour includes a group of uncommon benign non-neoplastic masses arising from the skeletal muscle. Several synonyms exist in human literature (Knight *et al.*, 2009), contributing to confusion surrounding the comprehension of this uncommon disease. This condition has been reported in humans and animals (horses, dogs and cats) with no particular age or sex incidence and with different localisations (Cooper and Valentine, 2002; van der Woerdt, 2008; Loderstedt *et al.*, 2010; Gude *et al.*, 2011; Segawa *et al.*, 2014).

In humans, clinical or subclinical muscle injury and denervation injury have been proposed as a possible aetiology, however such correlations have not been proved (Cooper and Valentine, 2002; The Armed Forces Institute of Pathology, 2007; Knight *et al.*, 2009). The lesion may grossly appear paler and firmer than the surrounding normal muscle tissue. Pain is not a usual feature of muscle pseudotumours. When possible, wide excision of the lesions can be curative but the mass may also recur (Cooper and Valentine, 2002; The Armed Forces Institute of Pathology, 2007). In this dog clinical signs caused by LP were the only signs associated with the presence of the mass. LP is more frequent in older dogs in its acquired form; congenital forms are uncommon and have been reported in certain breeds with usual onset of clinical signs at less than 1 year of age.

Causes of acquired LP can be several although in most dogs the cause remains undetermined and LP is classified as idiopathic (Millard and Tobias, 2009; MacPhail, 2014).

In this case report the patient was a young adult dog; the age was unusual for both a congenital or acquired form of LP. All the additional diagnostics were unremarkable except for the presence of a mass on the CT scan of the neck. The severe structural alteration of the larynx seen on laryngoscopy and caused by the presence of the mass justified the impairment of the physiological movement of the larynx. We could not exclude or confirm concomitant nerve damage; however the anatomical localisation of the mass was not compatible with compression of the recurrent laryngeal nerve. Unilateral cricoarytenoid lateralisation was performed to relieve respiratory signs because the clinical response to the surgical excision of the mass alone was unpredictable.

The lack of response to initial medical treatment could have been suggestive of a neoplastic mass rather than an inflammatory condition and may have mislead the decision making process. Although histology report from the initial biopsies was indicative of a non-neoplastic muscular lesion, the samples could have not been representative of the mass. In this case the type and extent of surgery was decided balancing preservation of function against completeness of excision. Surgical removal of the mass associated with surgical management of LP could be a viable and curative treatment for similar cases. In this case, at the 13 months follow-up, the dog remains well with no signs of recurrence. One limitation of this case is that re-evaluation on follow-up was only based on clinical and neurological examination, whilst a CT scan of the neck would have been a desirable option to assess any possible recurrence of the mass lesion.

Muscle pseudotumour associated with laryngeal paralysis in dogs has not been documented previously and, although a rare condition, it should be listed amongst the differential diagnosis of focal lesions and possible causes of LP in dogs.

Aknowledgements

The authors would like to acknowledge Dr Linda Mecattini from the Clinica Colombo for her assistance in performing endoscopy and Dr Simonetta Citi from the University of Pisa for her assistance in interpretation of the CT images. The authors confirm that all individuals personally acknowledged have given their permission to be listed.

Conflict of interest

The authors declare that there is no conflict of interests.

References

Cooper, B.J. and Valentine, B.A. 2002. Muscle Pseudotumors. In: Tumors in domestic animals, 4th ed, ed Meuten D. J., Iowa state press, Ames, IA, pp: 359-361.

Gude, D., Rayudu, R. and Bansal, D. 2011. How pseudo is an inflammatory pseudotumor? Indian J. Med. Paediatr. Oncol. 32, 204-206.

Kitshoff, A.M., Van Goethem, B., Stegen, L., Vandekerckhove, P. and de Rooster, H. 2013. Laryngeal paralysis in dogs: An update on recent knowledge. J. S. Afr. Vet. Assoc. 84, E1-E9.

Knight, C., Fan, E., Riis, R. and McDonough, S. 2009. Inflammatory myofibroblastic tumors in two dogs. Vet. Pathol. 46, 273-276.

Loderstedt, S., Walmsley, G.L., Summers, B.A., Cappello, R. and Volk, H.A. 2010. Neurological, imaging and pathological features of a meningeal inflammatory pseudotumour in a Maltese terrier. J. Small Anim. Pract. 51, 387-392.

MacPhail, C. 2014. Laryngeal disease in dogs and cats. Vet. Clin. North Am. Small Anim. Pract. 44, 19-31.

Millard, R.P. and Tobias, K.M. 2009. Laryngeal paralysis in dogs. Compend. Contin. Educ. Vet. 31, 212-219.

Segawa, Y., Yasumatsu, R., Shiratsuchi, H., Tamae, A., Noda, T., Yamamoto, H. and Komune, S. 2014. Inflammatory pseudotumors in head and neck. Auris Nasus Larynx. 3, 321-324.

The Armed Forces Institute of Pathology. 2007. Department of Veterinary Pathology. http://askjpc.org/wsco/wsc/wsc07/07WSC01.pdf

van der Woerdt, A. 2008. Orbital inflammatory disease and pseudotumor in dogs and cats. Vet. Clin. North Am. Small Anim. Pract. 38, 389-401.

22

Pulmonary ossification and microlithiasis in a bitch with multicentric mammary tumors

Mahir A.G. Kubba[*]

Department of Pathology and Clinical Pathology, Faculty of Veterinary Medicine, University of Tripoli, Libya

Abstract

Microliths and ossification were found in the lungs of a 12-year-old bitch suffering from compound mammary gland tumor which has disseminated in the inguinal lymph node glands and the lungs. Pulmonary ossification appeared grossly as irregular stony sharp particles which infiltrated the lung tissue and were readily recognizable from under the pleura as grayish sharp protruding particles. Microscopic examination revealed the existence of intra-alveolar single or multilobular particles of ossification which are formed of lamellated osseous substance with osteocytes in lacunae. Microlith particles were also seen and were smaller, usually solitary and less frequent. They comprised strongly basophilic smooth laminated spherical particles which may enclose faintly stained substances. Both structures were not associated with inflammatory response. Larger particles appeared as white miliary spots by radiography. This article documents for a very rare case of pulmonary microlithiasis and ossification in a dog.

Keywords: Multicentric mammary tumors, Pulmonary microlithiasis, Pulmonary ossification.

Introduction

The existence of mature bone fragments and calcium concretions in the pulmonary alveoli were described in man and animals. This condition was first described in man in 1918 and was termed "pulmonary alveolar microlithiasis" in 1938 (Bush *et al.*, 1976). In 2004, Mariotta *et al.* (2004) reviewed 576 cases which represented all the scientific literatures up to January 2003. In addition to others (Malhotra *et al.*, 2010; Devi *et al.*, 2011; Yin and Shen, 2011), they described the disease as a rare condition which occurs mostly in Europe and Asia.

The disease has familial and sporadic patterns, affects all ages and possesses no gender predilection. Pulmonary alveolar microlithiasis is even rarer in animals and the few available documents have reported it in sheep (Romboli and Del Bono, 1966), dogs (Liu *et al.*, 1969; Brix *et al.*, 1994; de Brot and Hilbe, 2013), a cat (Brummer *et al.*, 1989), and few exotic animals including binturong (Bush *et al.*, 1976), orange-utan (Kelly, 1976), Afghan pika (Madarame *et al.*, 1989), nacht mice (Starost *et al.*, 2002) and alpaca (Lee *et al.*, 2012). They described the affected lungs as having grainy consistency on palpation with gritty texture on cutting. Bush *et al.* (1976) demonstrated a pinpoint to 2 mm hard whitish foci distributed throughout the lungs in binturong. Microliths appeared microscopically as circular to irregularly shaped, slightly basophilic non-birefringent periodic acid-schiff- positive laminated concretions within alveolar walls or free in the alveoli. Mature bone concretions of variable size were also observed attached to the alveolar septa and often filled the alveolar spaces. They consisted of boney lamellae and osteocytes in lacunae arranged in concentric layers. Most investigations have ruled out associated inflammatory response. Radiographic findings have shown bilateral interstitial miliary pattern of increased pulmonary density with a 'snowstorm' or 'sandstorm' appearance (Bush *et al.*, 1976; Brix *et al.*, 1994). In man, these findings were often missed for miliary tuberculosis, silicosis, berylliosis, sarcoidosis, hemosiderosis, fungal infections and carcinomatosis (Malhotra *et al.*, 2010), while deep pulmonary mycosis and lymphosarcoma were missed for in dogs (Brix *et al.*, 1994).

In human, microliths are composed mainly of calcium phosphate (Schoenhals and Fishman, 1980; Brix *et al.*, 1994), while those assuming boney structure possess consistency equal to bone (Bush *et al.*, 1976). The etiology of the disease is unknown but many theories have been suggested. Possible etiologies include an inherited metabolic abnormality in the lung (Moran *et al.*, 1997), abnormalities in calcium and phosphorus metabolism (Arslan *et al.*, 1996), abnormalities in the immune system (Meyer *et al.*, 1956), environmental factors (Prakash *et al.*, 1983) and anatomic and physiologic abnormalities of the lung (Sosman *et al.*, 1957; Moran *et al.*, 1997). Recent investigations have identified gene SLC34A2 to be responsible (Gocmen *et al.*, 1992; Yin and Shen, 2011). The clinical signs associated with this condition ranged from asymptomatic to respiratory insufficiency. This article documents for a very rare case of pulmonary microlithiasis and ossification in a dog.

*Corresponding Author: Mahir Abdul Ghani Kubba. Former Professor at the Department of Pathology and Clinical Pathology, Faculty of Veterinary Medicine, University of Tripoli, Libya. Email: magkubba@yahoo.com

Case Details

A twelve years old bitch suffering from advanced multiple mammary gland tumors was euthanized because of poor prognosis. Postmortem examination revealed the involvement of three mammary glands with voluminous tumors in addition to dissemination in the inguinal lymph node glannd and the lungs. Both lungs harboured superficial and deeply seated tumor secondaries ranging from 0.5 - 6.0 cm in diameter. Both lungs were pale, not well inflated, anthracotic, with patchy emphysema. A peculiar finding was the existence of palpable foci of mineralization scattered under the pleura and deep in the parenchyma in both lungs. Those located superficially are protruding irregular grayish white stony masses of 1.0-5.0 mm in diameter with occasional boney spicules that perforate the pleura (Fig. 1and 2).

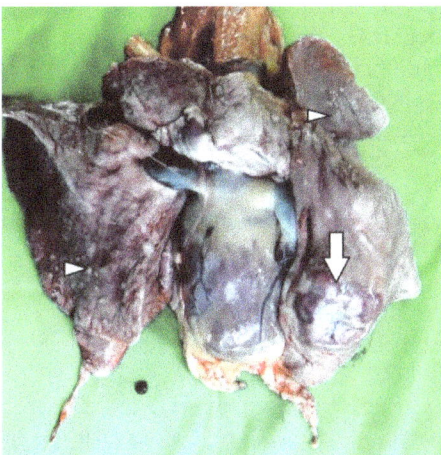

Fig. 1. Mineralization nodules are protruding from the sub-pleura (arrow heads). The right lung shows a large secondary tumor growth (arrow).

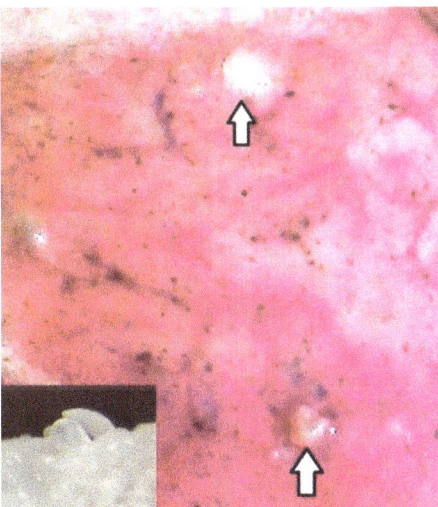

Fig. 2. Large irregular prominent white boney particles are seen through the lung surface (Arrows). Some boney spicules perforate to the lung surface through the pleura (Inset). Dark spots are Carbon particles.

The heart showed left ventricular hypertrophy and mild right ventricular dilatation. Other organs were obviously normal. Microscopic examination revealed the existence of two morphologically different tumors comprising cystic adenocarcinoma in two glands and mixed mammary tumor in the third gland. The secondary tumor growth in the inguinal glands and the lungs was that of solid adenocarcinoma. Both lungs -in addition- contained irregular single or multi-lobulated softly laminated masses of boney structure formed of osseous material and lacunated osteocytes. The outer lamellae often showed increased basophilia and numerous osteocytes while the centers had occasional areas of non-boney mineralization. Alveoli distended with such structures had their walls usually stretched or ruptured (Fig. 3 and 4).

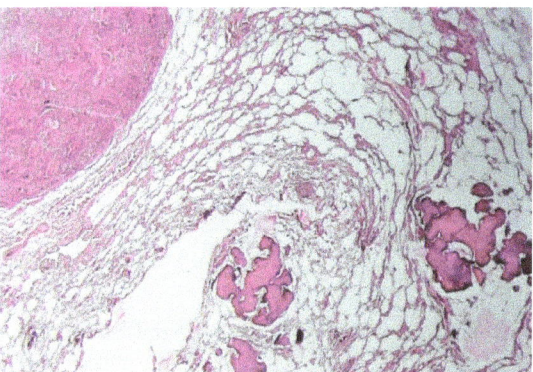

Fig. 3. Multiobular intra-alveolar mass of boney structure are seen. Part of the metastatic tumor is seen in the left upper corner. The lung is rather emphysematous (Magnification: X40).

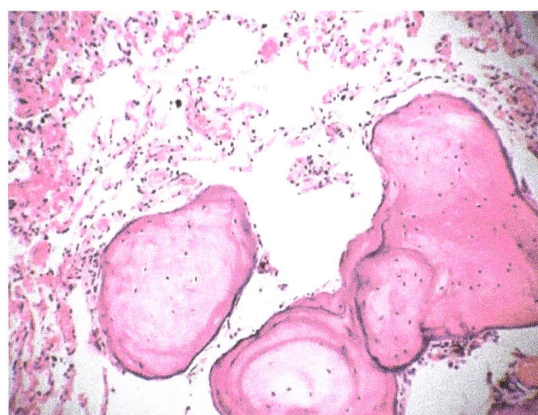

Fig. 4. Ossification lobules showing lamellated orientation with osteocytes in lacunae. They are surrounded by stretched alveolar wall membrane (Magnification: X100).

Other kind of less frequently noticed alveolar concretions has also existed. These are solitary measuring about 30 um and are formed of non-cellular deeply basophilic onion-like laminations which may enclose faint eosinophilic soft substance (Fig. 5).

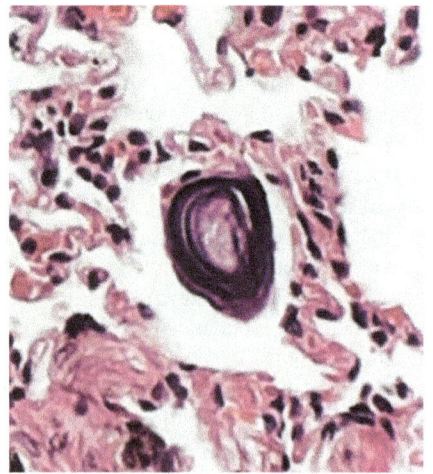

Fig. 5. Intra-alveolar onion-like concretion formed of strongly basophilic non-cellular lamination which encloses a faintly eosinophilic soft substance (Magnification: X400).

Both structures were not associated with local tissue inflammatory response. Exploration radiography has shown the ossified concretions as small whitish spots.

Discussion

Pulmonary alveolar microlithiasis is a rare pathological condition of man and animal whose etiology has not yet been resolved. Available literatures have so far reported this condition in three aged dogs of different sex, breed and diseases association. Liu *et al.* (1969) have reported the disease in an 11-year old Poodle with ruptured chordae tendineae of the mitral and tricuspid valves, while de Brot and Hilbe (2013) reported the disease in a 10-year-old female Bulldog with concurrent pleural mesothelioma. The third report was about a 9-year- old male English Setter dog with no history of associated disease (Brix *et al.*, 1994).

The nature of the alveolar concretions in those reports varied from microliths in one dog (de Brot and Hilbe, 2013) to boney nodules in another (Liu *et al.*, 1969) while the third dog possessed both kinds (Brix *et al.*, 1994). Many investigators have suggested that microliths may provide a nidus for bone formation and the presence of few small foci of non-bony mineralization in bony tissue may confirm that concept (Bush *et al.*, 1976; Brix *et al.*, 1994). Both kinds of concretions existed in the current report which investigates a 12-year-old local-breed female dog with concurrent mammary gland tumor that has disseminated in the inguinal glands and the lungs. Their structure, location and lack of associated inflammatory response are in accordance with those mentioned for previous investigations. The complexity of the bony particles noticed in this dog is unique among others and the multilobular intra-alveolar morphology probably indicates an expansive pattern of growth involving adjacent alveoli.

Having reviewed the literature, this study added another case of pulmonary microlithiasis in a bitch suffering this time from mammary tumor with pulmonary dissemination. The relationship between the two conditions could neither be established nor ruled out.

Conflict of interest

The authors declare that they have no competing interests.

References

Arslan, A., Yalin, T., Akan, H. and Belet, U. 1996. Pulmonary alveolar microlithiasis associated with calcification in the seminal vesicles. J. Belge. Radiol. 97, 118-119.

Brix, A.E., Latimer, K.S., Moore, G.E. and Roberts, R.E. 1994. Pulmonary alveolar microlithiasis in a dog. Vet. Pathol. 31, 382-385.

Brummer, D.G., French, T.W. and Cline, J.M. 1989. Microlithiasis associated with chronic bronchopneumonia in a cat. J. Am. Vet. Med. Assoc. 194, 1061-1064.

Bush, M., James, A.E., Montali, R.J. and Stitik, F.P. 1976. Pulmonary alveolar microlithiasis in a binturong (*Arctictis binturong*): a case report. J. Am. Vet. Radiol. Soc. 17, 157-160.

de Brot, S. and Hilbe, M. 2013. Pulmonary alveolar microlithiasis with concurrent pleural mesothelioma in a dog. J. Vet. Diag. Invest. 25, 798-802.

Devi, G., Rao, H.J.M., Prathima, K.N., Das, K.M. and Jayanth, K. 2011. Pulmonary alveolar microlithiasis. Lung India 28(2), 139-141.

Gocmen, A., Toppare, M.F., Kiper, N. and Buyukpamukcu, N. 1992. Treatment of pulmonary alveolar microlithiasis with diphosphonate-- preliminary results of a case. Respiration 59(4), 250-252.

Kelly, O.F. 1976. Pulmonary alveolar microlithiasis in the orange-utan (Pongo pymaeus). Acta Zool. Pathol. Antverb. 66, 53-57.

Lee, E.J., Dawood, K.E., Brudar, R. and Philbey, A.W. 2012. Pulmonary alveolar microlithiasis in an alpaca (*Vicugna pacos*). Aust. Vet. J. 90, 510-512.

Liu, S.K., Suter, P.F. and Ettinger, S. 1969. Pulmonary alveolar microlithiasis with ruptured chordae tendinae in mitral and tricuspid valves in a dog. J. Am. Vet. Med. Assoc. 155, 1692-1703.

Madarame, H., Kumaga, M., Suzuki, J., Watanabe, A. and Kanno, S. 1989. Pulmonary alveolar microlithiasis in Afghan pika (*Ochotona rufescens rufescens*). Vet. Pathol. 26, 333-337.

Malhotra, B., Sabharwal, R., Singh, M. and Singh, A. 2010. Pulmonary alveolar microlithiasis with calcified pleural plaques. Lung India 27, 250-252.

Mariotta, S., Ricci, A., Papale, M., Clementi, F., Sposato, B., Guidi, L. and Mannino, F. 2004. Pulmonary alveolar microlithiasis: report on 576 cases published in the literature. Sarcoidosis Vasculitis and Diffuse Lung Diseases 21(3), 173-181.

Meyer, N.H., Gilbert, E.S. and Kent, G. 1956. A clinical review of pulmonary microlithiasis. J. Am. Med. Assoc. 161, 1153-1157.

Moran, C.A., Hochholzer, L., Hasleton, P.S., Johnson, F.B. and Koss, M.N. 1997. Pulmonary alveolar microlithiasis. A clinicopathologic and chemical analysis of seven cases. Arch. Pathol. Lab. Med. 121, 607-611.

Prakash, U.B., Barham, S.S., Rosenow, E.C., Brown, M.L. and Payne, W.S. 1983. Pulmonary alveolar microlithiasis. A review including ultrastructural and pulmonary function studies. Mayo. Clin. Proc. 58, 290- 300.

Romboli, B. and Del Bono, G. 1966. Pneumopatia a microliti nell'ovino. Ann. Fac. Med. Vet. 19, 175-201.

Schoenhals, J.A. and Fishman, A.P. 1980. Pulmonary alveolar microlithiasis. In: Pulmonary diseases and disorders, ed. Fishman AP, 1st ed. McGraw-Hill, New York , NY, pp: 987-989.

Sosman, M.C., Dodd, G.D., Jones, W.D. and Pillmore, G.U. 1957. The familial occurrence of pulmonary alveolar microlithiasis. Am. J. Reontgenol. Radium. Ther. Nucl. Med. 77, 947-1012.

Starost, M.F., Benavides, F. and Conti, C.J. 2002. A variant of pulmonary alveolar microlithiasis in nacht mice. Vet. Pathol. 39, 390-392.

Yin, J. and Shen, K. 2011. Pulmonary alveolar microlithiasis in a child. N. Engl. J. Med. 364:e49. DOI: 10.1056/NEJMicm1002094.

23

Opioid-free anaesthesia in three dogs

Donna M. White*, Alastair R. Mair and Fernando Martinez-Taboada

Department of Anaesthesia and Analgesia, Veterinary Teaching Hospital, University of Sydney, Evelyn Williams Building B10, 65 Parramatta Road, Camperdown, NSW. 2050. Australia

Abstract

Opioid-free anaesthesia (OFA) is a relatively new and growing field in human medicine. There are multiple motivations behind this emerging practice with the recognition of several serious potential opioid-related adverse effects including opioid induced hyperalgesia, opioid tolerance and immunomodulatory effects of opioids. Opioids have long been the mainstay of veterinary anaesthesia and pain management practice. The feasibility of OFA in veterinary patients is presented here. A case series of three dogs that underwent OFA for canine ovariohysterectomy is reported. The authors conclude OFA is possible in veterinary medicine; however the move away from the familiar effects of opioids perioperatively is challenging. Gaining experience with these types of protocols for standard procedures in healthy animals, such as neutering, will provide the anaesthetist with the building blocks for more invasive surgeries.

Keywords: Anaesthesia, Analgesia, Dog, Pain.

Introduction

Opioids have long been a cornerstone of pain management in both human and veterinary anaesthesia. They provide analgesia, sedation and anaesthetic sparing effects, and often contribute significantly to haemodynamic stability during surgery and anaesthesia. Opioid use is not without side effects that can include well recognised clinically significant respiratory depression, ileus and potential for development of addiction and tolerance in both humans (Ronald and Kissin, 1998) and animals (Martin and Eades, 1961; Kissin et al., 1991). Currently there is a growing body of evidence, from both human and animal studies, supporting a condition of opioid-induced hyperalgesia OIH (Lee et al., 2011; Pasero and McCaffery, 2012). There has been a recognition of the negative immunomodulatory effects of some opioids (Sacerdote, 2006; Odunayo et al., 2010; Levite, 2012) and even an association of increased rates of cancer recurrence with opioid use (Cata et al., 2016).

Opioid-induced hyperalgesia can occur in a subset of patients, for currently undefinable reasoning. Increased post-operative pain scores and opioid requirements have been reported in people following administration of a single opioid-containing anaesthetic (Sukhani et al., 1996; Chia et al., 1999; Guignard et al., 2000; Bakan et al., 2015). Administration of opioids initially produces analgesia but after a period of time hyperalgesia may be induced (Angst and Clark, 2006). While the condition itself is still poorly understood, the seriousness of a hyperalgesic state for postoperative patients has provided the motivation for the fast growing practice of opioid-free anaesthesia (OFA) in human medicine. Additional reported benefits of OFA include reduced post-operative opioid requirements (Feld et al., 2003; Mansour et al., 2013; Bakan et al., 2015), reduced incidence of post-operative nausea and vomiting (Mather and Peutrell, 1995; Callesen et al., 1999; Ziemann-Gimmel et al., 2014; Bakan et al., 2015), reduced intraoperative hypotension (Jagannathan et al., 2007; Bakan et al., 2015), and reduced post-operative sedation levels (Feld et al., 2003). Opioids provide the mainstay of analgesia in a significant proportion of veterinary anaesthesia. Veterinarians are familiar with their use and perioperative effects. The use of OFA provides a difficult challenge with loss of this familiarity. However it is likely there is a subset of veterinary patients that are also susceptible to OIH and arguable that our oncologic and immunodeficient patients may also benefit from OFA (Celerier et al., 2000; Cabanero et al., 2009). OFA highlights the need for a multimodal drug approach to ensure the patient receives an opioid-free, but not analgesic-free, anaesthetic and post-anaesthetic experience. This report presents three cases that underwent successful OFA, with a protocol the authors consider an acceptable baseline for more invasive surgeries, and with a potential for prospective randomized studies.

Case details

All cases discussed were presented to the University Veterinary Teaching Hospital Sydney (UVTHS), for routine ovariohysterectomy, through the teaching neuter program.

***Corresponding Author:** Donna M. White. Department of Anaesthesia and Analgesia, Veterinary Teaching Hospital, University of Sydney, Australia. Email: donna.white@sydney.edu.au*

Case 1

A 6-month-old Bull Terrier was presented for ovariohysterectomy. The owner reported no current health concerns but noted a previous episode of conjunctivitis one month prior to presentation. The dog's physical examination findings were unremarkable. Her demeanour was noted to be quiet and friendly.

Case 2

A 2-year-old Shetland Sheepdog presented for ovariohysterectomy. The dog was current on her vaccination schedule with no ill-health reported by the owner. Physical exam of the dog revealed a grade II/VI heart murmur, with point of maximum intensity over the left heart base. The owner declined cardiac work up, however, reported no clinical signs of cardiac disease. The dog's demeanour was noted to be bright, alert and responsive.

Case 3

A 5-year-old Labrador was presented for ovariohysterectomy. The owner reported no health concerns. The dog had whelped three months prior to presentation. Physical examination was unremarkable. The dog was noted to be very timid and nervous of people.

Procedures

Dogs underwent the standard pre-anaesthetic protocol of the teaching hospital neuter clinic, performed by final year veterinary students during their anaesthesia clinical training rotation. This included physical examination, basic pre-anaesthetic blood testing (PCV/TP), preoperative behaviour scoring (Romano *et al*., 2015) and assignment of ASA health status score (Table 1).

Perioperative patient assessments included sedation scoring (Gurney *et al*., 2009), recovery scoring (Becker *et al*., 2013) and post-operative pain scoring (Reid *et al*., 2007), performed by students with guidance from an anaesthetist (Table 1).

The UVTHS neuter clinic protocol dictates that sedation scoring is performed immediately prior to induction. Recovery scoring is performed immediately after extubation. Post-operative pain scoring is initially performed when the dog is extubated and responsive, and thereafter hourly for three hours (by anaesthesia students). Once transferred to recovery ward dogs' pain was scored every four hours (by recovery ward nursing staff) until discharge time (the following morning).

The same anaesthetist managed all three cases. OFA was achieved with a pre-anaesthetic medication of varying doses of medetomidine (Domitor, Pfizer Animal Health, Australia), ketamine (Ceva Ketamine, Ceva Animal Health Pty Ltd, Australia) and acepromazine (A.C.P.2, Delvet, Australia). All drugs were mixed in a single syringe and administered intramuscularly.

Table 1. Pre-anaesthetic blood testing (PCV/TP), ASA health status score, perioperative sedation scoring, intraoperative anaesthetic complications, post-operative recovery scoring, and post- operative pain scoring for each case.

Parameter	Case 1	Case 2	Case 3
PCV/TP	51/66	43/60	58/62
ASA	1	2	1
Sedation Score (/15)	10	6	6
Anaesthetic complications	H.	SR (surgical). H.	SR (surgical). H.
Recovery Score (/4)	1	1	1
PS 1 (/25) (alert and response)	1	3	1
PS 2 (+60mins)	1	8	2 (4pm)
PS 3 (+120 mins)	3	4	2
PS 4 (+180mins)	2	0 (4pm)	2
PS 4pm	1	0	2
PS 8pm	2	0	6
PS12 midnight	1	1	2
PS 4am	2	0	2
PS 8am	0	0	2

(SR): intraoperative sympathetic response; (H): hypothermia (<37°C); (PS): Pain score.

Anaesthesia was induced intravenously with alfaxalone (Alfaxan, Jurox, Australia) or alfaxalone and lidocaine (Lignocaine Injection 2%, Pfizer Animal Health, Australia) co-induction. Anaesthesia was maintained with Isoflurane (Isothesia, Henry Schein, Australia) in oxygen.

Medetomidine and ketamine infusions were administered intraoperatively for analgesia and minimum alveolar concentration (MAC) sparing effects to improve the dogs' haemodynamics. Sympathetic response (dramatic or sustained increases in heart rate and blood pressure) was viewed as light plane of anaesthesia for the level of surgical stimulation and was treated with either adjustment in isoflurane concentration or intraoperative injection of analgesia (ketamine or lidocaine). Transversus abdominis plane (TAP) regional anaesthesia with bupivacaine (Bupivacaine Injection BP 0.5%, Pfizer Animal Health, Australia) 4mg/kg was performed in all cases. Carprofen (Carprieve, Norbrook Laboratories, Australia Ltd, Australia) 4mg/kg was administered subcutaneously and paracetamol (Paracetamol Kabi, Fresenius Kabi Australia Pty Ltd, Australia) 10mg/kg intravenously during the preoperative or intraoperative period.

Atracurium (Atracurium Besylate Injection, Hospira Australia Pty Ltd, Australia) was administered to one of the three cases (Case 2) as required to assist mechanical ventilation. All three cases were monitored with use of pulse oximetry, capnography, non-invasive (appropriately sized cuff placed on antebrachium) or invasive blood pressure (arterial catheter placed in dorsal pedal artery), volatile anaesthetic monitoring, intraoperative oesophageal and post-operative rectal temperatures. Animals were visually monitored continuously in recovery until alert and responsive, standing and having a rectal temperature above 37 degrees Celsius. Active warming was provided with a warm air blanket (Warm Air Blanket, Darvall Vet, Australia).

The protocol was varied with each case as indicated by individual patient factors and for improvement of the overall technique (Table 2).

Table 2. OFA protocol for each case.

Drugs	Case 1	Case 2	Case 3
Medetomidine (ug/kg) IM	10	5	10
Ketamine (mg/kg) IM	2	2	2
Acepromazine (mg/kg) IM	0.02	0.02	0.02
Alfaxalone (mg/kg) IV	0.4	2	2.7mg/kg
Lidocaine (mg/kg) IV	1	-	-
Isoflurane (ET%)	0.8-1.4	0.9-1.1	0.9-1.3
Ketamine CRI (ug/kg/min) /total dose (mg/kg)	10/0.8	5-10/1.2	10/1.3
Lidocaine CRI (ug/kg/min) /total dose (mg/kg)	50/1.3	-	-
Dex/Medetomidine CRI (ug/kg/hr) /total dose (ug/kg)	M2/2.4	M2/4.6	M2/4.4
Ketamine bolus IV /(total dose mg/kg)	N	N	Y (0.5)
Lidocaine bolus IV /(total dose mg/kg)	N	N	Y (2)
TAP block	Y	Y	Y

Case 1 received the highest sedation score of 10/15. It should be noted Case 1 was assessed to be quiet and friendly preoperatively compared with the following two cases that were noted to be bright, alert and responsive or nervous and timid preoperatively, and as such this difference in patient factors may have contributed to the heavier sedation level achieved. Case 1 utilised lidocaine as a co-induction agent and this likely contributed to a dose sparing effect of alfaxalone. For Case 2, the premedication dose of medetomidine was half that of Case 1 with no change to the dosing of ketamine or acepromazine. Although heavy sedation was achieved (sedation score 9/15) the dog was also noted to be dysphoric. Subsequent to this a high dose of alfaxalone was required to induce anaesthesia. Lower end-tidal isoflurane concentrations were used to maintain anaesthesia with no intraoperative analgesia boluses required.

However, Case 2 had the only pain score >5/24 in the first three hours post-operatively. Case 2 was administered methadone analgesia however the dog's pain score did not improve with this. The increased score was deemed to be primarily anxiety based and was successfully treated with acepromazine (0.01mg/kg) intravenously. In an attempt to eliminate the possibility of dysphoria Case 3 received a higher dose of medetomidine, as also previously given to Case 1. Although the dog did not appear dysphoric she did show muscle rigidity, suspected secondary to ketamine administration. Subsequently a higher dose of alfaxalone was required to induce anaesthesia. Postoperative pain scoring for Case 3 remained low with no post-operative opioids required.

Anaesthetic complications included increases in heart rate and blood pressure, and hypothermia (<37°C). No episodes of intraoperative hypotension occurred. Hypothermia resolved within two hours postoperatively in all dogs. The recovery scores of all dogs reflected excellent post-operative recoveries.

Discussion

OFA is possible for dogs undergoing routine ovariohysterectomy. OFA was achieved in a series of three cases using a multimodal drug approach including medetomidine, ketamine, carprofen, paracetamol and bilateral TAP regional anaesthesia with bupivacaine. The long-standing use of opioids in veterinary anaesthesia has led to a familiarity of their effects during anaesthesia. Opioids are potent analgesics with significant MAC sparing effects. The UVTHS neuter clinic utilises the MAC-sparing effects of opioids in the vast majority of anaesthetics. Loss of this familiarity with increasing use of OFA has brought with it several challenges. The use of a multidrug approach was deemed essential for OFA to ensure adequate analgesia. The protocol presented was developed based on currently used opioid-free protocols in human anaesthesia (Bakan et al., 2015; Mulier, 2016). With each case came increased familiarity of the drug combinations resulting in increased competence in performing OFA.

Medetomidine is a selective alpha-2 agonist drug providing analgesia, sedation and sympatholysis with significant opioid sparing effects (Blaudszun et al., 2012). Alpha-2 agonist analgesic doses can be variable and the duration of analgesia is unreliable (Sinclair, 2003). Medetomidine can be used in combination with an opioid, rather than a potential substitute, to improve its analgesic effects (Kuo and Keegan, 2003), providing a potential drawback of OFA. Alpha-2 agonist drugs are considered core components in many human OFA protocols (Bakan et al., 2015; Mulier, 2016). Ketamine is a dissociative agent with NMDA receptor antagonism and sympathomimetic effects (Peltoniemi et al., 2016). At low doses it provides analgesia, while also providing anaesthesia at high doses (Peltoniemi et al., 2016). It is thought to provide less intense analgesia than pure-μ opioids and is often used in combination with an opioid for multimodal analgesic effects (Carstensen and Moller, 2010; Gutierrez-Blanco et al., 2015).

Ketamine is a common component of OFA in people and has even been shown to reduce the development of OIH if administered prior to opioid treatment in animals (Celerier et al., 2000) and humans (Hong et al., 2011; Kaur et al., 2015). The dysphoria reported for Case 2 after premedication was believed to be secondary to ketamine administration. Continuation of ketamine intraoperatively may also have contributed to the post-operative anxiety shown by the dog. Subanaesthestic doses of ketamine have been shown to cause adverse behaviour changes in humans (Krystal et al., 1994).

Case 3 experienced muscle rigidity following premedication and this was again considered a side effect of ketamine administration. These side effects are potential drawbacks of utilizing ketamine within opioid free protocols. Ketamine is often omitted or used at lower doses when combined with opioids.

Intravenous lidocaine has been shown to have analgesic and anti-inflammatory effects (Rang et al., 2012). Intraoperative intravenous lidocaine infusion can reduce inhalational anaesthetic requirements, reduce post-operative pain scores and opioid requirements (McCarthy et al., 2010).

Carprofen and paracetamol have been used as adjunct analgesics in these cases. Although they do not contribute an anaesthetic sparing effect they add to the multimodal approach that is essential when considering OFA. Carprofen is a non-steroidal anti-inflammatory analgesic with COX-2 inhibitory effects. Carprofen has been shown to be safe and efficacious when given preoperatively to healthy animals undergoing fracture repair (Bergmann et al., 2005).

Paracetamol is a centrally acting analgesic with mild to moderate effects (Rang et al., 2012). Paracetamol is not commonly used in veterinary medicine compared to its use in human medicine, however it is widely used at the UVTHS. Species variation in use, and specifically acute toxicity effects in felines, and a lack of familiarity are likely significant contributors to the reduced use of paracetamol in veterinary medicine. Although not often used on its own paracetamol has been shown repeatedly to provide significant opioid-sparing effects in humans (Korpela et al., 1999; Remy et al., 2005; Sinatra et al., 2005; Maund et al., 2011). Mburu et al. (1988) reported a 33% reduction in post-operative surgical site swelling and 47% reduction in pain in dogs treated with paracetamol compared with placebo after undergoing experimental forelimb surgery. Paracetamol was well tolerated in the cases presented with no adverse effects seen.

When preparing an OFA technique, a great amount of effort must go into ensuring an effective multimodal approach is achieved, as one of the potential drawbacks associated with the practice of OFA is inadequate analgesia. Traditional opioid anaesthetic (OA) techniques for routine ovariohysterectomies at UVTHS involve the use of opioids and non-steroidal anti-inflammatories. Premedication is usually achieved with medetomidine and/or acepromazine, as done in this OFA technique. The addition of intraoperative constant rate infusions of medetomidine and ketamine, and lidocaine boluses were the mainstay of the OFA techniques presented. Regional anaesthesia in the form of TAP block with bupivacaine was viewed as only adjunctive analgesia and believed to likely be of greatest benefit post-operatively for the laparotomy wound.

There were notable differences of OFA to OA. The first occurred with premedication. A standard premedication for OA at the UVTHS involves use of a sedative and opioid. For these OFA cases the opioid was essentially substituted with ketamine and medetomidine. The dose of medetomidine required to achieve the same level of sedation that would be expected when combined with morphine was approximately double than when combined with ketamine and midazolam.

This highlighted the clinically significant synergistic effects of adding an opioid to medetomidine, especially when considering the lower level of sedation that is expected when morphine is given on its own. Acepromazine was administered to Case 2 post-operatively after the dog showed signs of anxiety on recovery and following no response to methadone analgesia trial bolus. It is unlikely the sedative effects of the ketamine and medetomidine were remaining during recovery, with acepromazine the only long-acting drug utilized in this protocol. This varies significantly from traditional OA techniques where longer acting opioids, such as morphine and methadone, are often given as part of the premedication, providing ongoing sedative effects and contributing to recovery quality.

The second notable difference, and arguably the most clinically relevant, was a lack of hypotension during OFA. Hypotension is one of the most common complications of anaesthesia (Gaynor et al. 1999). Increase in blood pressure can be a sign of sympathetic response to surgical stimulation. Initial management of dramatic or sustained increases in blood pressure included increasing anaesthetic depth or provision of an analgesic dose of ketamine intravenously. However a lack of response to such measures and lack of physical indicators of light plane of anaesthesia (eye position, jaw tone) resulted in recognition of blood pressure values in the high normal range to be secondary to our combination of anaesthetic drugs. Increasing the depth of anaesthesia of the dogs at this time resulted in physical indicators of deep anaesthesia (centrally placed eyes and lack of jaw tone).

The most likely contributor was the peripheral vascular effects of medetomidine with subsequent vasoconstriction. These results are consistent with those of Bakan *et al*. (2015) who compared OFA with propofol, dexmedetomidine and lidocaine infusions with opioid anaesthesia of propofol and remifentanil infusions and found the OFA group had only 3% of patients requiring use of ephedrine for treatment of hypotension compared with 20% of the OA group. Furthermore 28% of the OFA group actually required treatment for hypertension while none of the OA group did. As the authors' experience with OFA increased the recognition of increased blood pressure values as drug effects lead to greater comfort level with management of the anaesthesia and subsequently comfort in appropriately using lower inhalational levels.

All dogs had a smooth initial recovery with low recovery scores at extubation. Analgesia was administered to Case 2 to ensure pain was not a component of the anxious behaviour shown post-operatively (with no response). The lack of pain in all dogs on recovery was somewhat unexpected with an almost expected pain response in the face of opioid omission.

Use of OFA will continue to be a growing field in human medicine and will likely be of benefit to a particular subset of veterinary patients. Development of OFA protocols for more invasive, advanced surgeries can occur once the anaesthetist is comfortable performing OFA in less invasive, commonly performed surgeries such as ovariohysterectomy.

Conflict of interest

The Authors declare that there is no conflict of interest.

References

Angst, M.S. and Clark, J.D. 2006. Opioid-induced hyperalgesia; A qualitative systemic review. Anesthesiology 104, 570-587.

Bakan, M., Umutoglu, T., Topuz, U., Uysal, H., Bayram, M., Kadioglu, H. and Salihoglu, Z. 2015. Opioid- free total intravenous anaesthesia with propofol, dexmedetomidine and lidocaine infusions for laparoscopic cholecystectomy: a prospective, randomised, double-blind study. Rev. Bras. Anestesiol. 65(3), 191-199.

Becker, W.M., Mama, K.R., Rao, S., Palmer, R.H. and Egger, E.L. 2013. Prevalence of dysphoria after fentanyl in dogs undergoing stifle surgery. Vet. Surg. 42, 302-307.

Bergmann, H.M.L., Nolte, I.J.A. and Kramer, S. 2005. Effects of preoperative administration of carprofen on renal function and hemostasis in dogs undergoing surgery for fracture repair. Am. J. Vet. Res. 66(8), 1356-1363.

Blaudszun, G., Lysakowski, C., Elia, N. and Tramer, M.R. 2012. Effect of perioperative systemic α2 agonists on postoperative morphine consumption and pain intensity: systematic review and meta-analysis of randomized controlled trials. Anesthesiology 116(6), 1312-1322.

Cabanero, D., Campillo, A., Celerier, E., Romero, A. and Puig, M.M. 2009. Pronociceptive effects of remifentanil in a mouse model of postsurgical pain: effect of a second surgery. Anesthesiology 111, 1334-1345.

Callesen, T., Schouenborg, L., Nielsen, D., Guldger, H. and Kehlet, H. 1999. Combined epidural-spinal opioid-free anaesthesia and analgesia for hysterectomy. Br. J. Anaesth. 82(6), 881-885.

Carstensen, M. and Moller, A.M. 2010. Adding ketamine to morphine for intravenous patient-controlled analgesia for acute postoperative pain: a qualitative review of randomized trials. Br. J. Anaesth. 104(9), 401-406.

Cata, J.P., Bugada, D., Marchesini, M., De Gregor, M. and Allegri, M. 2016. Opioids and cancer recurrence: a brief review of the literature. Can. Cell Microenviron. 2016; 3: e1159. doi: 10.14800/ccm.1159.

Celerier, E., Rivat, C., Jun, Y., Laulin, J.P., Larcher, A., Reynier, P. and Simonnet, G. 2000. Long-lasting hyperalgesia induced by fentanyl in rats: Preventative effect of ketamine. Anesthesiology 92, 465-471.

Chia, Y.Y., Liu, K., Wang, J.J., Kuo, M.C. and Ho, S.T. 1999. Intraoperative high dose fentanyl induces postoperative fentanyl tolerance. Can. J. Anaesth. 46, 872-877.

Feld, J.M., Laurito, C.E., Beckerman, M., Vincent, J. and Hoffman, W.E. 2003. Non-opioid analgesia improves pain relief and sedation after gastric by-pass surgery. Can. J. Anaesth. 50(4), 336-341.

Gaynor, J.S., Dunlop, C.I., Wagner, A.E., Wertz, E.M., Golden, A.E. and Demme, W.C. 1999. Complications and mortality associated with anesthesia in dogs and cats. J. Am. Anim. Hosp. Assoc. 35(1), 13-17.

Guignard, B., Bossard, A.E., Coste, C., Sessler, D.I., Lebrault, C., Alfonsi, P., Fletcher, D. and Chauvin, M. 2000. Acute opioid tolerance: Intraoperative remifentanil increases postoperative pain and morphine requirement. Anaesthesiology 93, 409-417.

Gurney, M., Cripps, P. and Mosing, M. 2009. Subcutaneous pre-anaesthetic medication with acepromazine-buprenorphine is effective as and less painful than the intramuscular route. J. Small Anim. Pract. 50(9), 474-477.

Gutierrez-Blanco, E., Victoria-Mora, J.M., Ibancovichi-Camarillo, J.A., Sauri-Arceo, C.H., Bolio González, M.E., Acevedo-Arcique, C.M., Marin-Cano, G. and Steagall, P.V. 2015. Postoperative analgesic effects of either a constant rate infusion of fentanyl, lidocaine, ketamine, dexmedetomidine, or the combination lidocaine-ketamine-dexmedetomidine after ovariohysterectomy in dogs. Vet. Anaesth. Analg. 42(3), 309-318.

Hong, B.H., Lee, W.Y., Kim, Y.H., Yoon, S.H. and Lee, W.H. 2011. Effects of intraoperative low dose ketamine on remifentanil-induced hyperalgesia in gynecologic surgery with sevoflurane anesthesia. Korean J. Anesthesiol. 61(3), 238-243.

Jagannathan, V.K., Hariharan, A. and Yanny, H.F. 2007. Opioid-free anaesthesia: fracture neck of femur (DHS) surgery. Reg. Anesth. Pain Med. 32(Suppl. 1), 142.

Kaur, S., Saroa, R. and Aggarwal, S. 2015. Effect of intraoperative low-dose ketamine infusion of management of postoperative analgesia. J. Nat. Sci. Biol. Med. 6(2), 378-382.

Kissin, I., Brown, P.T., Robinson, C.A. and Bradley, E.L. 1991. Acute tolerance in morphine analgesia: continuous infusion and single injection in rats. Anesthesiology 74, 166-171.

Korpela, R., Korvenoja, P. and Meretoja, O. 1999. Morphine-sparing effect of acetaminophen in pediatric day-case surgery. Anesthesiology 8(91), 442-447.

Krystal, J.H., Karper, L.P., Seibyl, J.P., Freeman, G.K., Delaney, R., Bremner, J.D., Heninger, G.R., Bowers, M.B. and Charney, D.S. 1994. Subanesthetic Effects of the Noncompetitive NMDA Antagonist, Ketamine, in Humans. Arch. Gen. Psychiatry 51(3), 199-214.

Kuo, W.C. and Keegan, R.D. 2003. Comparative cardiovascular, analgesic, and sedative effects of medetomidine, medetomidine-hydromorphone, and medetomidine-butorphanol in dogs. Am. J. Vet. Res. 65(7), 931-937.

Lee, M., Silverman, S., Hansen, H., Patel, V. and Manchikanti, L. 2011. A Comprehensive review of Opioid-Induced Hyperalgesia. Pain Physician 14, 145-161.

Levite, M. 2012. The effects of opioids on immune cells, functions and diseases in Nerve Driven Immunity. Ed Ninkovic, J., Sabita, R., Springer Vienna, pp: 175-202.

Mansour, M.A., Mahmoud, A.A. and Geddawy, M. 2013. Non-opioid versus opioid-based general anaesthesia technique for bariatric surgery: A randomized double-blind study. Saudi J. Anaesth. 7(4), 387-391.

Martin, W.R. and Eades, C.G. 1961. Demonstration of tolerance and physical dependence in the dog following a short-term infusion of morphine. J. Pharmacol. Exp. Ther. 133, 262-270.

Mather, S.J. and Peutrell, J.M. 1995. Postoperative morphine requirement, nausea and vomiting following anaesthesia for tonsillectomy. Comparison of intravenous morphine and non-opioid analgesic techniques. Paediatr. Anaesth. 5, 185-188.

Maund, E., McDaid, C., Rice, S., Wright, K., Jenkins, B. and Woolacott, N. 2011. Paracetamol and selective and non-selective non-steroidal anti-inflammatory drugs for the reduction in morphine-related side-effects after major surgery: a systematic review. Br. J. Anaesth. 106(3), 292-297.

Mburu, D.N., Mbugua, S.W., Skoglung, L.A. and Lokken, P. 1988. Effects of paracetamol and acetylsalicylic acid on the post-operative course after experimental orthopaedic surgery in dogs. J. Vet. Pharmacol. Ther. 11(2), 163-171.

McCarthy, G.C., Megalla, S.A. and Habib, A.S. 2010. Impact of intravenous lidocaine infusion on postoperative analgesia and recovery from surgery: a systematic review of randomized controlled trials. Drugs 70(9), 1149-1163.

Mulier, J.P. 2016. Perioperative opioids aggravate obstructive breathing in sleep apnea syndrome: mechanisms and alternative anesthesia strategies. Curr. Opin. Anaesthesiol. 29(1), 129-133.

Odunayo, A., Podam, J.R., Kerl, M.R., DeClue and A.E. 2010. State-of-the-Art-Review: Immunomodulatory effects of opioids. J. Vet. Emerg. Crit. Care 20(4), 376-385.

Pasero, C. and McCaffery, M. 2012. Opioid-induced hyperalgesia. J. Perianesth. Nurs. 27(1), 46-50.

Peltoniemi, M.A., Hagelberg, N.M., Olkkola, K.T. and Teijo, S.I. 2016. Ketamine: A Review of Clinical Pharmacokinetics and Pharmacodynamics in Anesthesia and Pain Therapy. Clin. Pharmacokinet 55(9), 1059-1077.

Rang, H.P., Dale, M.M., Ritter, J.M., Flower, R.J. and Henderson, G. 2012. Rang and Dale's Pharmacology 7th Edition. Elsevier, Spain.

Reid, J., Nolan, A.M., Hughes, J.M.L., Lascelles, D., Pawson, P. and Scott, E.M. 2007. Development of the short-form Glasgow Composite Measure pain scale (CMPS-SF) and derivation of analgesic intervention score. Anim. Welf. 16, 97-104.

Remy, C., Marret, E. and Bonnet, F. 2005. Effects of acetaminophen on morphine side-effects and consumption after major surgery: meta-analysis of randomized controlled trials. Br. J. Anaesth. 94(4), 505-513.

Romano, M., Portela, D.A., Breghi, G. and Otero, P.E. 2015. Stress-related biomarkers in dogs administered regional anaesthesia or fentanyl for analgesia during stifle surgery. Vet. Anaesth. Analg. 43(1), 44-54.

Ronald, V.H. and Kissin, I. 1998. Rapid Development of Tolerance to Analgesia During Remifentanil Infusion in Humans. Anesth. Analg. 86(6), 1307-1311.

Sacerdote, P. 2006. Opioids and the immune system. Palliat. Med. 20, 9-15.

Sinatra, R.S., Jahr, J.S., Reynolds, L.W., Viscosi, E. R., Groudine, S.B. and Payen-Champenis, C. 2005. Efficacy and Safety of Single and Repeated Administration of 1 Gram Intravenous Acetaminophen Injection (Paracetamol) for Pain Management after Major Orthopedic Surgery. Anesthesiology 102, 822-831.

Sinclair, M.D. 2003. A review of the physiological effects of α2-agonists related to the clinical use of medetomidine in small animal practice. Can. Vet. J. 44(11), 885-897.

Sukhani, R., Vazquez, J. and Pappos, A.L. 1996. Recovery after propofol with and without intraoperative fentanyl in patients undergoing ambulatory gynecologic laparoscopy. Anesth. Analg. 83, 975-981.

Ziemann-Gimmel, P., Goldfarb, A.A., Koppman, J. and Marema, R.T. 2014. Opioid-free total intravenous anaesthesia reduces postoperative nausea and vomiting in bariatric surgery beyond triple prophylaxis. Br. J. Anaesth. 112(5), 906-911.

24

Multiple endocrine neoplasia similar to human subtype 2A in a dog: Medullary thyroid carcinoma, bilateral pheochromocytoma and parathyroid adenoma

E.A. Soler Arias[1,*], V.A. Castillo[1], R.H. Trigo[2] and M.E. Caneda Aristarain[3]

[1]Hospital Escuela, Unidad de Endocrinología, Area de Clínica Médica de Pequeños Animales, Fac. de Ciencias Veterinarias, UBA, Av. Chorroarín 280, Ciudad Autónoma de Buenos Aires, Argentina
[2]Catedra de Patología, Fac. de Ciencias Veterinarias, UBA, Av. Chorroarín 280, Ciudad Autónoma de Buenos Aires, Argentina
[3]Alumna de Programa de Investigación. Fac. de Ciencias Veterinarias, UBA, Chorroarín 280, Ciudad Autónoma de Buenos Aires, Argentina

Abstract

Human multiple endocrine neoplasia subtype 2A (MEN 2A) is characterized by medullary thyroid carcinoma, pheochromocytoma and parathyroid hyperplasia or adenoma in the same individual. In this report, a case of a female Rottweiler with medullary thyroid carcinoma, bilateral pheochromocytoma and parathyroid adenoma was described. Clinical manifestations of muscle weakness, polydipsia, polyuria, diarrhea and weight loss were observed. Two adrenal neoplasms were identified incidentally by ultrasonography, and tumor in the left thyroid lobe was identified by palpation. Primary hyperparathyroidism was diagnosed by biochemical testing. Histopathology report was consistent with diagnosis of bilateral pheochromocytoma and parathyroid adenoma. Immunohistochemical staining was positive for calcitonin and synaptophysin, and negative for thyroglobulin, which confirmed medullary thyroid carcinoma. This case in a dog is presenting neoplastic characteristics similar to human MEN 2A and emphasizing the importance of using immunohistochemistry for confirmation.

Keywords: Calcitonin, Immunohistochemistry, MEN 2A, Synaptophysin, Thyroglobulin.

Introduction

Human multiple endocrine neoplasia (MEN) is characterized by the development of two or more tumors in specific endocrine glands in the same individual. Two major forms are recognized: MEN 1 and MEN 2 (Table 1). MEN 2 is caused by a dominant autosomal mutation within the RET proto-oncogene (Brandi et al., 2001). MEN 2 is further divided into MEN 2A, MEN 2B and familial medullary thyroid carcinoma (FMTC). MEN 2A, or Sipple syndrome, is characterized by a phenotypic association that comprises medullary thyroid carcinoma (MTC), unilateral or bilateral pheochromocytoma (PCC) and parathyroid adenoma (PA) or parathyroid hyperplasia (Brandi et al., 2001). In dogs, several neoplastic associations have been described in endocrine organs (Reusch, 2015), but those types of neoplasia have seldom been found in the specific association described for human MEN. To the best of the authors' knowledge, only one case of neoplasic associations specific of human MEN 2A has been reported in the literature, in a 15-year old Fox Terrier diagnosed with MTC, unilateral PCC and hyperplasia in two parathyroid glands (Peterson et al., 1982). The purpose of this report is to analyze the neoplastic association that corresponds to human subtype MEN 2A in a dog and to emphasize the importance of immunohistochemistry (IHC) as a powerful tool for the diagnosis of this syndrome.

Case Details

A 32 kg, 11-year old neutered female Rottweiler was referred to the Endocrinology Unit at the hospital of Veterinary Medicine of the University of Buenos Aires. This case was referred due to the incidental finding of bilateral adrenal gland tumor during ultrasound examination and normal adrenocortical function (Table 2). The haematological investigation and biochemical tests results were within reference ranges, with the exception of total calcium (Ca) levels, 3.55 mmol/l (reference ranges: 2.25-3 mmol/l), phosphatemia (Pi), 0.56 mmol/l (reference ranges: 0.71-1.13 nmol/l) and serum alkaline phosphatase (SAP), 470 U/l (reference value: up to 250U/l). Few months before, the owner had taken the dog to the hospital with the complaint of chronic diarrhea and mild weight loss, progressive weakness, polyuria and polydipsia, which they were still present. On physical examination, a mass was palpated on the left side of the neck, consistent with anatomic location of the thyroid gland.

From the clinical signs and biochemical profiles, a presumptive diagnosis of primary

*Corresponding Author: Elber Alberto Soler Arias. Area de Clínica Médica de Pequeños Animales, Fac. de Ciencias Veterinarias, UBA, Av. Chorroarín 280, Ciudad Autónoma de Buenos Aires, Argentina. E-mail: mveterinario@yahoo.es

Table 1. Classification of Human Multiple Endocrine Neoplasia.

Neoplastic association	MEN 1	MEN 2		
		MEN 2A	MEN 2B	FMTC
Medullary thyroid carcinoma	---	100%	100%	100%
Pheochromocytoma	---	50%	50%	---
Adenoma/Parathyroid hyperplasia	Yes	20-30%	---	---
Pituitary adenoma	Yes	---	---	---
Pancreatic tumors	Yes	---	---	---
Mutated gene	MEN gene	RET gene		

Table 2. Endocrine biochemical tests results.

Biochemistry	Results	Reference ranges	Method
PTH 1-84	6.42	0.6-3.55 pmol/l	CL
Ca	3.55	2.25-3 mmol/l	SP
ICa	2.13	1.1-1.4 mmol/l	ISE
Pi	0.56	0.71-1.13 nmol/l	SP
SAP	470	Up to 250 U/l	SP
UC:Cr	7.0	< 10×10-6	CL/SP
Post-Dx UC:Cr	3.1	<50% of UC:Cr	CL/SP
Co	68.9	13.79-165.4 nmol/l	CL
Post-ACTH Co	344.8	165.4-441.4 nmol/l	CL
VMA	19	12.0 mg/l*	HPLC
Glucose	5.32	3.92-6.16 mmol/l	SP
Potassium	3.9	3.6-5.8 mmol/l	ISE
Sodium	142	140-155 mmol/l	ISE
TSH	0.19	0.03-0.35 ng/ml	CL
FT4	15.44	7.72-20.59 pmol/l	CL
TT4	28.3	12.87-38.1 nmol/l	CL

PTH: Parathyroid hormone; Ca: Total calcium; iCa: Ionized calcium; Pi: Inorganic phosphate; SAP: Serum alkaline phosphatase; UC:Cr: Urine cortisol-creatinine ratio; Post Dx UC:Cr: Post-dexamethasone urine cortisol-creatinine ratio; Co: Plasmatic cortisol; Post-ACTH Co: Post-ACTH (adrenocorticotrophic hormone) cortisol; VMA: vanillin-mandelic acid (*values obtained in the central laboratory of School Animals Veterinary Hospital, Faculty of Vet. Sciences from 8 normal dogs, unpublished data). TSH: Thyroid-stimulating hormone; FT4: Free thyroxine; TT4: Total thyroxine; CL: Chemiluminescence; HPLC: High-performance liquid chromatography; SP: Spectrophotometry. ISE: Ion-selective electrode.

hyperparathyroidism (PHPTH) was suspected. On the other hand, after hypercortisolism was discarded, suspected PCC as an option of bilateral adrenal neoplasia. Accordingly, following laboratory serum test were ordered: Parathyroid hormone (PTH) and ionized calcium (iCa) to confirm PHPTH; thyroid-stimulating hormone (TSH), total thyroxine (T4) and

free canine T4 to evaluate functionality of thyroid gland; 24-hour urine test: Vanillin-mandelic acid (VMA, catecholamines' degradation product) to reach the diagnose of PCC (Gilson et al., 1994). For this test, 24 hours urine was collected in a recipient with 6N hydrochloric acid (HCL6N); the animal was hospitalized and through a urinary catheter, urine sample was collected. Blood pressure was measured to complement the possible diagnosis of PCC. Ultrasound of thyroid, parathyroid and adrenal glands was also carried out.

Results showed increased levels of PTH, iCa and VMA (Table 2). Three serial blood pressure measurements were taken at three different time points using impulse oscillometry (petMAP classic, Ramsey Medical, Inc-Tampa, USA) showed a hypertensive state with an average systolic pressure 205 mm Hg (considered normal less than 150 mmHg) and an average diastolic pressure 95 mm Hg (considered normal less than 95 mm Hg) (Reusch, 2015).

By ultrasound, a neoplasm was observed in the left thyroid lobe with rounded shape (2 cm x 1.8 cm), and the right parathyroid gland was bigger (1.2 cm in diameter) and hypoechoic.

The ultrasound (prior to consultation) and Doppler ultrasound, performed in the hospital, have revealed an altered shape and size of the left adrenal gland (4.3 cm long x 2.2 cm wide); enlarged right adrenal gland (10.3 cm long x 5.4 cm wide) in proximity to caudal vena cava (CVC). Additionally, turbulent blood flow in the CVC due to neoplastic invasion intraluminal was present.

Elevated PTH and iCa confirmed the diagnosis of PHPTH; whereas, high blood pressure and VMA data were strongly compatible with PCC. Imaging studies supported the diagnosis of PHPTH possibly associated to bilateral PCC and thyroid neoplasic. Once diagnosis was established, owner did not return to the hospital, but two months later, the patient was admitted to the hospital service emergency with the complaint of tachypnea, tachycardia, hyperglycemia, fever and hypertension. The owner opted for humane euthanasia and authorized necropsy.

In this report, the case was diagnosed with medullary thyroid carcinoma (Fig. 1), bilateral pheochromocytoma (Fig. 2) and parathyroid adenoma (Fig. 3).

A 2 cm hard mass was noted with peripheral vascularization in the middle of the left thyroid lobe (Fig. 1A). The right adrenal gland was very large with irregular shape (10.3 cm long x 5.4 cm wide). The CVC was found displaced medially, while the right kidney was found displaced laterally. Abdominal phrenic vein (APV) and the CVC were being invaded by the neoplasia (Fig. 2A). Upon dissection, it appeared firm and hemorrhagic, and adrenal cortex area was not recognizable macroscopically (Fig. 2B).

The left adrenal gland was altered in shape and size (4.3 cm long and 2.2 wide), with APV invasion (Fig. 2C). Macroscopically, within the adrenal gland, noticeable hemorrhagic areas and thinning of the adrenal cortex were observed (Fig. 2D).

The right parathyroid gland, in cranial position, was larger than the rest (1.2 cm in diameter) with cystic appearance inside (Fig. 3A,B).

To perform IHC and histopathological procedures, samples of all the lesions were fixed in 10% buffered formalin and embedded in paraffin. Then, 3μm sections were cut, fixed on slides and stained with hematoxylin-eosin (HE) and appropriate antibodies.

IHC procedures were performed using the avidin-biotin complex (ABC) and the immunoperoxidase detection system (Millipore IHC Select®), while the chromogen 3.3'-diaminobenzidine (DAB) was used for development. Antibodies used are shown in Table 3.

Images were captured on a Leica DC160 digital camera connected to a trinocular microscope (Leica DM4000B led).

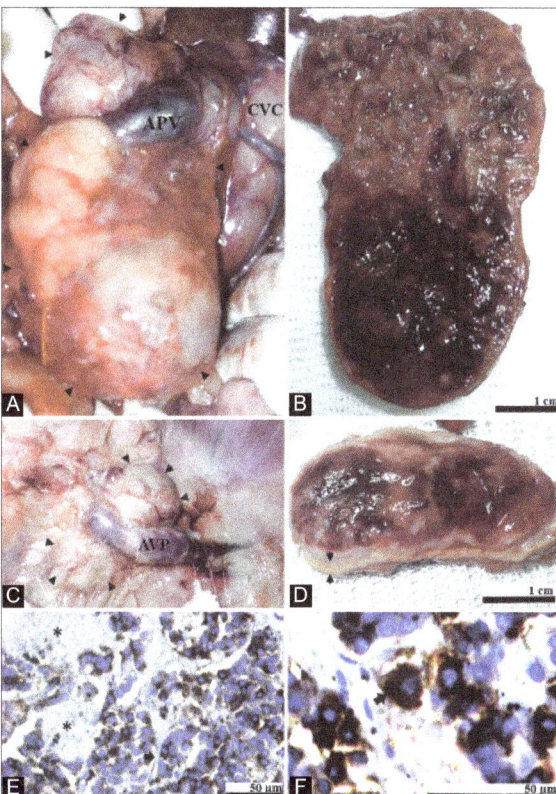

Fig. 2. (A-F) Pheochromocytoma. (A) Right adrenal gland, macroscopic appearance with abdominal phrenic vein (APV) and caudal vena cava (CVC) tumor invasion (B) Right adrenal gland, longitudinal section, neoplasia with congestive, hemorrhagic appearance. No cortical tissue observed macroscopically (Bar = 1 cm). (C) Left adrenal gland, macroscopic appearance with APV invasion (D) Left adrenal gland (macroscopic appearance) longitudinal section. Please note the hemorrhagic appearance of the neoplasia and thinning of the adrenal cortex (arrows) (Bar = 1 cm). (E) Positive cytoplasmic reaction of neoplastic cells with anti-synaptophysin antibody. Cells form nests delimited by fibrovascular septa (arrow), with vascular congestion (*) (Bar = 50 μm). (F) Polyhedral cells, cytoplasm reactive to anti-synaptophysin antibody (arrow). Cells with rounded nuclei, dispersed chromatin and small nucleoli (Bar = 50 μm).

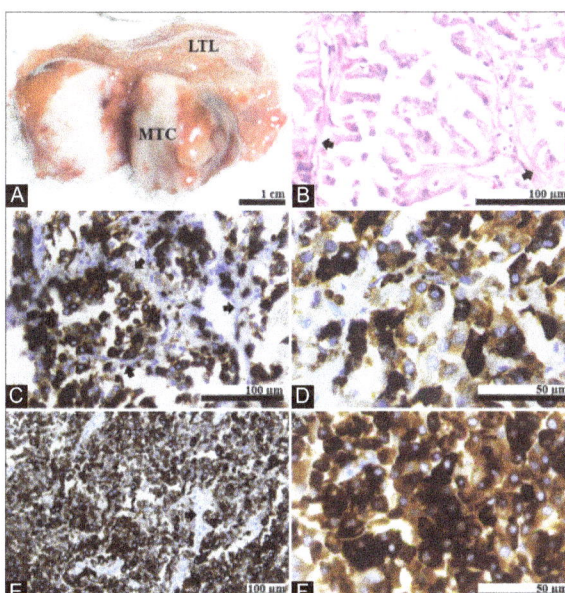

Fig. 1. (A-F) Medullary thyroid carcinoma. (A) Medullary thyroid carcinoma (MTC), macroscopic appearance. LTL: Left thyroid lobe (Bar = 1cm). (B) Structures of papillary appearance, formed by cubic and cylindrical cells with intensely acidophilic cytoplasm arranged over a fibrovascular stroma (arrows) (HE. Bar = 100μm). (C) Positive reaction of neoplastic cells with anti-calcitonin antibody, arranged in nests delimited by fibrovascular tissue septa (arrows) (Bar = 100μm). (D) Positive cytoplasmic reaction with anti-calcitonin antibody. Rounded nuclei and apparent nucleoli (Bar = 50μm). (E) Positive cytoplasmic reaction in neoplastic cells with anti-synaptophysin antibody. A fibrovascular tissue septum can be observed (arrow) (Bar = 100μm). (F) Positive cytoplasmic reaction of neoplastic cells with anti-synaptophysin antibody (Bar = 50 μm).

Quantification of the IHC staining was performed, semi-quantitatively, through the percentage of tumor cells stained positively/cells per field. Staining intensity was subjectively classified as mild, moderate and intense.

In the thyroid tissue we observed cubic and cylindrical cells proliferation, arranged over a delicate fibrovascular stroma; it also showed a pseudostratified lining with branching papillae. Morphologically, these cells were characterized by oval or rounded nuclei, moderate anisocariosis and variable quantities of acidophilic cytoplasm, which let to high anisocytosis. Mitotic figures were also observed (Fig. 1B). More than 60% of neoplastic cells showed intense positive cytoplasmic reaction to anti-calcitonin antibody (Fig. 1C,D). Cytoplasmic staining with anti-synaptophysin antibody was intensely positive in more than 90% of neoplastic cells (Fig. 1E,F).

Neoplastic cells stained negative for thyroglobulin (TG); only the areas of normal thyroid parenchyma stained positive. Cromogranin A (CgA) staining was also negative. Morphologically and immunohistochemically, the neoplasia was consistent with an MTC.

Adrenal cortex thinning was observed, caused by proliferation of polyhedral monomorphic cells originated from adrenal medullary. Morphologically, they consisted in rounded nuclei with dispersed chromatin, though some of them were hyperchromatic, with small nucleoli and acidophilic, finely granular and scarcely apparent cytoplasm. Cells were arranged in multiple narrow nests, delimited by the fibrovascular septa of the stroma surrounding the neoplasia. The lesion also showed intense vascular congestion and some necrosis areas (Fig. 2E). Cytoplasmic staining with anti-synaptophysin antibody was moderately positive in 60% of neoplastic cells (Fig. 2F). CgA staining was negative. Morphologically and immunohistochemically, the adrenal neoplastic tissue was consistent with bilateral PCC.

The parathyroid tissue showed a proliferative process formed by irregular cords of polyhedral cells with basophilic granular cytoplasm, with large rounded nuclei with dispersed chromatin and smaller eosinophilic cells with pyknotic nucleus (Fig. 3C,D). The diagnosis was consistent with chief cells parathyroid adenoma.

Discussion

This case report describes three types of neoplasia, each of which is, in itself, rare in dogs. The neoplastic association (phenotypic expression of RET proto-oncogen mutation) similar to MEN 2A in human, has only been reported in a 15-year old male neutered Fox Terrier (Peterson et al., 1982) diagnosed with MTC, unilateral PCC and chief cells hyperplasia in both parathyroid glands. Additionally, two previous reports with similar cases to subtype MEN 2 described an association of PA and PCC in a 13-year old Yorkshire Terrier (Wright et al., 1995) and FMTC in four mixed Alaskan Malamutes (Lee et al., 2006). In our case, the RET proto-oncogene mutation could not be analyzed (not available in Argentina), but the phenotypic expression (neoplastic association) was accurate to the MEN 2A in humans.

MTC is a neoplasia which originates from the C cells (or parafollicular cells) of the thyroid gland; in humans, it is first expressed in MEN 2A, because of its high penetrance 90%, followed by PCC 50% and, lastly, parathyroid gland lesions 20-30% (Brandi et al., 2001). Both in ours and Peterson's report (Peterson et al., 1982), thyroid function was preserved, the size and the macroscopic appearance of the MTC were similar, but the histopathological appearance was different.

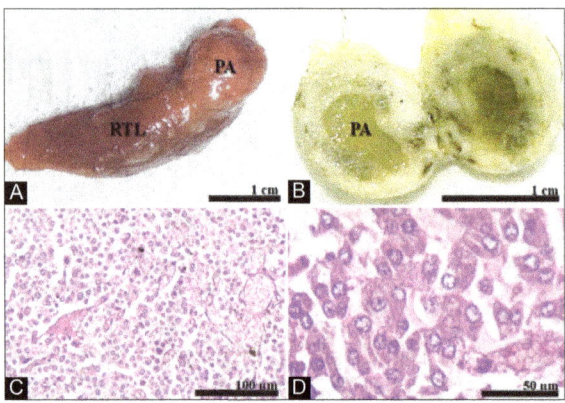

Fig. 3. (A-D) Parathyroid adenoma. (A) Parathyroid adenoma (PA) macroscopic appearance, next to the right thyroid lobe (RTL). (B) Parathyroid adenoma was dissected in half and fixed in 10% buffered formalin. (C) Chief cell adenoma parathyroid (HE. Bar = 100μm). (D) Irregular cords of polyhedral cells with basophilic granular cytoplasm, with large rounded nuclei with dispersed chromatin and smaller eosinophilic cells with pyknotic nucleus (HE. Bar = 50μm).

Table 3. Antibodies used for immunohistochemical staining of medullary thyroid carcinomas and pheochromocytoma, and the canine tissues used as positive controls.

Primary antibody	Type of antibody	Dilution	Positive control
Thyroglobulin	Monoclonal mouse*	1:50	Thyroid (follicular cells)
Calcitonin	Polyclonal rabbit**	1:200	Thyroid (parafollicular cells)
Chromogranin A	Polyclonal goat*	1:50	Adrenal (medullar cells)
Synaptophysin	Monoclonal mouse*	1:50	Adrenal (medullar cells)

Negative control was performed by removing primary antibody; Santa Cruz Biotechnology*; Roche Laboratory**.

Although the MTC has certain histopathological features that make it recognizable (polygonal cells arranged in nests delimited by fibrovascular septa), some cases have shown an architectural pattern similar to that of papillary or follicular carcinomas (Hedinger *et al.*, 1989). In our case, histopathological findings indicated the presence of follicular thyroid carcinoma, but IHC procedures were done when we suspected MEN 2A. The fact that the thyroid lesion stained positive for calcitonin (CT) and synaptophysin (SYN) antibodies supported the diagnosis of MTC, while the negative immunoreactivity for TG ruled out follicular thyroid carcinoma. In the immunohistochemical diagnosis of MTC, CT is the most specific and reliable marker for this type of tumor (Patnaik and Lieberman, 1991; Rigopoulou *et al.*, 2008), while SYN, in determining its neuroendocrine origin, is the perfect complement (Gould *et al.*, 1987). In this case, the combination of the three markers confirmed the diagnosis of MTC.

In human medicine, plasma calcitonin is used as a diagnostic marker of MTC (Toledo *et al.*, 2009). In Peterson's case (Peterson *et al.*, 1982), increased levels, compared to human normal reference values, contributed to the diagnosis of MTC; in the current case study their determination was not considered due to lack of reference values for dogs and association studies linking it with MTC.

In the specific case of calcitonin, its role in inducing hypocalcemia within the PHPTH context is not well-known (Feldman, 2015), while hypocalcemia within the context of MTC is infrequent (Patnaik *et al.*, 1978). In our case, hypercalcemia generated by PHPTH had a clear influence on calcium levels.

On the other hand, chronic diarrhea may be attributed to a rise in plasma calcitonin secretion, considering that in humans 30% of patients with MTC show increased levels (Moline and Eng, 2011) and in dogs the infusion of calcitonin generated diarrheal episodes due to increased motility and a decrease in intestinal water absorption (Cox *et al.*, 1979).

PCC is a functional paraganglioma that originates from adrenal medullary chromaffin cells. In humans, 27% of PCC are hereditary and associated with mutations in several genes, of which RET proto-oncogene is responsible for MEN 2 (Subramaniam, 2011).

In dogs, PCC presentation is sporadic and its finding is usually incidental, as in our case (ultrasound). Reported cases of PCC with a possible hereditary component reduce to subtypes MEN 2A (Peterson *et al.*, 1982) and MEN 2 (Wright *et al.*, 1995) already mentioned in the MTC discussion. Other possible associations found in dogs are PCC and pituitary tumor (Von Dehn *et al.*, 1995; Bennett and Norman, 1998) and PCC, adrenal cortical tumor and pituitary tumor (Thuróczy *et al.*, 1998).

PCC malignancy criteria remain controversial, in human FCC malignancy is currently defined by the presence of metastasis, not local invasion; in dogs, however, either local invasion or distant metastasis usually qualifies for definition of malignancy (Reusch, 2015). Histologically, it may be difficult to distinguish benign from malignant PCC (Reusch, 2015). However, we define malignancy PCC based on local vascular invasion and through the scale PASS (Pheochromocytoma of the Adrenal Gland Scaled Score) used in human medicine; foci of necrosis, vascular invasion, monomorphic growth, nuclear hyperchromatism and cells arranged in nests (Parenti *et al.*, 2012).

Clinical signs in patients with PCC are usually nonspecific, but they can be explained considering the type of catecholamine and its actions, quantities, type of secretion (continuous or episodic), location and type of receptor on which they have effect (Sako *et al.*, 2001). In dogs with PCC, noradrenaline is the predominant catecholamine, and the one that appeared to increase systolic blood pressure in our case. Some dogs showed an increased secretion of adrenaline that may potentiate cardiorespiratory signs (tachycardia, tachypnea) and metabolic signs (hyperglycemia), and PCC may secrete other peptides that cause other signs, such as interleukin-6 (fever) and VIP (diarrhea). Muscle weakness, weight loss, polyuria and polydipsia are signs attributed both to PCC and PHPTH (Feldman, 2015; Reusch, 2015).

Although the dog presented a large tumor with CVC and APV invasion, no local signs (such as ascites, hind-limb edema or abdominal distension) were observed.

It was initially suspected as bilateral PCC, after discarding the hypercortisolism by assessing urinary cortisol pre- and post-oral dexamethasone, inhibition test plasma cortisol pre- and post-intravenous dexamethasone and ACTH stimulation test (Behrend, 2015). Although the determination of the relationship normetanephrine urine/urine creatinine (degradation product of noradrenaline) proved to be best method for the diagnosis of pheochromocytoma in dogs, in this case we considered the use of vanillin-mandelic acid (VMA) because in our country at the time of diagnosis, it was the only tool available for PCC diagnosis in veterinary practice. The value obtained was above reference value of the central laboratory of the Hospital School, Small Animals, Faculty of Veterinary Sciences, UBA (Unpublished data). VMA in dogs, in absence of reference values, was used, as reported by Gilson *et al.* (1994) (13.2 mg/l); similar reference value obtained in our hospital. Sustained hypertension was a fact important for suspected PCC.

Finally, histopathology and IHC confirmed the definitive diagnosis of PCC. We opted for an IHC procedure with SYN antibody (reliable marker for normal and tumoral neuroendocrine cells) (Buffa *et al.*,

1987). Though CgA is the most specific tumor marker for neuroendocrine differentiation, in our case, all types of neoplasia stained negative for CgA. In this respect, it should be noted that its sensitivity depends on granular density, which in turn depends on the degree of tissue differentiation; it is also worth mentioning that in this case the contents of presynaptic vesicles (they contain CgA) may have been emptied during the crisis that affected the patient before euthanasia.

PHPTH, present in 20 to 30% of patients with human MEN 2A, is usually mild and encompasses a number of conditions, from a solitary adenoma to hyperplasia in one or more parathyroid glands. Within the context of MEN 2A, most cases of PHPTH do not manifest clinical symptoms; however, hypercalciuria and renal lithiasis can be observed (Brandi et al., 2001). Hypercalcemia, hypophosphatemia and increase PTH, were decisive finding in diagnosis of PHPTH (Feldman, 2015). Solitary adenoma of parathyroid gland was present in our case, while hyperplasia in two parathyroid gland was reported by Peterson. The absence of lithiasis suggests the adenoma grew rapidly in the last stages of the animal's life (the last neoplasia to appear), and the clinical manifestations were more accentuated near the time the disease was diagnosed. However, in this case we believe it is hard to attribute the predominance of signs to one of the three types of neoplasia, since it is the three combined that defined the diverse manifestations observed in the animal. Histopathology confirmed PA, because of its morphological features.

By conclusion, definitive diagnosis of thyroid neoplasia required routinely use of IHC to avoid errors in classification, treatment and follow-up of MTC. When a PCC is found, it is of vital importance to rule out the presence of thyroid or parathyroid tumor; likewise, in the presence of MTC, it is advisable to rule out PCC.

Finally, we would like to highlight the importance of IHC; without it, the diagnosis of MTC and its phenotypic association with MEN 2A would not have been possible.

Conflict of interest
The authors declare that there is no conflict of interest

References

Behrend, E.N. 2015. Canine hyperadrenocorticism, in: Feldman, E.C., Nelson, R.W., Reusch C.E., Scott-Moncrieff, J.C.R. and Behrend, E.N. Canine & Feline Endocrinology, fourth edition, Elsevier, pp: 377-451.

Bennett, P.F. and Norman, E.J. 1998. Mitotane (o'p'-DDD) resistance in a dog with pituitary-dependent hyperadrenocorticism and phaeochromocytoma. Aust. Vet. J. 76(2), 101-103.

Brandi, M.L., Gagel, R.F., Angeli, A., Bilezikian, J.P., Beck-Peccoz, P., Bordi, C., Conte-Devolx, B., Falchetti, A., Gheri, R.G., Libroia, A., Lips, C.J., Lombardi, G., Mannelli, M., Pacini, F., Ponder, B.A., Raue, F., Skogseid, B., Tamburrano, G., Thakker, R.V., Thompson, N.W., Tomassetti, P., Tonelli, F., Wells, S.A.Jr. and Marx, S.J. 2001. Guidelines for diagnosis and therapy of MEN type 1 and type 2. J. Clin. Endocrinol Metab. 86(12), 5658-5671.

Buffa, R., Rindi, G., Sessa, F., Gini, A., Capella, C., Jahn, R., Navone, F., De Camilli, P. and Solcia, E. 1987. Synaptophysin immunoreactivity and small clear vesicles in neuroendocrine cells and related tumours. Mol. Cell Probes. 1(4), 367-381.

Cox, T.M., Fagan, E.A., Hillyard, C.J., Allison, D.J. and Chadwick, V.S. 1979. Role of calcitonin in diarrhoea associated with medullary carcinoma of the thyroid. Gut 20(7), 629-633.

Feldman, E.C. 2015. Hypercalcemia and primary hyperparathyroidism, in: Feldman, E.C., Nelson, R.W., Reusch C.E., Scott-Moncrieff, J.C.R. and Behrend, E.N. Canine & Feline Endocrinology, fourth edition, Elsevier, pp: 579-624.

Gilson, S.D., Withrow, S.J., Wheeler, S.L. and Twedt, D.C. 1994. Pheochromocytoma in 50 dogs. J. Vet. Intern. Med. 8(3), 228-232.

Gould, V.E., Wiedenmann, B., Lee, I., Schwechheimer, K., Dockhorn-Dworniczak, B., Radosevich, J.A., Moll, R. and Franke, W.W. 1987. Synaptophysin expression in neuroendocrine neoplasms as determined by immunocytochemistry. Am. J. Pathol. 126(2), 243-257.

Hedinger, C., Williams, E.D. and Sobin, L.H. 1989. The WHO histological classification of thyroid tumors: A commentary on the second edition. Cancer 63(5), 908-911.

Lee, J.J., Larsson, C., Lui, W.O., Höög, A. and Von Euler, H. 2006. A dog pedigree with familial medullary thyroid cancer. Int. J. Oncol. 29(5), 1173-1182.

Moline, J. and Eng, C. 2011. Multiple endocrine neoplasia type 2: An overview. Genet. Med. 13(9), 755-764.

Parenti, G., Zampetti, B., Rapizzi, E., Ercolino, T., Giachè, V. and Mannelli, M. 2012. Updated and new perspectives on diagnosis, prognosis and therapy of malignant pheochromocytoma/paraganglioma. J. Oncol. Article ID 872713. doi:10.1155/2012/872713.

Patnaik, A.K., Lieberman, P.H., Erlandson, R.A., Acevedo, W.M. and Liu, S.K. 1978. Canine medullary carcinoma of the thyroid. Vet. Pathol. 15(5), 590-599.

Patnaik, A.K. and Lieberman, P.H. 1991. Gross, histologic, cytochemical, and immunocytochemical study of medullary thyroid carcinoma in sixteen dogs. Vet Pathol, 28(3), 223-233.

Peterson, M.E., Randolph, J.F., Zaki, F.A. and Heath, H. 3rd.1982. Multiple endocrine neoplasia in a dog. J.

Am. Vet. Med. Assoc. 180(12), 1476-1478.

Reusch, C.E. 2015. Pheochromocytoma and multiple endocrine neoplasia, in: Feldman, E.C., Nelson, R.W., Reusch, C.E., Scott-Moncrieff, J.C.R. and Behrend, E.N. Canine & Feline Endocrinology, fourth edition, Elsevier, pp: 521-551.

Rigopoulou, D., Gómez Lobo, I., Guadalix Iglesias, S. and Calatayud Gutiérrez, M. Carcinoma de tiroides. 2008. Clasificación. Manifestaciones Clínicas. Diagnóstico. Actitudes terapéuticas. TSHrh y tiroglobulina sérica en el manejo del carcinoma diferenciado tiroideo. Medicine 10(14), 904-913.

Sako, T., Kitamura, N., Kagawa, Y., Hirayama, K., Morita, M., Kurosawa, T., Yoshino, T. and Taniyama, H. 2001. Immunohistochemical Evaluation of a Malignant Pheochromocytoma in a Wolfdog. Vet. Pathol. 38(4), 447-450.

Subramaniam, R. 2011. Pheochromocytoma-Current concepts in diagnosis and management. Trends Anaesth. Crit. Care 1(2), 104-110.

Thuróczy, J., Van Sluijs, F.J., Kooistra, H.S., Voorhout, G., Mol, J.A., van der Linde-Sipman, J.S. and Rijnberk, A. 1998. Multiple endocrine neoplasias in a dog: Corticotrophic tumour, bilateral adrenocortical tumours, and pheochromocytoma. Vet Q. 20(2), 56-61.

Toledo, S.P.A., Lourenço, D.M.Jr., Santos, M.A., Tavares, M.R., Toledo, R.A. and Correia-Deur, J.E. 2009. Hypercalcitoninemia is not pathognomonic of medullary thyroid carcinoma. Clinics (Sao Paulo) 64(7), 699-706.

Von Dehn, B.J., Nelson, R.W., Feldman, E.C. and Griffey, S.M. 1995. Pheochromocytoma and hyperadrenocorticism in dogs: Six cases (1982-1992). J. Am. Vet. Med. Assoc. 207(3), 322-324.

Wright, K.N., Breitschwerdt, E.B., Feldman, J.M., Berry, C.R., Meuten, D.J. and Spodnick, G.J. 1995. Diagnostic and therapeutic considerations in a hypercalcemic dog with multiple endocrine neoplasia. J. Am. Anim. Hosp. Assoc. 31(2), 156-162.

25

Analysis of serum magnesium ions in dogs exposed to external stress

Izumi Ando[1], Kaoru Karasawa[1,2], Shinichi Yokota[3], Takao Shioya[4], Hiroshi Matsuda[1,3] and Akane Tanaka[1,2,*]

[1]*Cooperative Major in Advanced Health Science, Graduate School of Bio-Applications and System Engineering, Tokyo University of Agriculture and Technology, Tokyo 183-8509, Japan*
[2]*Laboratory of Comparative Animal Medicine, Division of Animal Life Science, Institute of Agriculture, Tokyo University of Agriculture and Technology, Tokyo 183-8509, Japan*
[3]*Laboratory of Veterinary Molecular Pathology and Therapeutics, Division of Animal Life Science, Institute of Agriculture, Tokyo University of Agriculture and Technology, Tokyo 183-8509, Japan*
[4]*The Eye Mate Inc., Tokyo 177-0051, Japan*

Abstract
Magnesium ions (Mg^{2+}) are essential for various enzymatic reactions in the body associated with energy production and activation of the muscles and nerves. Mg^{2+} is also involved in blood pressure regulation, maintenance of body temperature, and glucose metabolism. Although various factors including foods and physical conditions have been reported to change serum Mg^{2+} status in humans, serum Mg^{2+} in dogs exposed to external stress has been unclear. In this study, we examined serum levels of Mg^{2+} in dogs at different conditions using the guide dog candidates for the blind. Serum Mg^{2+} was decreased in winter and increased in summer. Guide dog candidates in an elementary class of the training showed markedly lower levels of serum Mg^{2+}, compared with that of dogs in an advanced class. When healthy adult dogs were subjected to forced exercise using a treadmill, a significant reduction in serum Mg^{2+} levels was observed, particularly in winter. These findings suggest that serum levels of Mg^{2+} may be influenced by weather fluctuation such as air temperature, nervousness in unaccustomed situations, age, and physical stress induced by exercise. The results indicate that Mg^{2+} supplementation should be considered for working dogs, dogs moving or traveling to a new environment, and dogs during winter.
Keywords: Exercise, Guide dogs, Seasonality, Serum magnesium ions, Training.

Introduction

Magnesium ions (Mg^{2+}) are one of the essential minerals necessary to maintain life. Most Mg^{2+} is stored in the cells of organs and tissues, particularly in the bones and teeth. Small amounts of Mg^{2+} are present in extracellular spaces, where Mg^{2+} binds with either proteins or anions. Mg^{2+} is needed to generate energy by assisting in the reaction of various enzymes with Mg^{2+} binding sites in their active region (Cowan, 2002). Mg^{2+} is necessary for the synthesis of proteins, energy metabolism (Pfeiffer and Barnes, 1981; He *et al.*, 2006), contraction of the muscles (Altura and Altura, 1981), blood pressure regulation (Resnick *et al.*, 2000; He *et al.*, 2005), and modulating blood glucose levels (Dominguez *et al.*, 1998; Singh *et al.*, 1998), as well as a considerable number of enzymatic reactions within the body (Cowan, 2002). Lack of Mg^{2+} induces deterioration in energy production, leading to fatigue (Lukaski and Nielsen, 2002). Mg^{2+} deficiency also causes poor concentration, chronic fatigue, loss of appetite, and cardiovascular abnormalities in humans (Bohl and Volpe, 2002). Concentration of Mg^{2+} in blood is regulated by the interaction of several

hormones, including, noradrenaline, parathyroid hormone, glucagon, and cortisol (Soria *et al.*, 2014). Intravenous injection of catecholamine induced a marked increase of Mg^{2+} excretion in the urine (Rayssiguier, 1977; Joborn *et al.*, 1985), suggesting catecholamine may reduce blood Mg^{2+} levels. In humans, abnormalities in serum Mg^{2+} levels have been reported in various diseases (Elin, 1988; Rude and Gruber, 2004; Sinert *et al.*, 2005; Baltaci *et al.*, 2013), and, interestingly, the morbidity of these diseases has been reported to correlate with Mg^{2+} intake (Elin, 1988; Singh *et al.*, 1997; Eby and Eby, 2006). However, the dietary intake of Mg^{2+} reduces with age (Bazzarre *et al.*, 1993; Durlach *et al.*, 1993; Tucker *et al.*, 1999). The market for Mg^{2+} supplements has expanded for prophylactic amelioration of lifestyle related diseases (Seelig and Altura, 1997). In addition, Mg^{2+} supplementation in training athletes has also increased (Haymes, 1991). Moreover, reduction in Mg^{2+} intake has been reported to be associated with severity of depression and anxiety in community-dwelling adults, and administration of Mg^{2+} to patients improved their conditions (Jacka *et al.*, 2009).

*****Corresponding Author:** Akane Tanaka. Tokyo University of Agriculture and Technology, Tokyo 183-8509, Japan. Email: *akane@cc.tuat.ac.jp*

Changes in the serum Mg^{2+} levels of dogs have not been fully explored. The aim of this study was to analyze changes in serum Mg^{2+} levels of dogs before and after a training or exercise load.

Materials and Methods

Animals

All animal experiments complied with the standards specified in the guidelines of the University Animal Care and Use Committee of the Tokyo University of Agriculture and Technology as well as the guidelines for the use of laboratory animals provided by the Science Council of Japan. The procedures conducted were approved by the University Animal Care and Use Committee of the Tokyo University of Agriculture and Technology (No. 27-62; July, 27, 2015). For blood collection from guide dog candidates, all procedures were informed approved by The Eye Mate Inc. (Tokyo, Japan). Young Labrador retrievers (aged from 17 to 35 months, mean age was 23 ± 0.8 months old.) that had been selected as candidates for guide dogs for the blind were subjected to the measurement of serum Mg^{2+} in the experiment 1 (12 dogs) and 2 (24 dogs). They were housed in individual cages in a room illuminated daily from 6:00–21:00 with a temperature of $15–25 \pm 3°C$. The room temperature of the kennel was set according to that of the outside, because the training of the dog was carried out in city areas. They were fed with appropriate food once a day at 7:00 and were given water ad libitum. They were all neutered and belonged to The Eye Mate Inc. The Eye Mate Inc. has the longest history of dog training in Japan and provides the largest number of well-trained guide dogs to the blind. Healthy Labrador retrievers that worked as guide dogs for the blind (mean age was 6.9 ± 0.4 years old, 6 neutered males and 8 neutered females) were subjected to the measurement of serum Mg^{2+} in the experiment 2 (14 dogs). They were all neutered and belonged to their user. They were fed by their users. Three of them were fed in the morning and 11 of them were fed in the night. All the guide dog candidates and guide dogs were fed with the same food.

In the experiment 3, we used 6 laboratory dogs. They were housed in individual cages in a room illuminated daily from 7:00–19:00 with a temperature of $21 \pm 4°C$. They were fed with appropriate food once a day at 19:00 and were given water ad libitum. They were allowed to take a walk or free exercise at the outside of their facilities with animal care staffs for 30–60 min in one day for their welfare, except the day of the experiment. They were all neutered, fed with the same food, and managed in the same circumstances.

Foods supplied to dogs used in the current study are shown in Table 1. Natural Harvest Maintenance (13–15 g/kg body weight/day) (Vanguard International Foods Co., Chiba, Japan) was given to guide dog candidates and guide dogs for the blind, and Acana Pacifica for

dogs (15–20 g/kg body weight/day) (Champion Pet Foods Ltd., AB, Canada) was given to laboratory dogs.

Dogs used in each experiment

In the experiment 1, 12 guide dog candidates in the advanced classes (aged from 21 to 35 months) were used to confirm seasonal changes of serum Mg^{2+} levels. The advanced class is a final stage of their training. Blood samples collected in January, May, and August from different dogs in the advanced class at each month, and serum Mg^{2+} levels were analyzed. Each group was consisted of 4 dogs (1 neutered male and 3 neutered females). In Eye Mate Inc., 4 dogs finish their trainings every month and start working as mature guide dogs for the blind.

In the experiment 2, the total of 24 guide dog candidates and 14 working guide dogs were used to measure serum Mg^{2+} levels. Training phases of those candidates are divided into three classes as described below. The elementary training class included dogs that could walk with their instructor on their leads for 10–15 min. The intermediate class included dogs that could wear harnesses to walk under the simple commands of their instructor on an empty street for 20–30 min. The advanced class included dogs that could wear harnesses to walk under the commands of their instructor on a busy street for 40–50 min. Six dogs (the mean age was 19.8 ± 0.8 months old, 1 neutered male and 5 neutered females) in the elementary class, 10 dogs (the mean age was 21.1 ± 0.9 months old, 4 neutered males and 6 neutered females) in the intermediate class, and 8 dogs (the mean age was 26.5 ± 1.5 months old, 2 neutered males and 6 neutered females) in the advanced class were subjected to the study. Fourteen healthy Labrador retrievers that worked as guide dogs for the blind (mean age was 6.9 ± 0.4 years old, 6 neutered males and 8 neutered females) were subjected to the measurement of serum Mg^{2+} in the experiment 2 under the informed consent of their owners as adult controls.

In the experiment 3, we used a treadmill to test the effects of forced exercise. In this experiment, three healthy mixed breed dogs (aged from 5 to 6 years), one Beagle dog (6 years old), one Jack Russell Terrier (6 years old) and one Miniature Dachshund (9 years old), belonging to the colony of our laboratory were used. They included 3 neutered males and 3 neutered females. Before and after the treadmill training performed in January and August, blood samples were collected. To assess the effects of forced exercise on serum Mg^{2+} levels, laboratory dogs undertook 20 min of physical exercise on a treadmill that was set at 3–6.5 km/h. The speed of the treadmill was set according to the physical ability of each dog.

Blood sampling

To investigate serum Mg^{2+} levels of dogs, guide dog candidates at different phases of training were examined. We collected blood samples from dogs in the elementary and intermediate classes on the first day of their training. We collected blood samples from dogs in the advanced class on the day that the training was completely over. Blood samples (1.5 mL/dog) of laboratory dogs were collected at each time point of their exercise. Samples were taken from the cephalic vein by experienced veterinarians and were collected into serum-separator tubes (SST II; Becton, Dickinson & Co.). The tubes were allowed to stand for 30 min at room temperature and were then centrifuged for 10 min at 425 g. Separated serum was collected and stored at -30°C until use.

Measurement of serum Mg^{2+} levels

Serum Mg^{2+} was measured by the quantitative colorimetric determination method using the QuantiChrom Magnesium Assay Kit (DIMG-250; BioAssay Systems, Hayward, CA), according to the manufacturer's protocol. Using the assay kit, we can directly measure magnesium ions in serum samples without any pretreatment. All assays were performed in flat-bottom 96 well plates (Nunc PolySorp®; Thermo Fisher Scientific, Inc., Tokyo, Japan). A calmagite dye used in the assay kit forms a colored complex specifically with magnesium ions. The absorbance values were measured at 500 nm using a micro plate reader (ImmunoMini (NJ-2300); BioTec, Suffolk, UK). Serum Mg^{2+} values were expressed as the mean of triplicate measurements.

Measurement of plasma adrenaline and noradrenaline levels

Previous studies have described that increase in blood levels of adrenaline might associate with of hypomagnesemia in humans and ewes (Rayssiguier, 1977; Joborn et al., 1985). Since exercise stress induces increase in blood catecholamine levels, we measured adrenalin and noradrenalin after exercise loads and tried to delineate possible association of those markers in blood Mg^{2+} levels. Plasma of each dog was isolated using EDTA-2Na and stored at -30°C until use as described above. Plasma adrenaline and noradrenaline levels were measured by using the high-speed liquid chromatography systems (Shimadzu Corp., Kyoto, Japan) in SRL Inc. (Tokyo, Japan).

Statistical analysis

Data were analyzed using IBM SPSS Statistics ver. 22.0. In the experiment 1, the comparison between three groups was analyzed using multiple comparisons with Bonferroni correction ($P < 0.05/3$ was estimated as a level of significance). In the experiment 2, the comparison between four groups was analyzed using a one-way ANOVA and Dunnett test ($P < 0.05$). In the experiment 3, the influences of seasonal variation, and before and after the exercise load, were analyzed using a two-way ANOVA within-participant design ($P < 0.05$). Serum Mg^{2+} levels were quoted as median and interquartile ranges in all figures.

Results

Experiment 1; Seasonality of serum Mg^{2+} levels

To examine the serum Mg^{2+} levels of dogs with very few individual differences due to their environments and foods, we used guide dog candidates with the agreement of The Eye Mate Inc., a Japanese public incorporated foundation that raises guide dogs. Since serum Mg^{2+} levels are influenced by temperature and the seasons in humans (Owaki et al., 1996), we first assessed seasonal variations of serum Mg^{2+} levels in dogs. We collected blood samples from the guide dog candidates in the advanced class in January (winter, average temperature for the last five years in Tokyo, Japan is 5.7°C), May (spring, 19.4°C), and August (summer, 28.6°C). The serum Mg^{2+} levels of January, May, and August were 16.7 ± 0.2 µg/mL (the median is 16.9 µg/mL), 20.7 ± 0.3 µg/mL (the median is 21.0 µg/mL), and 21.2 ± 0.2 µg/mL (the median is 21.7 µg/mL), respectively (Fig. 1a). Serum Mg^{2+} levels of dogs in the advanced class were significantly lower in winter. On the other hand, serum Mg^{2+} levels increased in summer.

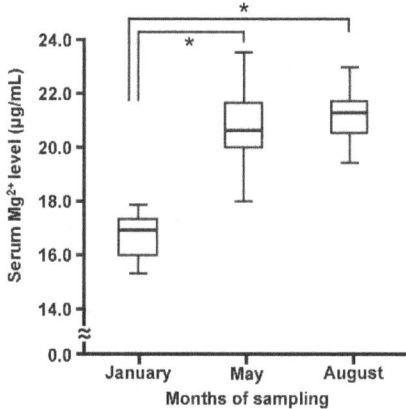

Fig. 1a. Seasonal variation in serum Mg^{2+} levels of guide dog candidates in the advanced class. The median values of serum Mg^{2+} levels are indicated by the bar within each box. The statistical significance of differences between the three groups was tested using Bonferroni correction. n = 4 in each group. (* $P < 0.05$).

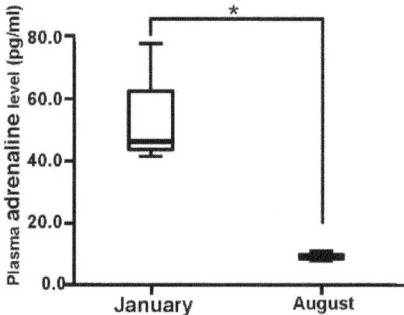

Fig. 1b. Seasonal variation in plasma adrenaline levels of guide dog candidates in the advanced class. The statistical significance of differences between January and August was tested using paired t-test. n = 4 in each group. (* $P < 0.05$).

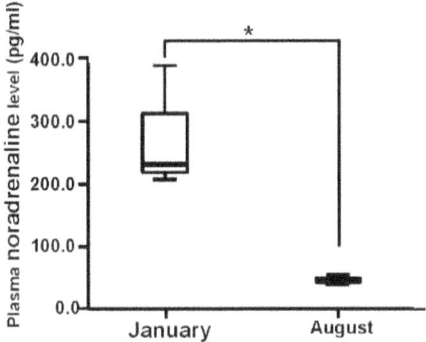

Fig. 1c. Seasonal variation in plasma noradrenaline levels of guide dog candidates in the advanced class. The statistical significance of differences between January and August was tested using paired t-test. n = 4 in each group. (* P < 0.05).

Table 1. Foods supplied to dogs in the current study

Calorie and components	Natural Harvest Maintenance*	Acana Pacifica for dogs**
Metabolic calorie (kJ/g food)	13.4	14.7
Crude protein (% wt.)	18	33
Crude fat (% wt.)	9.5	17
Crude fiber (% wt.)	4	5
Moisture (% wt.)	10	10
Minerals		
Magnesium (% wt.)	0.1	0.1
Calcium (% wt.)	1.6	1.5
Sodium (% wt.)	0.36	0.6
Chloride (% wt.)	0.57	1.1
Potassium (% wt.)	1.0	1.0
Iron (mg/kg food)	265	170
Zinc (mg/kg food)	404	230
Copper (mg/kg food)	23.8	20
Manganese (mg/kg food)	51.2	23
Iodine (mg/kg food)	4.6	1.8
Selenium (mg/kg food)	0.34	1.5

*Natural Harvest was given to guide dog candidates and guide dogs for the blind. **Acana Pacifica was given to laboratory dogs used in the treadmill experiment.

In the previous studies, it mentioned that intravenous injection of adrenaline decreased blood levels of Mg^{2+} in humans (Joborn *et al.*, 1985) and ewes (Rayssiguier, 1977), and that the consequent increase in adrenaline induced magnesium loss (Seelig, 1994). Therefore, we examined adrenaline and noradrenaline levels in winter and summer (Fig. 1b, Fig. 1c). Plasma adrenaline and noradrenaline levels were higher in winter; on the other hand, they became lower in summer, showing the inverse correlation with serum Mg^{2+} levels.

Experiment 2; Serum Mg^{2+} levels of guide dog candidates in different training phases

To investigate serum Mg^{2+} levels of dogs exposed to different amounts of external stress, we selected dogs in elementary, intermediate, and advanced training classes. These different training stages were classified according to the total of training hours and days. Serum samples were collected from May to August and Mg^{2+} levels were measured. The steady state levels of serum Mg^{2+} of dogs in elementary, intermediate, and advanced classes were 13.0 ± 0.3 µg/mL (the median is 13.0 µg/mL), 19.3 ± 0.9 µg/mL (the median is 19.9 µg/mL), 21.5 ± 0.5 µg/mL (the median is 21.7 µg/mL), respectively. Serum Mg^{2+} levels were lower in dogs in the elementary class than those of dogs in other classes (Fig. 2).

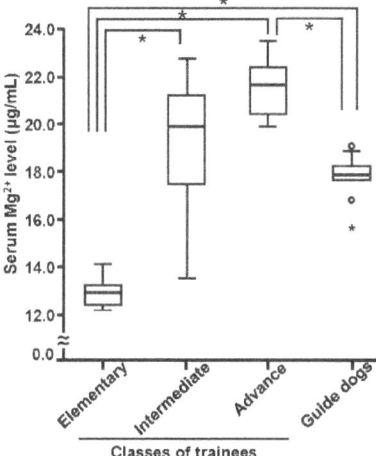

Fig. 2. Serum Mg^{2+} levels of guide dog candidates in different stages of training. The medians of serum Mg^{2+} levels measured in samples collected from May to August are indicated by the bar within each box. The statistical significance of differences between classes was tested using a one way ANOVA Dunnet. Elementary class, n = 6; intermediate class, n = 10; advanced class, n = 8; healthy adult guide dogs for the blind, n = 14. (* P < 0.05).

On the other hand, serum Mg^{2+} levels were significantly higher in dogs in the advanced class comparing to those of dogs in the elementary class (Fig. 2). Interestingly, serum Mg^{2+} levels of dogs in the intermediate class showed intermediate levels with some variation (Fig. 2).

Serum Mg^{2+} levels of working guide dogs for the blind were markedly higher than those of guide dog candidates in the elementary class, but lower than those of dogs in the advanced class. The right column of Fig. 2 shows the serum Mg^{2+} levels of healthy guide dogs for the blind without any clinical abnormalities. The serum samples were collected in May. Serum Mg^{2+} levels of mature guide dogs for the blind were 17.8 ± 0.7 µg/mL (the median is 17.9 µg/mL), and no individual differences were observed.

Means of serum Mg^{2+} levels of each group with or without breakfast were 17.5 ± 0.4 µg/mL and 17.9 ± 0.3 µg/mL respectively, and there was no the statistical significant difference (t = -0.676, df = 12, p > 0.05). In the mature guide dogs, the Mg^{2+} value of female dogs was 17.7 ± 0.4 µg/mL and that of male dogs was 17.9 ± 0.3µg/mL, and no significant difference due to the distinction of sex was observed (t = 0.456, df = 12, p > 0.05). All dogs used were clinically healthy throughout the experiment 1 and 2.

Experiment 3; Serum Mg²⁺ levels after exercise loads
To investigate the effect of physical exercise on serum Mg^{2+} levels, dogs were subjected to forced exercise using a treadmill for 20 min in the morning, and Mg^{2+} levels were measured in January (winter) and August (summer).

As shown in Fig. 3, serum Mg^{2+} levels of dogs after forced exercise were significantly lower than those of dogs before exercise in both January (before; 16.6 ± 0.4 µg/mL and after; 10.8 ± 0.4 µg/mL) and August (before; 18.2 ± 0.5 µg/mL and after; 12.5 ± 0.5 µg/mL). All dogs used were clinically healthy throughout the experiment 3.

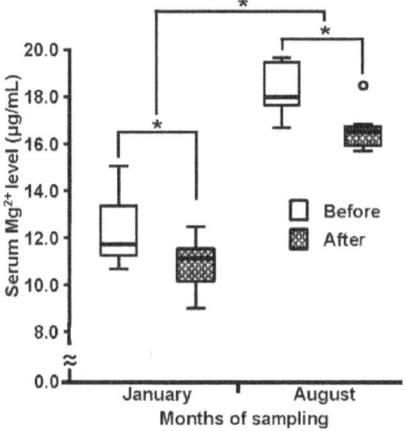

Fig. 3. Serum Mg^{2+} levels before and after treadmill exercise in winter and summer. The medians of serum Mg^{2+} levels of each group of dogs (n = 6) measured before and after treadmill exercise are indicated by the bar within each box. The statistical significance of differences between the each groups were analyzed using a two-way ANOVA within-participant design (P < 0.05).

Discussion

Recently, decrease in blood Mg concentrations has been reported to associate with urinary Mg excretion (Disashi *et al*., 1996; Nielsen and Lukaski, 2006; Belluci *et al*., 2011). Moreover, abnormalities in Mg concentrations in both blood and urine have been identified in patients with neoplastic disorders (Wilhelm *et al*., 2002) and athletes (Nuviala *et al*., 1999; Nielsen and Lukashi, 2006), proposing the significance of Mg supplementation in some cases (Haymes, 1991; Bazzarre *et al*., 1993; Toba *et al*. 2000;

Volpe, 2015). Although dogs have long history as good partners of humans, we found very few report on changes in Mg concentrations of dogs induced by external stress. In the current study, we focused on serum Mg^{2+} levels as one of biomarkers fluctuated by external stress. Since examination of urine during dogs' training or working without contamination was quite difficult, we tried to evaluate serum Mg^{2+} levels before and after external stress.

First, by using young-adult guide dog candidates, we measured serum Mg^{2+} levels of dogs in January (winter), May (spring), and August (summer) to check seasonal changes. Serum Mg^{2+} levels were lower in winter; on the other hand, they became higher in summer. In previous research on humans, blood Mg^{2+} levels became lower in winter because the Mg^{2+} content of food was decreased during this season (Owaki *et al*., 1996). Dogs used in our study were the same breed, fed with the same dog food throughout the year in the quite similar environment. Therefore, the observed reduction in serum Mg^{2+} levels of dogs in winter is likely to have been caused by the effects of climatic changes, such as low temperature and the atmospheric pressure fluctuation, rather than the content of their diet. Since mammals need to maintain their body temperature during the winter, Mg^{2+} may be important for sustaining metabolic processes including enzymatic reactions.

Adrenaline decreased blood levels of Mg^{2+} in humans (Joborn *et al*., 1985) and exes (Rayssiguier, 1977), and induced magnesium loss (Seelig, 1994). Moreover, in humans, plasma free normetanephrine levels were higher in winter than summer (Pamporaki *et al*., 2014). Therefore, we checked levels of catecholamines and found that plasma adrenaline and noradrenaline levels were higher in winter than summer. Inversely, serum Mg^{2+} levels were higher in summer than winter, suggesting a possibility that the seasonal changes of serum Mg^{2+} levels were influenced by the increase in adrenaline and noradrenaline concentrations due to vasoconstriction and vasodilation in winter (Bolli *et al*., 1984).

Next, we measured serum Mg^{2+} levels of guide dog candidates at different stages in their training in order to evaluate the effects of mental and physical stress. Interestingly, serum Mg^{2+} levels were higher in dogs of the advanced class, compared to that of the elementary and intermediate classes. Since Mg^{2+} is necessary to protect individuals from environmental, physical, and mental stress (Golf *et al*., 1998; Soldatovic *et al*., 1998; Zieba *et al*., 2000), Mg^{2+} might have been applied to biologic reaction of cells and tissues in dogs in the elementary class, leading to the reduction of serum Mg^{2+} levels observed. In contrast, since dogs in the advanced class were accustomed to their situation, Mg^{2+} might have been maintained at a higher level. The average serum Mg^{2+} level of healthy adult guide dogs for the blind was 17.8 ± 0.7 µg/mL. In a previous study, the mean serum Mg^{2+} level in adult dogs was 18.8 ± 1 µg/mL (Bailie et al., 1988), which is similar to our finding. In addition, the normal reference range for canine serum Mg^{2+} described in Veterinary Drug Handbook (Plumb, 1999) and the list of a biochemical examination for dogs by LSI Medience Co. (Tokyo, Japan) is 17–27 µg/mL. However, sex, breeds, age, and seasons when Mg^{2+} levels were measured were not mentioned. Since the guide dogs in the present study were fed with the same food as the guide dog candidates (Table 1), the differences between the groups have not resulted from their diet, but may have been due to the higher age of the guide dogs when compared to the guide dog candidates.

Finally, we found that the exercise load using a treadmill reduced serum Mg^{2+} levels of subjected dogs in both winter and summer. In experiment 3, seasonal variation between winter and summer of serum Mg^{2+} levels was remarkable, which is similar to results obtained in experiment 1. Since the laboratory dogs used were all fed with the same food, as indicated in Table 1, the influence of diet on serum Mg^{2+} levels could be excluded. Forced exercise might reduce serum Mg^{2+} levels because of activation of the muscles and nerves. These results suggest that serum Mg^{2+} levels are influenced by external physical stress.

In the current study, we demonstrated for the first time that serum Mg^{2+} levels of dogs might be influenced by air temperature, environment, age, and exercise load. Serum Mg^{2+} levels in dogs were reduced in winter, and they became higher in summer. Serum Mg^{2+} levels of guide dog candidates were lower in the elementary class.

As the training proceeds, serum Mg^{2+} levels were increased. Serum Mg^{2+} levels of dogs after the forced exercise were significantly lower than those before the exercise in both winter and summer. Further experiments with more dogs must take place; however, the variation of serum Mg^{2+} levels of dogs may become one of biomarkers that reflect physical status of dogs.

Previous research has shown that pigs became healthier after administration of the Mg^{2+} supplement (O'Driscoll et al., 2013). Supplementation of Mg^{2+} in healthy dogs with vigorous exercise or training regimes must be discussed for animal welfare. Mg^{2+} supplementation may also be necessary for aged dogs and beneficial for dogs that are subjected to new environments. Moreover, in winter, Mg^{2+} supplementation may be needed not only for working dogs but also for companion dogs, particularly those suffering from disease.

Acknowledgments

We would like to appreciate Assoc. Prof. Hideyuki Tanaka for his advice on the statistical analysis, and thank Dr. Akira Matsuda, Dr. Kumiko Oida, Dr. Yosuke Amagai, Dr. Hyosun Jang, Dr. Saori Ishizaka, and Ms Juri Toyama (Tokyo University of Agriculture and Technology) for their supports and animal care. This work was partially supported by a joint research grant (No. 26-619) from Tateho Chemical Industries Co., Ltd. (Hyogo, Japan).

Conflict of interest
The authors declare that there is no conflict of interest.

References

Altura, B.M. and Altura, B.T. 1981. Magnesium ions and contraction of vascular smooth muscles: relationship to some vascular diseases. Fed. Proc. 40(12), 2672-2679.

Bailie, D.S., Inoue, H., Kaseda, S., Ben-David, J. and Zipes, D.P. 1988. Magnesium suppression of early after depolarizations and ventricular tachyarrhythmias induced by cesium in dogs. Circulation 77(6), 1395-1402.

Baltaci, A.K., Mogulkoc, R. and Belviranli, M. 2013. Serum levels of calcium, selenium, magnesium, phosphorus, chromium, copper and iron-their relation to zinc in rats with induced hypothyroidism. Acta Clin. Croat. 52, 151-156.

Bazzarre, T.L., Scarpino, A., Sigmon, R., Marquart, L.F., Wu, S.M. and Izurieta, M. 1993. Vitamin-mineral supplement use and nutritional status of athletes. J. Am. Coll. Nutr. 12(2), 162-169.

Belluci, M.M., Gior, G., del Barrio, R.A., Pereira, R.M., Marcantonio, E. Jr. and Orrico, S.R. 2011. Effects of magnesium intake deficiency on bone metabolism and bone tissue around osseointegrated implants. Clin. Oral Implants Res. 22(7), 716-721.

Bohl, C.H. and Volpe, S.L. 2002. Magnesium and exercise. Crit. Rev. Food Sci. Nutr. 42(6), 533-563.

Bolli, P., Erne, P., Ji, B.H., Block, L.H., Kiowski, W. and Buhler, F.R. 1984. Adrenaline induces vasoconstriction through post-junctional alpha 2 adrenoceptors and this response is enhanced in patients with essential hypertension. J. Hypertens. Suppl. 2(3), S115-118.

Cowan, J.A. 2002. Structural and catalytic chemistry of magnesium-dependent enzymes. Biometals. 15(3), 225-235.

Disashi, T., Iwaoka, T., Inoue, J., Naomi, S., Fujimoto, Y., Umeda, T. and Tomita, K. 1996. Magnesium metabolism in hyperthyroidism. Endocr. J. 43(4), 397-402.

Dominguez, L.J., Barbagallo, M., Sowers, J.R. and Resnick, L.M. 1998. Magnesium responsiveness to insulin and insulin-like growth factor I in erythrocytes from normotensive and hypertensive subjects. J. Clin. Endocrinol. Metab. 83, 4402-4407.

Durlach, J., Durlach, V., Bac, P., Rayssiguier, Y., Bara, M. and Guiet-Bara, A. 1993. Magnesium and ageing II. Clinical data: aetiological mechanisms and pathophysiological consequences of magnesium deficit in the elderly. Magnes. Res. 6(4), 379-394.

Eby, G.A. and Eby, K.L. 2006. Rapid recovery from major depression using magnesium treatment. Med. Hypotheses 67(2), 362-370.

Elin, R.J. 1988. Magnesium metabolism in health and disease. Dis. Mon. 34(4), 161-218.

Golf, S.W., Bender, S. and Gruttner, J. 1998. On the significance of Magnesium in extreme physical stress. Cardiovasc. Drugs Ther. 12(2), 197-202.

Haymes, E.M. 1991. Vitamin and mineral supplementation to athletes. Int. J. Sport Nutr. 1(2), 146-169.

He, K., Liu, K., Daviglus, M.L., Morris, S.J., Loria, C.M., Van Horn, L., Jacobs D.R. and Savage, P.J. 2006. Magnesium intake and incidence of metabolic syndrome among young adults. Circulation 113(13), 1675-1682.

He, Y., Yao, G., Savoia, C. and Touyz, R.M. 2005. Transient receptor potential melastatin 7 ion channels regulate magnesium homeostasis in vascular smooth muscle cells: Role of angiotensin II. Circ. Res. 96(2), 207-215.

Jacka, F.N., Overland, S., Stewart, R., Tell, G.S., Bjelland, I. and Mykletun, A. 2009. Association between magnesium intake and depression and anxiety in community-dwelling adults: the Hordaland Health Study. Aust. N. Z. J. Psychiatry 43(1), 45-52.

Joborn, H., Akerstrom, G. and Ljunghall, S. 1985. Effects if exogenous catecholamines and exercise on plasma magnesium concentrations. Clin. Endocrinol. 23(3), 219-226.

Lukaski, H.C. and Nielsen, F.H. 2002. Dietary Magnesium Depletion Affects Metabolic Responses during Submaximal Exercise in Postmenopausal Women. J. Nutr. 132(5), 930-935.

Nielsen, F.H. and Lukaski, H.C. 2006. Update on the relationship between magnesium and exercise. Magnes. Res. 19(3), 180-189.

Nuviala, R.J., Lapieza, M.G. and Bernal, E. 1999. Magnesium, Zinc, and copper status in women involved in different sports. Int. J. Sport Nutr. 9(3), 295-309.

O'Driscoll, K., O'Gorman, D.M., Taylor, S. and Boyle, L.A. 2013. The influence of a magnesium-rich marine extract on behaviour, salivary cortisol levels, and skin lesions in growing pigs. Animal 7(6), 1017-1027.

Owaki, A., Takatsuka, N., Kawakami, N. and Shimizu, H. 1996. Seasonal Variations of Nutrient Intake Assessed by 24-Hour Recall Method. J. Nutr. 54(1), 11-18.

Pamporaki, C., Bursztyn, M., Reimann, M., Ziemssen, T., Bornstein, S.R., Sweep, F.C., Timmers, H., Lenders, J.W. and Eisenhofer, G. 2014. Seasonal variation in plasma free normetanephrine concentrations: implications for biochemical diagnosis of pheochromocytoma. Eur. J. Endocrinol. 170(3), 349-357.

Pfeiffer, C.C. and Barnes, B. 1981. Role of zinc, manganese, chromium, and vitamin deficiencies in birth defects. Int. J. Environ. Stud. 17(1), 43-56.

Plumb, D.C. 1999. Veterinary drug handbook, Third Edition. Iowa State Press, Ames, Iowa, USA, pp: 812.

Rayssiguier, Y. 1977. Hypomagnesemia resulting from adrenaline infusion in ewes: its relation to lipolysis. Horm. Metab. Res. 9(4), 309-314.

Resnick, L.M., Oparil, S., Chait, A., Haynes, R.B., Kris-Etherton, P., Stern, J.S., Clark, S., Holcomb, S., Hatton, D.C., Metz, J.A., McMahon, M, Pi-Sunyer, F.X. and McCarron, D.A. 2000. Factors affecting blood pressure responses to diet: the Vanguard study. Am. J. Hypertens. 13(9), 956-965.

Rude, R.K. and Gruber, H.E. 2004. Magnesium deficiency and osteoporosis: Animal and human observations. J. Nutr. Biochem. 15(12), 710-716.

Seelig, M. and Altura, B.M. 1997. How best to determine magnesium requirement: need to consider cardiotherapeutic drugs that affect its retention. J. Am. Coll. Nutr. 16(1), 4-6.

Seelig, M.S. 1994. Consequences of magnesium deficiency on the enhancement of stress reactions; preventive and therapeutic implications. J. Am. Coll. Nutr. 13(5), 429-446.

Sinert, R., Spektor, M., Gorlin, A., Doty, C., Rubin, A., Altura, B.T. and Altura, B.M. 2005. Ionized magnesium levels and the ratio of ionized calcium to magnesium in asthma patients before and after treatment with magnesium. Scand. J. Clin. Lab. Invest. 65(8), 659-670.

Singh, R.B., Beegom, R., Rastogi, S.S., Gaoli, Z. and Shoumin, Z. 1998. Association of low plasma concentrations of antioxidant vitamins, magnesium and zinc with high body fat percent measured by bioelectrical impedance analysis in Indian men. Magnes. Res. 11(1), 3-10.

Singh, R.B., Niaz, M.A., Moshiri, M., Gaoli, Z. and Shoumin, Z. 1997. Magnesium status and risk of coronary artery disease in rural and urban populations with variable magnesium consumption. Magnes. Res. 10(3), 205-213.

Soldatovic, D., Matovic, V., Vujanovic, D. and Stojanovic, Z. 1998. Contribution to interaction between magnesium and toxic metals: the effect of prolonged cadmium intoxication on magnesium metabolism in rabbits. Magnes. Res. 11, 283-288.

Soria, M., Gonzalez-Haro, C., Anson, M.A., Inigo, C., Calvo, M.L. and Escanero, J.F. 2014. Variations in serum magnesium and hormonal levels during incremental exercise. Magnes. Res. 27(4), 155-164.

Toba, Y., Kajita, Y., Masuyama, R., Takada, Y., Suzuki, K. and Aoe, S. 2000. Dietary magnesium supplementation affects bone metabolism and dynamic strength of bone in ovariectomized rats. J. Nutr. 130(2), 216-220.

Tucker, K.L., Hannan, M.T., Chen, H., Cupples, L.A., Wilson, P.W. and Kiel, D.P. 1999. Potassium, magnesium, and fruit and vegetable intakes are associated with greater bone mineral density in elderly men and women. Am. J. Clin. Nutr. 69(4), 727-736.

Volpe, S.L. 2015. Magnesium and the Athlete. Curr. Sports Med. Rep. 14(4), 279-283.

Wilhelm, Z., Kleinova, J. and Kalábová, R. 2002. Effect of magnesium administration on urinary ion excretion in healthy subjects and cancer patients. Scr. Med. (Brno). 75(5), 231-238.

Zieba, A., Tata, R., Dudek, D., Schlegel-zawadzka, M. and Nowak, G. 2000. Serum trace elements in animal models and human depression: Part III. Magnesium. Relationship with copper. Hum. Psychopharmacol. 15(8), 631-635.

26

Direct evidence of *Rickettsia typhi* infection in *Rhipicephalus sanguineus* ticks and their canine hosts

Karla Dzul-Rosado*, Cesar Lugo-Caballero, Raul Tello-Martin, Karina López-Avila and Jorge Zavala-Castro

Center of Research and Regional Studies Dr Hideyo Noguchi, Autonomous University of Yucatan. Av. Itzáes and 59th street, number490, Mérida, Yucatán. Postal code 97000, Mexico

Abstract

Murine typhus is a rickettsiosis caused by *Rickettsia typhi,* whose transmission is carried out by rat fleas in urban settlements as classically known, but it also has been related to cat fleas in a sub-urban alternative cycle that has been suggested by recent reports. These studies remarks that in addition to rats, other animals like cats, opossums and dogs could be implied in the transmission of *Rickettsia typhi* as infected fleas obtained from serologically positive animals have been detected in samples from endemic areas. In Mexico, the higher number of murine typhus cases have been detected in the Yucatan peninsula, which includes a great southeastern region of Mexico that shows ecologic characteristics similar to the sub-urban alternative cycle recently described in Texas and California at the United States. To find out which are the particular ecologic characteristics of murine typhus transmission in this region, we analyzed blood and *Rhipicephalus sanguineus* ticks obtained from domestic dogs by molecular approaches, demonstrating that both samples were infected by *Rickettsia typhi*. Following this, we obtained isolates that were analyzed by genetic sequencing to corroborate this infection in 100% of the analyzed samples. This evidence suggests for the first time that ticks and dogs could be actively participating in the transmission of murine typhus, in a role that requires further studies for its precise description.

Keywords: Dogs, Murine typhus, *Rhipicephalus sanguineus*, *Rickettsia typhi*, Vector.

Introduction

Murine typhus is a human rickettsiosis caused by *Rickettsia typhi,* that is characterized by fever, headache, arthralgia, hepatomegaly, neurological deficits and a mortality rate close to 4% (Civen and Ngo, 2008). This disease has been typically concentrated in urban environments, in which the rat flea *Xenopsylla cheopis* and rats (*Rattus rattus, Rattus norvegicus*) are implied in its transmission. In addition, recent studies have demonstrated that in sub-urban areas with no rat presence, murine typhus transmission is related to a link between cats (*Felis catus*), dogs (*Canis familiaris*), opossums (*Didelphis virginiana*) and the flea *Ctenocephalides felis* that requires further research for a clearer description (Civen and Ngo, 2008; Blanton *et al.*, 2016).

The highest number of human murine typhus reports in Mexico are from the Yucatan peninsula, in which the characteristics of peridomiciliary areas, weather and ecology, create suitable environments for the transmission of this illness however, the dynamics of its transmission remain unclear (Zavala-Castro *et al.*, 2009, 2014; Dzul-Rosado *et al.*, 2013a; Labruna, *et al.*, 2011b). On this last subject, recent molecular evidence supports the existence of rickettsemia caused by *Rickettsia typhi* in dogs and rats from rural and suburban communities from Yucatan, but there are no data regarding a potential arthropod vector, the possible existence of a sylvatic cycle and, if this is the case, the possible connection with the urban and sub-urban cycles (Peniche-Lara *et al.*, 2015; Martinez-Ortiz *et al.*, 2016). Considering that previous studies found that *Rhipicephalus sanguineus* is the most prevalent tick among dogs in our region (Rodriguez-Vivas *et al.*, 2016), and the close contact that people have with these animals, we analyzed ticks infesting domestic dogs from a rural community that has shown cases of murine typhus in Mexico, in order to find out the possible role of ticks in the transmission pathway of this disease.

Materials and Methods

Dog blood and tick DNA extraction

Ticks and blood were collected from 10 infested dogs from Teabo (20.4001° N, 89.2830° W) during the month of April from 2015 (dry season), which is a rural community in Mexico where human cases of rickettsiosis have been diagnosed. Population of Teabo includes 6,205 people distributed among 1,380 households which are occupying an area of 261, 87 Km². This town is a sub humid zone surrounded by mid-elevation semi-deciduous jungle. The average annual temperature is 26.3 °C and the average annual rainfall is 65.7 millimeters (rainy season occurs from June to October). This community was selected because there have been human cases of rickettsiosis,

*Corresponding Author: Karla Dzul-Rosado. Center of Research and Regional Studies Dr Hideyo Noguchi, Autonomous University of Yucatan, Mérida, Yucatán, Mexico. Email: karla.dzul@correo.uady.mx

people has a very close contact to dogs due to its different daily activities, its accessibility to the research center, and the good disposition of the people for working with the team.

Dog blood obtained by venous puncture in the forearm, was processed with the DNeasy Blood & Tissue Kit (Qiagen, Germantown MD, USA) following manufacturer directions and stored until its use. In the other hand, ticks that were identified as *Rhipicephalus sanguineus* adult males by taxonomical keys (Alekseev *et al.*, 2001; Guzmán-Cornejo and Robbins, 2010), were employed for DNA extraction, using the ammonium hydroxide technique as described elsewhere (Guy and Stanek, 1991).

For this, ticks were disinfected with a mixture of 0.15M Iodine-70% ethanol for 15 minutes and washed with sterile water to remove iodine. Half of each tick was macerated and resuspended in 100 ul of 0.7M ammonium hydroxide to free the DNA, and after being cooled, the tubes were heated for 20 minutes at 90°C to evaporate the ammonia.

The resulting DNA was used for PCR or stored at -70°C until its use; the remaining half body was conserved for future isolation. We also inspected the dogs for fleas but none was found.

PCR and RFLPs reactions set up

The amplification of *gltA* was used as a first approach to identify infected ticks and dogs with the primers Rpcs877fw (5'-GGGGGCCTGCTCACGGCGG-3') and Rpcs1258rv (5'-ATTGCAAAAAGTACAGTGAACA-3') using Platinum Taq (Invitrogen) as described previously (Regnery *et al.*, 1991; Dzul-Rosado *et al.*, 2013b). For the follow up and identification of positive controls we amplified *17kDa* with the primers: 17kDa1Fw (5'-GCTCTTGCAACTTCTATGTT-3') and 17kDa1Rv (5'- CATTGTTCGTCAGGTTGGCG-3'); and *OmpB* with a nested reaction using the primers: rOmpBfw (5'- GCTTAGAATCAACTGATACAG-3') and rOmpBrv (5'-GCTTTATAACCAGCTAAACCACC-3') for the first round, followed by a second one with primers: rOmpBTGIfw (5'-AAGATCCTTCTGATGTTGCAACA-3') and rOmpBTHIrv (5'-GGTTTGGCCCATATACCATAAG-3').

PCR products were analyzed in BrEt stained gels of polyacrylamide (Webb *et al.*, 1990). As a first and fast approach to identify the agents that could be infecting ticks prior to start the isolation steps, RFLP analysis were performed as described in a previous work (Zavala-Castro *et al.*, 2009), using 1.2 UI of AluI and 50ng of the *17kDa* PCR product overnight; and then the bands were analyzed expecting 200bp and 250bp fragments (Zavala-Castro *et al.*, 2009). RFLP analysis were also useful to fast track the isolation experiments

prior the corroboration of the isolates through DNA sequencing.

Rickettsia typhi isolation from Rhipicephalus sanguineus

As reported previously (Dzul-Rosado *et al.*, 2013b), a total of 50,000 Vero cells were grown in 6 separated wells of a 24 well cell culture plate (Corning Inc, Corning NY USA) with Dulbecco's modified eagle medium (DMEM) supplemented with 10% fetal bovine serum (FBS) (Caisson Labs, Smithfield UT, USA), with 5% CO2, 37°C for 48 hours or until 95% confluence was achieved. The remaining half body from positive male ticks was macerated and resuspended in microtubes containing 600ul of brain heart infusion (BHI).

DMEM medium was carefully removed, and wells were refilled with 300 ul of each tick suspension; then the plate was covered with parafilm and centrifugued at 700g, 22°C, for 60 minutes. Finally, the supernatant was removed and wells were refilled with 1ml of DMEM supplemented with 4% FCS, 100 U of penicillin, 100 μg of streptomycin and 250 ng of amphotericin B (Sigma-Aldrich, St Louis MO, USA); then the plates were incubated at 33°C with 5% CO2. From this point, the medium was changed every 3 days using DMEM without antibiotics and supplemented with 5% of FCS and the supernatants were screened using Gimenez stain to verify the status of the infection on days 9 and 15 (Gimenez, 1964).

On the day 15, cells from positive wells were scrapped and transferred into 5 ml of DMEM to culture flasks (25cm^2) that was changed every 3 days. Cultures were scrapped for DNA extraction using the kit DNeasy Blood and Tissue on day 15 according manufacturer (Qiagen, Germantown MD, USA). Species identification was performed by the amplification of *17kDa*, *gltA* and *OmpB*, followed by RFLP analysis for *17kDa* as it has been described. Finally, three PCR amplicons of *17kDa* and *OmpB* from every positive well were fully sequenced by Sanger at the Biotechnology Institute (UNAM, Cuernavaca Morelos, Mexico), and compared with other sequences in the GenBank.

Results

Blood samples were obtained from 10 domestic dogs that roam freely in the town and act as companions to their owners in activities that take place in the surrounding jungle like agriculture or hunt. No tick co-infestation was observed. Additionally, we obtained a random number of *Rhipicephalus sanguineus* ticks from these dogs. DNA obtained from both kind of samples was subjected to conventional PCR and RFLP analysis, obtaining a 100% of ticks and dogs infected with *Rickettsia typhi* (Data not shown).

Six adult ticks positive to *Rickettsia typhi* were randomly selected for isolation, using a 24-well culture plate technique previously established by our group for the infection of Vero cells (Dzul-Rosado *et al.*, 2013b). The infected monolayers were followed up by Gimenez stain and PCR/RFLP analysis (Fig. 1 and Fig. 2); after 3 passages, amplicons of *OmpB* and *17kDa* obtained from the scrapping of the positive wells were fully sequenced in the Biomedical Institute of the National Autonomous University of Mexico (IBT-UNAM), and compared with sequences reported at the GenBank (NCBI). Amplicons showed 100% of identity with the *OmpB* (RT0699) and *17kDa* genes (RT0821) *of Rickettsia typhi* str. Wilmington (Access Number AE017197.1).

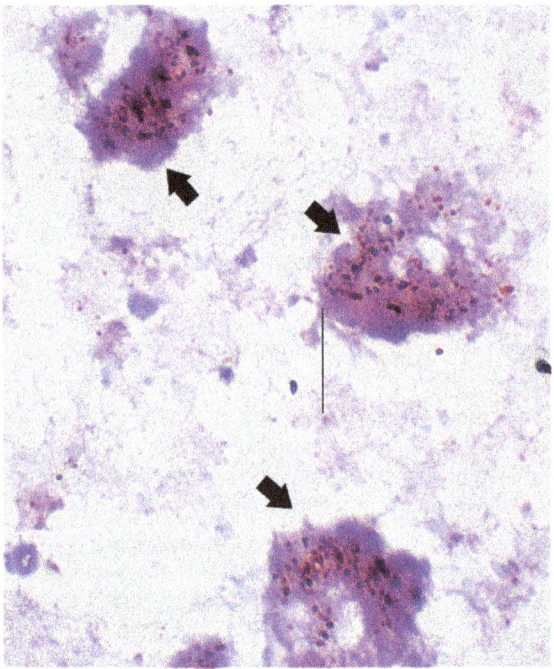

Fig. 1. Gimenez stain of isolates. Representative micrograph showing the follow up of isolates by Gimenez stain. Arrows shows infected Vero cells.

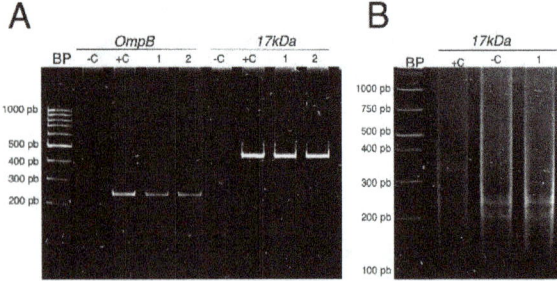

Fig. 2. PCR and RFLP analysis of isolates. Representative acrylamide gel electrophoresis showing how every isolate obtained from infected ticks was subjected to PCR amplification of *OmpB* and *17kDa* (A), using previously characterized positive controls. PCR products were obtained according to expected;17kDa amplicon was subjected to further analysis by AluI RFLPs (B), obtaining fragments according to the molecular pattern expected for *R. typhi*.

Discussion

The importance of rickettsiosis for the public health in Mexico has begun to be showed by several epidemiologic studies but the ecologic characteristics of its transmission have not been deeply explored. It is classically known that *Rickettsia typhi* transmission to humans requires fleas (*Xenopsylla cheopis*) that acquire the bacteria from rats and mice in urban settlements, being the main route of infection worldwide. However, it is also recognized than some sub-urban regions like southern states of America, the cat flea (*Ctenocephalides felis*) and opossums are highly effective for the transmission and maintenance of murine typhus (Civen and Ngo, 2008). This last alternate cycle was described during epidemic outbreaks of murine typhus, in communities from Texas and California that were not in touch with the classic transmission, however, data supported the infection of fleas by *Rickettsia typhi* but no rickettsemia in opossums, only anti-*Rickettsia typhi* antibodies. (Blanton *et al.*, 2016; Maina *et al.*, 2016). Other studies have demonstrated that dogs can play an important role in the transmission of murine typhus, as high antibody titers against *Rickettsia typhi* and rickettsemia have been demonstrated by IFA and PCR/sequencing in dog blood samples from different world regions including Yucatan; however, its potential as reservoirs remains to be assessed (Nogueras *et al.*, 2013; Martinez-Ortiz *et al.*, 2016). Those studies have not described the participation of an arthropod as a possible vector which, considering the classic cycle could be a flea. Here, we show molecular and cellular evidence that the most abundant ticks in dogs of southeastern Mexico (*Rhipicephalus sanguineus*) could have an important role in the life cycle of *Rickettsia typhi*. To our knowledge extent, this is the first report of *Rhipicephalus sanguineus* ticks infected with *Rickettsia typhi*, which alongside with the demonstration of rickettsemia from the same species in their dogs hosts, highlights that vectorial competence and animal transmission studies are needed to a better understanding of the life cycle of *Rickettsia typhi* in our region, where several studies have demonstrated a close contact among ticks and humans in communities that have had positive cases of rickettsiosis (Martinez-Ortiz *et al.*, 2016; Rodriguez-Vivas *et al.*, 2016). These studies should include tests on the capacity of the vector to become infected from an animal source, the transovarian transmission of the pathogen and the capabilities of nymphs to infect healthy animals, as it has been done in recent studies (Labruna *et al.*, 2011a; Levin *et al.*, 2017). Murine typhus is a public health problem in our region that, for its control, needs a deeper understanding of its ecologic characteristics. Here we show the first molecular and cellular evidence of *Rickettsia typhi* infecting *Rhipicephalus sanguineus* ticks from dogs that are in close contact with humans. Although additional experiments would be necessary to a better understanding of this phenomena, we could suggest that ticks, and not only fleas, could be participating in the transmission of this disease.

Acknowledgements
This work was supported by a grant of the Mexican National Council for Science and Technology (Conacyt FOSIS 261885) to Dra. Karla Dzul-Rosado. The authors would also express their gratitude for the people of Teabo, Yucatan and to the people that supported us for data acquisition.

Conflict of interest
The authors declare that there is no conflict of interests.

References

Alekseev, A.N., Dubinina, H.V., Van De Pol, I. and Schouls, L.M. 2001. Identification of Ehrlichia spp. and Borrelia burgdorferi in Ixodes ticks in the Baltic regions of Russia. J. Clin. Microbiol. 39, 2237-2242.

Blanton, L.S., Idowu, B.M., Tatsch, T.N., Henderson, J.M., Bouyer, D.H. and Walker, D.H. 2016. Opossums and Cat Fleas: New Insights in the Ecology of Murine Typhus in Galveston, Texas. Am. J. Trop. Med. Hyg. 95, 457-461.

Civen, R. and Ngo, V. 2008. Murine typhus: an unrecognized suburban vectorborne disease. Clin. Infect. Dis. 46, 913-8.

Dzul-Rosado, K., Gonzalez-Martinez, P., Peniche-Lara, G., Zavala-Velazquez, J. and Zavala-Castro, J. 2013a. Murine typhus in humans, Yucatan, Mexico'. Emerg. Infect. Dis. 19, 1021-1022.

Dzul-Rosado, K., Peniche-Lara, G., Tello-Martin, R., Zavala-Velazquez, J., Pacheco Rde, C., Labruna, M.B., Sanchez, E.C. and Zavala-Castro, J. 2013b. Rickettsia rickettsii isolation from naturally infected Amblyomma parvum ticks by centrifugation in a 24-well culture plate technique. Open Vet. J. 3, 101-105.

Gimenez, D.F. 1964. Staining rickettsiae in yolk-sac cultures. Stain. Technol. 39, 135-140.

Guy, E.C. and Stanek, G. 1991. Detection of Borrelia burgdorferi in patients with Lyme disease by the polymerase chain reaction. J. Clin. Pathol. 44, 610-611.

Guzmán-Cornejo, C. and Robbins, R.G. 2010. The genus Ixodes (Acari: Ixodidae) in Mexico: adult identification keys, diagnoses, hosts, and distribution. Revista mexicana de biodiversidad 81, 289-298.

Labruna, M.B., Ogrzewalska, M., Soares, J.F., Martins, T.F., Soares, H.S., Moraes-Filho, J., Nieri-Bastos, F.A., Almeida, A.P. and Pinter, A. 2011a. Experimental infection of Amblyomma aureolatum ticks with Rickettsia rickettsii, Emerg. Infect. Dis. 17, 829-834.

Labruna, M.B., Mattar, S.V., Nava, S., Bermudez, S., Venzal, J.M., Dolz, G., Katia, A., Romero, L., de Sousa, R., Oteo, J. and Zavala-Castro, J. 2011b. Rickettsioses in Latin America, Caribbean, Spain and Portugal. Revista MVZ Córdoba, 16, 2435-2457.

Levin, M.L., Zemtsova, G.E., Killmaster, L.F., Snellgrove, A. and Schumacher, L.B.M. 2017. Vector competence of Amblyomma americanum (Acari: Ixodidae) for Rickettsia rickettsii. Ticks Tick Borne Dis. 8, 615-622.

Maina, A.N., Fogarty, C., Krueger, L., Macaluso, K.R., Odhiambo, A., Nguyen, K., Farris, C.M., Luce-Fedrow, A., Bennett, S., Jiang, J., Sun, S., Cummings, R.F. and Richards, A.L. 2016. Rickettsial Infections among Ctenocephalides felis and Host Animals during a Flea-Borne Rickettsioses Outbreak in Orange County, California. PLoS One 11: e0160604. http://doi.org/10.1371/journal.pone.0160604.

Martinez-Ortiz, D., Torres-Castro, M., Koyoc-Cardena, E., Lopez, K., Panti-May, A., Rodriguez-Vivas, I., Puc, A., Dzul, K., Zavala-Castro, J., Medina-Barreiro, A., Chable-Santos, J. and Manrique-Saide, P. 2016. Molecular evidence of Rickettsia typhi infection in dogs from a rural community in Yucatan, Mexico. Biomedica 36, 45-50.

Nogueras, M.M., Pons, I., Pla, J., Ortuno, A., Miret, J., Sanfeliu, I. and Segura, F. 2013. The role of dogs in the eco-epidemiology of Rickettsia typhi, etiological agent of Murine typhus. Vet. Microbiol. 163, 97-102.

Peniche-Lara, G., Dzul-Rosado, K., Perez-Osorio, C. and Zavala-Castro, J. 2015. Rickettsia typhi in rodents and R. felis in fleas in Yucatan as a possible causal agent of undefined febrile cases. Rev. Inst. Med. Trop. Sao Paulo 57, 129-132.

Regnery, R.L., Spruill, C.L. and Plikaytis, B.D. 1991. Genotypic identification of rickettsiae and estimation of intraspecies sequence divergence for portions of two rickettsial genes. J. Bacteriol. 173, 1576-1589.

Rodriguez-Vivas, R.I., Apanaskevich, D.A., Ojeda-Chi, M.M., Trinidad-Martinez, I., Reyes-Novelo, E., Esteve-Gassent, M.D. and Perez de Leon, A.A. 2016. Ticks collected from humans, domestic animals, and wildlife in Yucatan, Mexico. Vet. Parasitol. 215, 106-113.

Webb, L., Carl, M., Malloy, D.C., Dasch, G.A. and Azad, A.F. 1990. Detection of murine typhus infection in fleas by using the polymerase chain reaction. J. Clin. Microbiol. 28, 530-534.

Zavala-Castro, J.E., Zavala-Velazquez, J.E. and Sulu Uicab, J.E. 2009. Murine typhus in child, Yucatan, Mexico. Emerg. Infect. Dis. 15, 972-974. http://doi.org/10.3201/eid1506.081367.

Zavala-Castro, J.E., Dzul-Rosado, K.R., Peniche-Lara, G., Tello-Martín, R. and Zavala-Velázquez, J.E. 2014. Isolation of Rickettsia typhi from Human, Mexico. Emerg. Infect. Dis. 20, 1411-1412.

27

In vivo fluoroscopic kinematography of dynamic radio-ulnar incongruence in dogs

Thomas Rohwedder[1,*], Martin Fischer[2] and Peter Böttcher[1]

[1]Department of Small Animal Medicine, University of Leipzig, An den Tierkliniken 23, 04103 Leipzig, Germany
[2]Institute of Systematic Zoology and Evolutionary Biology with Phyletic Museum, Friedrich-Schiller-University, Jena, Germany

Abstract

Aim of the study was to investigate dynamic radio-ulnar incongruence (dRUI) in the canine elbow joint comparing orthopedic healthy and dysplastic dogs in a prospective in vivo study design. In 6 orthopedic sound elbow joints (5 dogs, median age 17 months & mean body weight 27.9 kg) and 7 elbow joints with medial coronoid disease (6 dogs, median age 17.5 months & mean body weight 27.6 kg) 0.8 mm Ø tantalum beads were surgically implanted into radius, ulna and humerus for dynamic radiosteriometric analysis (RSA) using high-speed biplanar fluoroscopy with the dogs walking on a treadmill. dRUI, in the form of proximo-distal translation of the radius relative to the ulna, was measured for the first third of stance phase and compared between groups using unpaired t-testing. Healthy elbow joints exhibited a relative radio-ulnar translation of 0.7 mm (SD 0.31 mm), while dysplastic joints showed a translation of 0.5 mm (SD 0.30 mm). No significant difference between groups was detected (p = 0.2092, confidence interval - 0.6 – 0.2). Based on these findings dRUI is present in every canine elbow joint, as part of the physiological kinematic pattern. However, dysplastic elbow joints do not show an increased radio-ulnar translation, and therfore dRUI cannot be considered causative for medial coronoid disease.

Keywords: Canine, Elbow dysplasia, Fluoroscopy, Gait analysis, Radio-ulnar incongruence.

Introduction

Developmental elbow disease is one of the most frequent causes of front limb lameness especially in young dogs, being bilateral in up to 35% (Kirberger and Fourie, 1998; Morgan *et al.*, 1999). Radio-ulnar incongruence (RUI) has been reported to occur concomitant to medial coronoid disease in up to 60% of clinical cases and has been shown to be related to the severity of medial compartment pathology (Eljack and Bottcher, 2015). Traditionally RUI has been defined as two forms of incongruence: (1) an abnormal shape of the trochlear notch of the ulna, leading to humero-ulnar incongruence (Wind, 1986; Wind and Packard, 1986) or (2) a step formation between the articular surfaces of the radius and ulna (short ulna or short radius), leading to radio-ulnar incongruence and secondary to this humero-ulnar conflict. Based on an ex vivo study we assume that under physiologic conditions joint forces are equally distributed between the radial head and the medial coronoid process (Mason *et al.*, 2005). A static positive radio-ulnar incongruence (short radius) induces load shift from the radial head to the medial coronoid process (Krotscheck *et al.*, 2014b; McConkey *et al.*, 2016), with the consequence of mechanical overload of the medial joint compartment and degenerative changes such as fragmentation of the medial coronoid process (Samoy *et al.*, 2006; Gemmill

and Clements, 2007). According to Eljack and Bottcher (2015) we refer to RUI as "axial radio-ulnar incongruence", in contrast to local positive radio-ulnar incongruence at the tip of the medial coronoid process. Axial static RUI is thought to develop because of asynchronous growth between the radius and ulna (Samoy *et al.*, 2006; Lau *et al.*, 2015; Nemanic *et al.*, 2016). However, in a significant number of dogs with medial coronoid disease RUI is not present (Gemmill *et al.*, 2005; Kramer *et al.*, 2006; Eljack and Bottcher, 2015). This might be due to transient RUI during growth, with incongruence having resolved by the time of clinical presentation, which is usually months later. Alternatively, RUI might occur dynamically when the joint is loaded during physical activity, resulting in false findings when the joint is evaluated for RUI in unloaded state, which is usually the case with dogs under anesthesia. There are two possible dynamic RUI scenarios: a radio-ulnar joint cup being congruent while unloaded becomes incongruent under load, and on the other hand, static RUI might become equalized when loaded. Both have been theorized by numerous investigators but remained unproven, until Guillou *et al.* (2011) confirmed in vivo dynamic axial radio-ulnar translation of up to 0.93 mm in sound canine elbow joints while the dogs were walking and trotting on a treadmill. Expecting a higher degree of dynamic RUI

---

*Corresponding Author: Dr. Thomas Rohwedder. Department of Small Animal Medicine, University of Leipzig, An den Tierkliniken 23, 04103 Leipzig, Germany. Email: *thomas.rohwedder@kleintierklinik.uni-leipzig.de*

necessary to cause fissuring or fragmentation of the medial coronoid process in dysplastic dogs, we hypothesized that dynamic axial RUI will be siginificantly greater in dysplastic elbow joints when compared to normals. Therfore, it was the aim of the current study to compare the amount of dynamic RUI in orthopedic healthy and dysplastic canine elbow joints while the dogs were walking on a treadmill using three-dimensional fluoroscopic kinematography.

Materials and Methods

Animals

Only orthopedic healthy, adult, mid to large breed dogs (20 – 35 kg) were included in the control group. Dogs were defined to be undiseased if no history of lameness was present, complete orthopedic examination, biplanar radiographs and computed tomography (CT) of both elbow joints were inconspicuous of any pathology. Radiographs were assessed according to the International Elbow Working Group (IEWG) protocol (Ohlerth et al., 2016). By definition, the IEWG score had to be zero, without any evidence of subtrochlear sclerosis.

Similar to the control group only mid to large breed dogs (20 – 35 kg) with closed physis were considered for the dysplastic group. Dogs had to be lame because of elbow pain, either uni- or bilaterally. Orthopedic and radiologic examination had to confirm evidence of medial coronoid disease for further enrollment. As for the control dogs, radiographic assessment of elbow pathology was done according to the IEWG protocol. Any orthopedic abnormality other than medial coronoid disease (not including OCD) was defined to be an exclusion criteria as well as any abnormal finding during physical examination other than elbow pain and effusion. Exclusion and inclusion criteria had to be confirmed by CT and arthroscopy of the index joint(s). Radiographic and CT findings indicative for medial compartment disease on the contralateral elbow in case of unilateral lameness did not result in exclusion of the patient. The decision to include both or only one elbow joint in the study was based solely on clinical indication for arthroscopic evaluation and treatment, which was defined to be bilateral or unilateral elbow lameness, respectively.

All owners were informed about the purpose of the study and had to provide signed consent. The study was further approved by the local governmental ethical committee for animal welfare (Reg.Nr.: 15-105/08).

Advanced Imaging

Axial CT was performed to quantify RUI on virtual 3D bone models using the sphere fitting technique (Eljack et al., 2013) and to confirm absence of any joint pathology in the control group. Using the sphere fitting technique static RUI was measured at the base of the medial coronoid process. For 3D modeling, radius and ulna were manually separated from each other in the

axial CT images using the open source image processing software MeVisLab (MeVis Medical Solutions AG, Bremen, Germany). This allowed generation of separate 3D surface renderings of isolated bone segments using dedicated image analysis software (VTK 3.0, Kitware Inc., NY, USA). Further enhancement, as well as inspection of the 3D models and quantification of RUI were performed using ParaView (Kitware, Inc., NY, USA). For CT scanning dogs were positioned in dorsal recumbence with both elbow joints extended at ~135°. Spiral CT imaging was performed with a slice thickness of 1 mm and an overlapping increment of 0.5 mm (Philips Brilliance, Philips, Netherlands).

Only the dogs in the dysplastic group were further assessed using elbow arthroscopy, using standard medial portals and a 1.9 mm fore-oblique scope (Storz Endoskope, Tuttlingen, Germany). Medial compartment pathology was scored based on a modified Outerbridge scale (Fitzpatrick et al., 2009; Goldhammer et al., 2010) and fragmentation/fissuring of the medial coronoid process was assessed using palpation. Intraarticular treatment consisted solely of fragment removal. No further surgical treatment was performed, especially no resection of medial coronoid bone other than the fragment(s). Dogs were discharged the same day and oral non-steroidal anti-inflammatory drugs (NSAID) were prescribed for 1 week.

Fluoroscopic Kinematography

Along the CT scanning and/or arthroscopy, percutaneous implantation of 0.8 mm tantalum beads (Tantalum Beads, X-Medics Scandinavia, Frederiksberg, Denmark) into radius and ulna and humerus was performed. A minimum of 3 markers were placed into each bone. Implantation was performed with a bone marrow cannula (MarrowCut, Somatex Medical Technology, Teltow, Germany). After a small cutaneous stab incision with an 11 scalpel blade, the cannula was advanced into the cortex. The tantalum bead was inserted into the cannula and pushed into the bone tunnel created by the trocar of the cannula. Proper marker position was evaluated intraoperatively using a C-arm. After implantation of all beads, CT scanning was repeated using the same settings as for the pre-operative CT imaging.

Three weeks after bead implantation biplanar fluoroscopic kinematography of the index joint(s) was performed. By that time, none of the dogs was under NSAID or other medication. Synchronized biplanar high-speed x-ray movies of the elbow joint were taken while the dog was walking on a treadmill (Fig. 1A, B) (Jog A Dog, LLC, Michigan, USA). The bi-planar fluoroscopic setup (Fig. 2) consisted of two high-powered x-ray tubes (Philips Medio 65 CP-H X-Ray Generator, Philips, Netherlands) and two fluoroscopic image intensifiers (Philips Typ BX 3i-2123, Philips,

Netherlands) with coupled digital high-speed video cameras (Optronis Cam Record CR600x2, Kehl, Germany). The system operated at 50-77 kV and 50-80 mA with an inter-beam angle of 60°. Video sequences of six seconds were taken at 500 frames per second, 0.5 ms shutter and a resolution of 1024 x 1024 pixels. The x-ray source-to-image intensifier distance was 1.4 m.

A third synchronized high-speed video camera recorded the life video of the patient walking on the treadmill (Fig. 1C). The life video was later used to determine ground contact. At least three steps were recorded and stored using dedicated software (TimeBench, Optronis GmbH, Kehl, Germany). Every video sequence was cut to a length of 150 frames, starting 30 frames before ground contact. The remaining 120 frames represent the first 30% of stance phase.

Image distortion was corrected using a perforated steel sheet with a defined hole-diameter in XrayProject (XrayProject, Brown University, Providence, Rhode Island, USA) (Gatesy *et al.*, 2010). Calibration of the experimental setup within the three dimensional space was also performed with XrayProject using a specified cube consisting of four layers of acrylic sheets with 64 radio-opaque markers embedded with uniform spacing (Brainerd *et al.*, 2010).

Virtual 3D Animation of elbow joint kinematics

Tracking of 3D joint movement was performed using XrayProject. The software measures marker trajectories representing motion of the implanted markers over time by tracking the tantalum beads in both x-ray videos. Together with the bead coordinates extracted from the CT data, 6-degree rigid-body motion (3 x translation and 3 x rotation) of radius and ulna in 3D space were calculated (Knörlein *et al.*, 2016). Within Autodesk Maya® (Autodesk Inc., San Rafael, CA, USA), a 3D computer animation software, the calculated rigid-body motion was then applied to the previously generated CT bone models of radius and ulna, resulting in a 3D animation of radius and ulna which precisely mirrors the kinematics of both bones when the dog was walking on the treadmill. Finally, global radial and ulnar motions in 3D space were converted to radial movement relative to the ulna, with the ulna remaining still.

Measurement of dynamic RUI

Within Maya, a Cartesian 3D joint coordinate system was defined (Fig. 3) with the z-axis orientated along the caudal border of the proximal ulna, the x-axis perpendicular to the z-axis and through the tip of the anconeal process and the y-axis perpendicular to the first two. Dynamic RUI was defined as any radial motion along the z-axis in relation to the ulna. Measurement of dynamic RUI started at frame 30, marking ground contact, and stopped at frame 150.

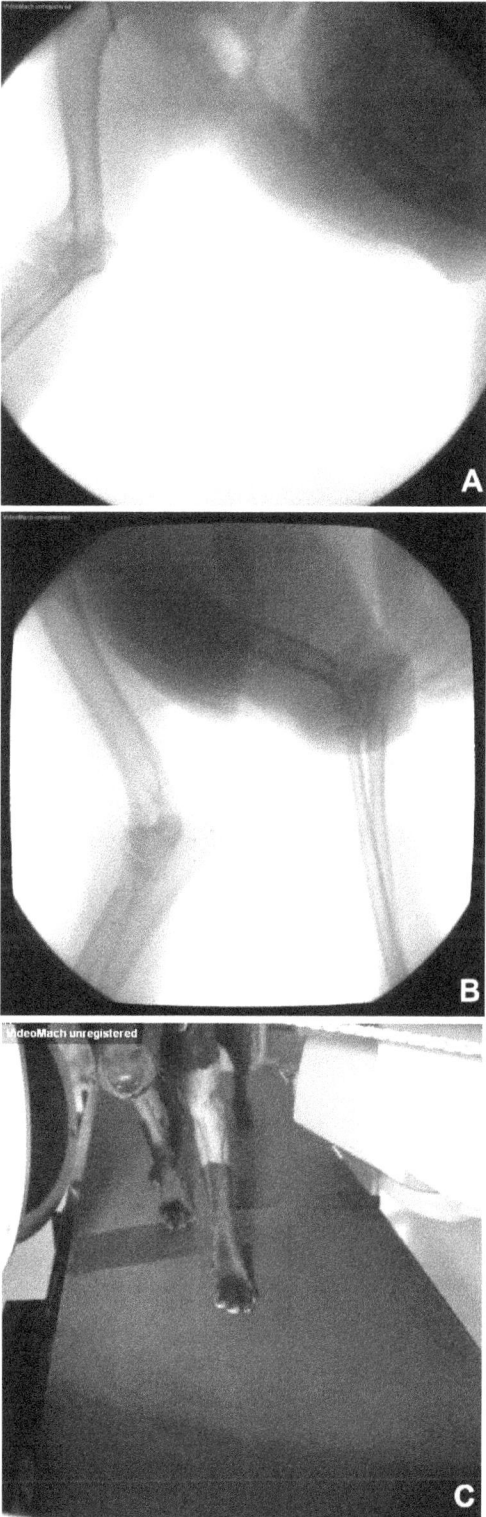

Fig. 1. Corresponding image set of synchronized bi-planar fluoroscopic high-speed video sequences **(A, B)** and live image camera just at the beginning of stance phase **(C)** for the left front limb. Implanted tantalum beads are clearly visible. All cameras operated at a frame rate of 500/sec, 0.5 ms shutter and a resolution of 1024 x 1024 pixels.

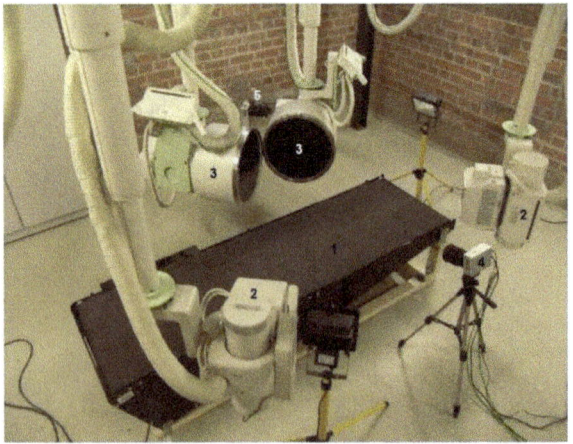

Fig. 2. Setup for high-speed bi-planar fluoroscopic kinematography. **(1):** treadmill; **(2):** x-ray tube assembly; **(3):** image intensifier; **(4):** digital high-speed video camera for live image capturing; **(5):** digital high-speed video cameras coupled to the image intensifier. The inter-beam angel is ~60° and the x-ray source-to-image intensifier distance 1.4 m.

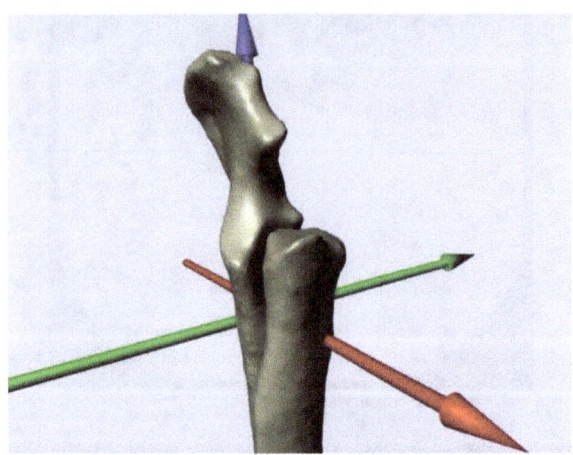

Fig. 3. Virtual bone model of the radius and ulna with embedded Cartesian joint coordinate system (cranio-medial view, left elbow joint). The z-axis (blue) is orientated along the caudal border of the proximal ulna. The x-axis (red) is orientated along the long axis of the anconeal process and the y-axis (green) is perpendicular to the first two axes. Dynamic radio-ulnar incongruence, expressed as axial proximo-distal translation of the radius relative to the ulna was measured along the blue axis.

The magnitude of dynamic RUI was expressed in form of the maximal amplitude of relative radio-ulnar translation (AmpRUI). For final data analysis, AmpRUI was averaged for the three step cycles of each joint (Fig. 4).

Statistical analysis

Standard descriptive statistic was performed on epidemiological data, static RUI derived from the 3D models as well as AmpRUI, and expressed as mean and standard deviation, or median and interquartile range, in case Kolmogorov-Smirnov-testing rejected the hypothesis of normality. Group wise comparison of age

was done using the Mann-Whitney-U-test, while body weight, static RUI and AmpRUI were compared using an unpaired t-test. For all tests α was set to 0.05. In case of significant difference, the 95% confidence interval for that difference was calculated. A software package (MedCalc, MedCalc Software, Belgium) was used to perform all analyses.

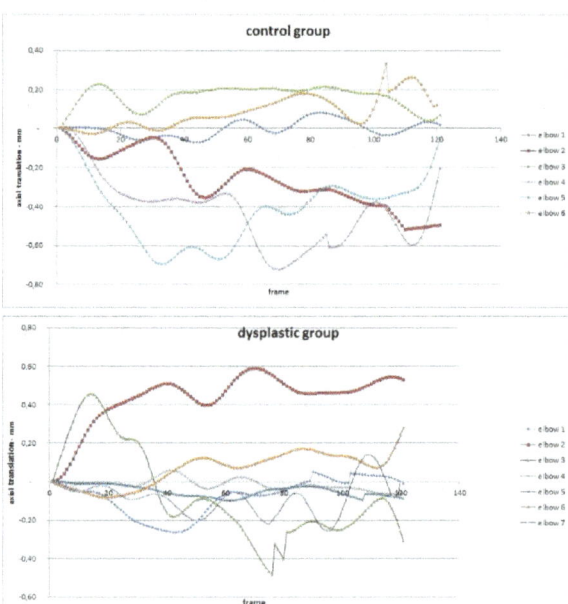

Fig. 4. Graphic depiction of axial radio-ulnar translation over 120 frames of stance phase, in healthy (control group) and dysplastic elbow joints. Frame 1 represents moment of weight bearing, defined as point zero of measurement.

Results

Animals

Five undiseased (two spayed and one intact female; two castrated males) and six dysplastic dogs (two spayed and two intact females; one castrated and one intact male) were recruited. Dogs in the control group had a median age of 17 months (IQR: 14.8 – 33.8) and the dysplastic dogs a median age of 17.5 months (IQR: 15.0 – 21.0), not being significantly different from each other (p = 0.8551). No significant difference was detected for body weight between groups (p = 0.8551; control: mean 27.9 kg [SD: 4.76]; dysplastic: 27.6 kg [SD: 3.98]). In the control group dog breeds included two mixed breed, and one each of Australian Shepard, Labrador retriever, and Eurasian. The dysplastic group consisted of two Labrador retriever and two mixed breed dogs, as well as one German Shepard and one Bernese mountain dog.

Only for the first dog in the control group both elbow joints where implanted with tantalum beads. This was abandoned afterwards, because time for bilateral implantation was felt to prolong anesthesia disproportionally. Overall, this led to three left and three right implanted elbow joints for the control group.

Side of implantation was chosen by alternating left and right. For the dysplastic group, four left and three right elbow joints where recruited, as only one dog appeared to be lame on both front limbs.

Clinical Data

According to the study protocol, all control dogs were free of lameness and any pathological findings on orthopedic examination, radiographs and CT. The primary indications for general anesthesia, which was also used for tantalum bead implantation in these dogs, were castration and/or dental care.

Five of the six dysplastic dogs showed a unilateral lameness of two to eight weeks prior to presentation. The remaining dog showed lameness on both front limbs lasting already ten months. All dogs within the dysplastic group where referred to the clinic because of suspected developmental elbow disease, which was confirmed by orthopedic examination, radiography and CT of the affected elbow(s), as well as arthroscopy.

Imaging Findings

Radiography and CT

IEWG score for the seven dysplastic joints ranged from 1 to 3, with loss of the cranial contour of the medial coronoid process in six of seven joints. CT findings included mild to moderate osteophytosis and fragmentation/fissuring of the medial coronoid process in six of seven joints.

Mean static RUI, measured in 3D bone models based on the pre-operative CT scans, was 0.2 mm (SD 0.30 mm) in control joints, with four/six elbow joints showing no detectable RUI. The two remaining joints had a positive RUI of 0.3 mm and 0.7 mm, respectively. All seven dysplastic elbow joints had at least mild positive RUI (minimum: 0.2 mm) with a mean RUI of 1.4 mm (SD 0.72 mm). The bilaterally affected dog had an RUI of 1.9 mm on both sides. The highest RUI measured in the dysplastic group was 2.2 mm. Overall, RUI in the dysplastic elbow joints was significantly greater than in the control elbows (p = 0.0044, 95% CI: 0.5 – 1.9).

Arthroscopy

Arthroscopy confirmed medial coronoid disease in all seven joints with fragmentation/fissuring of the medial coronoid process being evident in six joints. Three joints where free of any further medial compartment pathology, except for mild synovialitis. Three other joints where affected by Outerbridge grade 2 to 3 cartilage damage on the medial coronoid process (± humeral trochlea). Only one joint showed advanced medial compartment disease with grade 3 to 4 cartilage pathology at the medial coronoid process and humeral trochlea.

Dynamic RUI

In sound elbow joints, dynamic RUI, expressed as AmpRUI, averaged 0.7 mm (SD 0.31 mm), while the dysplastic joints showed a mean AmpRUI of 0.5 mm (SD 0.30 mm). Even though AmpRUI was smaller in the affected elbow joints, this difference was not significant (p = 0.2092).

Discussion

The current study confirms the findings of Guillou et al. (2011), who described dynamic RUI in healthy elbow joints, also using roentgen stereophotogrammetric analysis. Their reported amplitude of dynamic axial translation appears to be slightly higher (0.9 mm vs. 0.7 mm in the current study), which could be attributed to the fact that they measured axial radio-ulnar translation along a slightly different axis and/or that they investigated dynamic RUI along the entire gait cycle, while we investigated only the first 30% of stance phase.

Irrespectively, with a standard deviation of 0.3 mm in the current and 0.16 mm in the aforementioned study with similar sample sizes, we conclude that dynamic axial radio-ulnar shift of about 0.5 to 1 mm can generally be expected in normal adult dogs of 20 – 35 kg, while walking or trotting. While we did not investigate trotting in the current study, Guillou et al. (2011) were unable to find significant differences between walking and trotting, which suggests that radio-ulnar motion measured at the walk could be extrapolated to trotting activity.

Our results are also in accordance with the amount of radio-ulnar translation reported in a cadaveric model of simulated triceps pull (Might et al., 2011). Therefore, the widely suspected dynamic radio-ulnar step creation during weight bearing activity (Gemmill et al., 2005; Kramer et al., 2006; Gemmill and Clements, 2007; Fitzpatrick and Yeadon, 2009, Fitzpatrick et al., 2009, 2016; Smith et al., 2009; Might et al., 2011; Gutbrod and Guerrero, 2012; Starke et al., 2013, 2014; Krotscheck et al., 2014a; Mariee et al., 2014; Eljack and Bottcher, 2015) is a consistent physiological pattern of elbow kinematic in dogs.

While the results of the current data prove the presence of dynamic RUI in canine elbow joints, the amplitude of dynamic translation was not different between normal and dysplastic joints. Therefore, excessive dynamic deformation of the radio-ulnar joint cup is unlikely to play a role in the pathogenesis of medial coronoid disease, rejecting our working hypothesis. In conclusion, dynamic RUI is truly occurring in any canine elbow joint under load, but it cannot be considered causative for the pathological changes in dysplastic elbow joint, as the amplitude of relative axial radio-ulnar translation equals the one in sound, unaffected elbow joints, at least in the first 30 % of stance phase. In consequence, the discussion on dynamic RUI as the primary factor in the development of medial coronoid disease will have to be re-directed to alternative biomechanical mechanisms as an explanation for the obvious supraphysiological loading of the medial joint compartment in dysplastic elbow joints.

With a mean static RUI of 1.4 mm in the dysplastic group, we failed at recruiting two groups of dogs being comparable in every aspect considered relevant to the study. Certainly, it would have been desirable that the dysplastic dogs would have had congruent elbow joints, but on the other hand, this allows us to speculate on the significance of RUI measurement without joint load, which is inherent to the established clinical CT scanning protocols. Both normal and dysplastic elbow joints exhibit dynamic deformation of the radio-ulnar transition, but the amount of axial radio-ulnar translation did not differ in respect to the degree of static RUI. Therefore, equalization of severe static RUI during weight bearing activity appears to be unlikely. The same applies to congruent joints, which do not show dynamic RUI different to the incongruent once, and therefore can´t be considered to develop a pronounced, clinically relevant incongruence throughout the weight-bearing period. In the future, more elaborated analysis of static RUI and the pattern of dynamic change will be necessary for conclusion.

Limitations

Only the first third of stance phase was evaluated in the present study, which might have resulted in loss of significant kinematic data occurring at another time point of the gait cycle, including swing phase. Limiting data analysis to the first 120 frames after foot drop was due to the fact that later during stance phase, superimposition of both elbow joints and the thoracic wall occurred at least in one fluoroscopic plane. Superimposition of both joints and the thoracic wall produced very low fluoroscopic image quality, rendering marker tracking unreliable. Nevertheless, we consider the first 30% of stance phase to be the most relevant when investigating dynamic RUI, because maximal peak vertical force in the front limbs occurs early during stance phase (Corbee *et al.*, 2014). Therefore, we expect axial radio-ulnar translation reaching its maximum within the first third of stance phase, when the limb is maximally loaded. Another argument, further strengthening our confidence to present relevant data, is the close similarity of our kinematic findings with the one of Guillou *et al.* (2011), who measured axial radio-ulnar translation along the entire gait cycle, including both stance and swing phase.

Measuring only maximal amplitude (AmpRUI) of relative radio-ulnar translation, independent from the direction of radial motion, limits the prediction of the effect of radio-ulnar motion onto joint cup conformation. Proximal radial translation would result in a different radio-ulnar joint conformation than distally orientated translation. Despite no significant difference in AmpRUI values between normal and dysplastic elbow joints in the current study, individual motion patterns need to be further investigated to clarify the in vivo radio-ulnar joint cup conformation during stance phase.

Kinematic studies using treadmill walking may not mirror over ground motion, because of influence on gait pattern (Fredricson *et al.*, 1983; Buchner *et al.*, 1994). In humans, familiarization to the treadmill after 6 to 8 minutes has been reported. After that, gait pattern normalizes and does no longer differ from the gait on a flat underground (Schieb, 1986; Matsas *et al.*, 2000). There are multiple studies investigating the process of familiarization to treadmill walking in dogs (Vilensky *et al.*, 1994a, b; Owen *et al.*, 2004; Fanchon *et al.*, 2006) and 2 minutes turned out to be sufficient. (Owen *et al.*, 2004) Based on this, an individual time of at least two minutes was conceded to every dog before data collection. Because dynamic RUI is assumed to be dependent on joint load, not only kinematics on the treadmill should mimic the once during over ground activity, but also the kinetics. The latter has been confirmed by Brebner *et al.* (2006) who documented a good correlation of ground reaction forces on an instrumented treadmill and the one with a force plate embedded in the floor.

In conclusion, the results of this study show that the concept of in vivo dynamic RUI applies to both normal and dysplastic canine elbow joints. However, dynamic RUI is not different in dysplastic joints compared to normal, and therefore cannot be considered relevant for the development of medial compartment disease. In addition, compensation of severe static radio-ulnar incongruence in dysplastic elbow joints as well as the dynamic induction of radio-ulnar incongruence in statically congruent joints seems unlikely. However, this latter statement will need verification using more elaborated kinematic analysis as presented in the actual study.

Acknowledgments

The authors would like to thank the medical as well as the technical stuff of both, the imaging and aesthesia service, for their generous support throughout the study.

Conflict of interest

The authors declare that there is no conflict of interests.

References

Brainerd, E.L., Baier, D.B., Gatesy, S.M., Hedrick, T.L., Metzger, K.A., Gilbert, S.L. and Crisco, J.J. 2010. X-ray reconstruction of moving morphology (XROMM): precision, accuracy and applications in comparative biomechanics research. J. Exp. Zool. A. Ecol. Genet. Physiol. 313, 262-279.

Brebner, N.S., Moens, N. and Runciman, J. 2006. Evaluation of a treadmill with integrated force plates for kinetic gait analysis of sound and lame dogs at a trot. Vet. Comp. Orthop. Traumatol. 19, 205-212.

Buchner, H.H., Savelberg, H.H., Schamhardt, H.C., Merkens, H.W. and Barneveld, A. 1994. Kinematics of treadmill versus overground locomotion in horses. Vet. Q. 16(Suppl 2), S87-90.

Corbee, R.J., Maas, H., Doornenbal, A. and Hazewinkel, H.A.W. 2014. Forelimb and hindlimb ground reaction forces of walking cats: Assessment and comparison with walking dogs. Vet. J. 202, 116-127.

Eljack, H. and Bottcher, P. 2015. Relationship between axial radioulnar incongruence with cartilage damage in dogs with medial coronoid disease. Vet. Surg. 44, 174-179.

Eljack, H., Werner, H. and Bottcher, P. 2013. Sensitivity and specificity of 3D models of the radioulnar joint cup in combination with a sphere fitted to the ulnar trochlear notch for estimation of radioulnar incongruence in vitro. Vet. Surg. 42, 365-370.

Fanchon, L., Valette, J.P., Sanaa, M. and Grandjean, D. 2006. The measurement of ground reaction force in dogs trotting on a treadmill: an investigation of habituation. Vet. Comp. Orthop. Traumatol. 19, 81-86.

Fitzpatrick, N. and Yeadon, R. 2009. Working algorithm for treatment decision making for developmental disease of the medial compartment of the elbow in dogs. Vet. Surg. 38, 285-300.

Fitzpatrick, N., Smith, T.J., Evans, R.B. and Yeadon, R. 2009. Radiographic and arthroscopic findings in the elbow joints of 263 dogs with medial coronoid disease. Vet. Surg. 38, 213-223.

Fitzpatrick, N., Garcia, T.C., Daryani, A., Bertran, J., Watari, S. and Hayashi, K. 2016. Micro-CT Structural Analysis of the Canine Medial Coronoid Disease. Vet. Surg. 45, 336-346.

Fredricson, I., Drevemo, S., Dalin, G., Hjerten, G., Bjorne, K., Rynde, R. and Franzen, G. 1983. Treadmill for equine locomotion analysis. Equine Vet. J. 15, 111-115.

Gatesy, S.M., Baier, D.B., Jenkins, F.A. and Dial, K.P. 2010. Scientific rotoscoping: a morphology-based method of 3-D motion analysis and visualization. J. Exp. Zool. A Ecol. Genet. Physiol. 313, 244-261.

Gemmill, T.J. and Clements, D.N. 2007. Fragmented coronoid process in the dog: is there a role for incongruency? J. Small Anim. Pract. 48(7), 361-368.

Gemmill, T.J., Mellor, D.J., Clements, D.N., Clarke, S.P., Farrell, M., Bennett, D. and Carmichael, S. 2005. Evaluation of elbow incongruency using reconstructed CT in dogs suffering fragmented coronoid process. J. Small Anim. Pract. 46, 327-333.

Goldhammer, M.A., Smith, S.H., Fitzpatrick, N. and Clements, D.N. 2010. A comparison of radiographic, arthroscopic and histological measures of articular pathology in the canine elbow joint. Vet. J. 186, 96-103.

Guillou, R.P., Déjardin, L.M., Bey, M.J. and McDonald, C.P. 2011. Three Dimensional Kinematics of the Normal Canine Elbow at the Walk and Trot. 2011 American College of Veterinary Surgeons Veterinary Symposium November 3-5, Chicago, Illinois. Vet. Surg. 40, E17-E42.

Gutbrod, A. and Guerrero, T.G. 2012. Effect of external rotational humeral osteotomy on the contact mechanics of the canine elbow joint. Vet. Surg. 41, 845-852.

Kirberger, R.M. and Fourie, S.L. 1998. Elbow dysplasia in the dog: pathophysiology, diagnosis and control. J. South African Vet. Assoc. 69, 43-54.

Knorlein, B.J., Baier, D.B., Gatesy, S.M., Laurence-Chasen, J.D. and Brainerd, E.L. 2016. Validation of XMALab software for marker-based XROMM. J. Exp. Biol. 219, 3701-3711.

Kramer, A., Holsworth, I.G., Wisner, E.R., Kass, P.H. and Schulz, K.S. 2006. Computed tomographic evaluation of canine radioulnar incongruence in vivo. Vet. Surg. 35, 24-29.

Krotscheck, U., Bottcher, P.B., Thompson, M.S., Todhunter, R.J. and Mohammed, H.O. 2014a. Cubital subchondral joint space width and CT osteoabsorptiometry in dogs with and without fragmented medial coronoid process. Vet. Surg. 43, 330-338.

Krotscheck, U., Kalafut, S., Meloni, G., Thompson, M.S., Todhunter, R.J., Mohammed, H.O. and van der Meulen, M.C.H. 2014b. Effect of Ulnar Ostectomy on Intra-Articular Pressure Mapping and Contact Mechanics of the Congruent and Incongruent Canine Elbow Ex Vivo. Vet. Surg. 43, 339-346.

Lau, S.F., Hazewinkel, H.A. and Voorhout, G. 2015. Radiographic and computed tomographic assessment of the development of the antebrachia and elbow joints in Labrador Retrievers with and without medial coronoid disease. Vet. Comp. Orthop. Traumatol. 28, 186-192.

Mariee, I.C., Gröne, A. and Theyse, L.F.H. 2014. The role of osteonecrosis in canine coronoid dysplasia: Arthroscopic and histopathological findings. Vet. J. 200, 382-386.

Mason, D.R., Schulz, K.S., Fujita, Y., Kass, P.H. and Stover, S.M. 2005. In vitro force mapping of normal canine humeroradial and humeroulnar joints. Am. J. Vet. Res. 66, 132-135.

Matsas, A., Taylor, N. and McBurney, H. 2000. Knee joint kinematics from familiarised treadmill walking can be generalised to overground walking in young unimpaired subjects. Gait Posture 11, 46-53.

McConkey, M.J., Valenzano, D.M., Wei, A., Li, T., Thompson, M.S., Mohammed, H.O., van der Meulen, M.C.H. and Krotscheck, U. 2016. Effect of the Proximal Abducting Ulnar Osteotomy on Intra-Articular Pressure Distribution and Contact Mechanics of Congruent and Incongruent Canine Elbows Ex Vivo. Vet. Surg. 45, 347-355.

Might, K.R., Hanzlik, K.A., Case, J.B., Duncan, C.G., Egger, E.L., Rooney, M.B. and Duerr, F.M. 2011. In Vitro Comparison of Proximal Ulnar Osteotomy and Distal Ulnar Osteotomy with Release of the Interosseous Ligament in a Canine Model. Vet. Surg. 40, 321-326.

Morgan, J.P., Wind, A. and Davidson, A.P. 1999. Bone dysplasias in the labrador retriever: a radiographic study. J. Am. Anim. Hosp. Assoc. 35, 332-340.

Nemanic, S., Nixon, B.K. and Baltzer, W. 2016. Analysis of risk factors for elbow dysplasia in giant breed dogs. Vet. Comp. Orthop. Traumatol. 29, 369-377.

Ohlerth, S., Tellhelm, B., Amort, K. and Ondreka, N. 2016. Explanation of the IEWG grading system, In: 30th annual meeting of the INTERNATIONAL ELBOW WORKING GROUP, Vienna, Austria.

Owen, M., Richards, J., Clements, D., Drew, S., Bennett, D. and Carmichael, S. 2004. Kinematics of the elbow and stifle joints in greyhounds during treadmill trotting–An investigation of familiarisation. Vet. Comp. Orthop. Traumatol. 17, 141.

Samoy, Y., Van Ryssen, B., Gielen, I., Walschot, N. and van Bree, H. 2006. Review of the literature:

elbow incongruity in the dog. Vet. Comp. Orthop. Traumatol. 19, 1-8.

Schieb, D.A. 1986. Kinematic accommodation of novice treadmill runners. Res. Q. Exerc. Sport 57, 1-7.

Smith, T.J., Fitzpatrick, N., Evans, R.B. and Pead, M.J. 2009. Measurement of Ulnar Subtrochlear Sclerosis Using a Percentage Scale in Labrador Retrievers with Minimal Radiographic Signs of Periarticular Osteophytosis. Vet. Surg. 38, 199-208.

Starke, A., Bottcher, P. and Pfeil, I. 2013. Radiologic quantification of the elbow conformation with a new method for acquiring standardized x-rays under load. Reference valus for medium sized and large dogs without dysplasia of the elbow joint. Tierarztliche Praxis. Ausgabe K, Kleintiere/Heimtiere 41, 145-154.

Starke, A., Bottcher, P. and Pfeil, I. 2014. Comparative radiologic examination of the canine elbow with and without elbow dysplasia under standardized load. Tierarztliche Praxis. Ausgabe K, Kleintiere/Heimtiere 42, 141-150.

Vilensky, J.A., O'Connor, B.L., Brandt, K.D., Dunn, E.A. and Rogers, P.I. 1994a. Serial kinematic analysis of the trunk and limb joints after anterior cruciate ligament transection: Temporal, spatial, and angular changes in a canine model of osteoarthritis. J. Electromyogr. Kinesiol. 4, 181-192.

Vilensky, J.A., O'Connor, B.L., Brandt, K.D., Dunn, E.A., Rogers, P.I. and Delong, C.A. 1994b. Serial kinematic analysis of the unstable knee after transection of the anterior cruciate ligament: temporal and angular changes in a canine model of osteoarthritis. J. Orthop. Res. 12, 229-237.

28

Investigation of manganese homeostasis in dogs with anaemia and chronic enteropathy

Marisa da Fonseca Ferreira[*], Arielle Elizabeth Ann Aylor, Richard John Mellanby, Susan Mary Campbell and Adam George Gow

Hospital for Small Animals, The Royal (Dick) School of Veterinary Studies, The University of Edinburgh, UK

Abstract

Lethargy is a frequent and important clinical feature of anaemia; however, it does not absolutely correlate with the severity of anaemia. Manganese is efficiently absorbed through the gastrointestinal tract via divalent metal transporter 1 (DMT1), which is also responsible for iron transport. DMT1 is upregulated in iron deficiency (ID). Increased manganese concentrations are reported in ID anaemia (IDA) in various species. Manganese is neurotoxic and therefore may contribute to lethargy observed in some anaemic patients. In addition, anaemia and ID are common in human inflammatory bowel disease. Little is known about how anaemia influences manganese metabolism in veterinary patients and how common is anaemia in dogs with chronic enteropathy (CE). If elevated manganese concentrations are found, then potentially neurotoxicity may be contributing to morbidity in these cases. The objectives of this study were to investigate the hypothesis that whole blood manganese concentrations would be increased in dogs with anaemia, particularly in dogs with confirmed IDA, and that anaemia would be common in canine CE. Medical records from 2012-2016 were reviewed for dogs with CE that were anaemic, as well as dogs with confirmed IDA, where a sample suitable for manganese analysis was held in an archive. Manganese concentration was measured in whole blood from: 11 anaemic dogs with CE, 6 dogs with IDA, 9 non-anaemic ill controls, and 12 healthy controls. Mann-Whitney U and Kruskal-Wallis tests with post-test Dunn's multiple comparisons tests were performed, with $P<0.05$ considered significant. The prevalence of anaemia in canine CE was 20.6% (33/160). Manganese concentrations were significantly different between all groups ($P=0.0001$) and higher in non-anaemic than anaemic dogs ($P=0.0078$). Manganese concentrations were also higher in healthy compared to ill controls ($P<0.0001$), anaemic dogs with CE ($P=0.0056$) and to dogs with IDA ($P=0.0001$). No differences were observed between anaemic dogs with CE, IDA and ill controls. Although anaemia was frequently observed in canine CE, the hypothesis that dogs with anaemia would have increased manganese concentrations, possibly contributing to a lethargic state was not supported. Further research is warranted to understand the influence of anaemia on whole blood manganese.

Keywords: Inflammatory bowel disease, Iron, Trace element.

Introduction

Lethargy is a common clinical sign in anaemia. Although the reduction in haemoglobin concentration results in decreased delivery of oxygen to tissues, lethargy does not always correlate with anaemia severity (Chervier *et al.*, 2012; Bager, 2014). Therefore, it is possible that other factors might be contributing to lethargy. In humans with iron deficiency anaemia (IDA), increased intestinal iron absorption also results in increased absorption of other trace elements including manganese (Mn) (Meltzer *et al.*, 2010). Manganese is an essential trace element and a necessary cofactor for a few enzymes and metabolic pathways. Manganese is efficiently absorbed from the gastrointestinal tract via divalent metal transporter 1 (DMT1), which is concurrently responsible for iron transport (Au *et al.*, 2008).

Iron deficiency (ID) causes upregulation of DMT1 and has been associated with increased Mn concentrations in many species (Kim and Lee, 2011; Smith *et al.*, 2013).

Manganese is neurotoxic when present in excessive concentrations (Racette *et al.*, 2017). The mechanism of neurotoxicity appears multifactorial. Astrocytic dysfunction occurs due to their high affinity transport system accumulating high intracellular concentrations of Mn (Yin *et al.*, 2008). Manganese also causes microglial activation by induction of cytokines and reactive oxygen species (Dodd and Filipov, 2011), as well as causing disruption of several neurotransmitters and mitochondrial dysfunction, culminating in neuronal apoptosis (Smith *et al.*, 2017).

Hyperintensity of the basal ganglia on magnetic resonance imaging (MRI) is pathognomonic for Mn deposition in humans, correlating with neurological signs and fatigue in human cirrhosis as well as blood Mn concentrations (Burkhard *et al.*, 2003; Forton *et al.*, 2004). Hyperintensity in focal areas of the basal ganglia

*Corresponding Author: Marisa da Fonseca Ferreira. Easter Bush Campus, Roslin, EH25 9RG, UK.
Email: *marisa.ferreira@ed.ac.uk*

has also been shown in canine and feline congenital portosystemic shunts, which contained increased concentrations of Mn on post-mortem examination (Torisu *et al.*, 2008).

Iron deficiency has been linked with Mn accumulation within the brain, and increased uptake by astrocytes, mediated by DMT1 upregulation, in the absence of Mn overexposure (Erikson and Aschner, 2006). The presence of clinical Mn neurotoxicity with concurrent ID, and without Mn exposure, has been suggested in developing mice and confirmed in one child (Kwik-Uribe *et al.*, 1999; Brna *et al.*, 2011).

Anaemia is one of the most common extra-intestinal clinicopathological abnormalities in human inflammatory bowel disease (IBD), associated with a multifactorial aetiology, however over half of the cases demonstrated ID (Filmann *et al.*, 2014). Notably, ID is suggested to affect quality of life in human IBD, even in the absence of anaemia (Herrera-deGuise *et al.*, 2016).

There are only a few studies examining Mn homeostasis in human IBD. One report demonstrated higher whole blood Mn levels in 5/55 patients with ulcerative colitis, not associated with clinical or MRI evidence of toxicity, with 2/5 cases confirming low ferritin levels (El Muhtaseb *et al.*, 2007). The remaining studies have shown no differences, though all reports were based in serum or plasma Mn (Whineray *et al.*, 2000; Ma *et al.*, 2013). More importantly, none have concentrated specifically on anaemic, or iron deficient subjects.

Chronic enteropathies (CE) are a common cause of morbidity and mortality in dogs (Allenspach *et al.*, 2016). Metabolic complications are well described in dogs with CE, notably hypoalbuminaemia, hypocobalaminaemia and altered vitamin D status (Allenspach *et al.*, 2007; Gow *et al.*, 2011). Canine CE appears to share similarities to human IBD (Cerquetella *et al.*, 2010). Surprisingly, studies characterising anaemia in canine CE are scant, although a prevalence is reported of between 12-18% in studies with relatively small numbers (Craven *et al.*, 2004; Marchetti *et al.*, 2010). Essential trace elements in canine CE are even less well studied, with only one abstract reporting plasma Mn concentrations, showing no difference compared to laboratory beagle controls (Yokoyama *et al.*, 2016).

Given the high prevalence of anaemia in human IBD, the aim of this study was to investigate the prevalence of anaemia in a larger number of cases of canine CE, and to then establish whether anaemia is associated with increased Mn concentrations. An additional aim was to assess if confirmed absolute IDA, regardless of underlying aetiology, is associated with higher Mn concentrations. Non-anaemic controls, both ill and healthy, served as cohorts for comparison.

Materials and Methods

Samples

The small animal teaching hospital archive, at the authors' institution, was used to retrieve the samples for the study. The archive database of -80°C stored residual samples previously taken for clinical diagnostic purposes, with informed consent from the owners, was searched for ethylenediaminetetraacetic acid (EDTA) samples from January 2012 to January 2016.

Inclusion criteria

Using the corresponding patients' case numbers, a retrospective search using the hospital's electronic record system was undertaken to retrieve clinical information that would match inclusion criteria for each group: anaemic dogs with a clinical diagnosis of CE, either food responsive, antibiotic responsive or idiopathic, confirmed histologically from endoscopic or full thickness surgical gastric and/or intestinal biopsies; dogs with absolute IDA; ill dogs with normal haematology; and healthy dogs based on history and physical examination, with a normal packed cell volume (PCV). Mn analysis was performed on small cohorts of the first and last two groups, and on all patients with confirmed IDA.

Analyses

Gastrointestinal histology and haematology analyses were performed by the institution's pathology laboratory, with results confirmed by board-certified veterinary pathologists and clinical pathologists, respectively. Histological results confirming a diagnosis of CE would need to include mild, moderate or marked mucosal infiltration by inflammatory cells (lymphocytes, plasma cells, eosinophils). Anaemia was defined by a PCV below the lower limit of the laboratory reference range (0.39 L/L). Iron status analyses were performed by an external laboratory and diagnosis of absolute ID was defined by serum iron below the reference interval, combined with transferrin saturation below the reference interval and a normal total iron binding capacity (TIBC).

Manganese concentrations were prospectively determined at an external laboratory, by graphite furnace atomic absorption spectrometry (1100 Spectrometer, PerkinElmer Life and Analytical Sciences, Milan, Italy), in whole blood anticoagulated with EDTA, after dilution with Triton X-100 solution (Sigma-Aldrich, St. Louis, MO). All samples had been frozen within 4 hours of collection, archived as abovementioned, and subsequently shipped in dry ice to the reference laboratory. The assay had a limit of quantitation of 16nmol/L, an inter-assay coefficient of variation (CV) of 3.1% and an intra-assay CV of 5.4%.

Statistical analysis

Assessment for normality was performed with the Kolmogorov-Smirnov test for each group and the overall population regarding Mn concentrations, PCV and age. As not all groups were normally distributed in each of the three categories, nonparametric tests were therefore used for statistical analysis throughout, with data expressed as median (minimum/maximum ranges). Mann-Whitney U and Kruskal-Wallis tests with post-test Dunn's multiple comparisons tests were performed for assessment of differences in between groups. The correlation between Mn concentration and PCV was assessed by the Spearman's rank correlation coefficient (r_s). Statistical significance level was set at $P < 0.05$. Statistical analysis was performed with two commercial software packages (GraphPad InStat, version 3.10, GraphPad Software Inc.; and Minitab®, version 17.1.0, Minitab Inc.).

Results

A total of 1847 whole blood EDTA samples were available, from which 160 (8.7%) corresponded to dogs with histologically confirmed CE. Of these, anaemia was present in 33 (20.6%), with one patient being microcytic and hypochromic, and four normocytic and hypochromic. A cohort of the most anaemic dogs with CE (n = 11) was selected for Mn analysis, of which four had iron status results available, confirming absolute IDA in two, and anaemia of chronic disease (ACD) with relative IDA (low serum iron with normal transferrin saturation and low TIBC) in another two.

Within the archived available whole blood EDTA samples, six corresponded to cases from which an iron status confirmed absolute ID. Of these, two dogs were in the previously selected CE group, and the remaining had an underlying diagnosis each of: intestinal lymphoma, immune-mediated haemolytic anaemia, urinary bladder mass, or suspected disseminated histiocytic neoplasia.

Including the non-anaemic ill (n = 9, Table 1) and healthy (n = 12) cohort controls, a total of 36 samples were then prospectively analysed for Mn concentration. No differences were seen between groups with regard to age ($P = 0.2025$) or gender ($P = 0.1025$). Eight individuals were crossbreeds and the most commonly represented breeds included: Labrador Retriever (n = 6), Cocker Spaniel (n = 4), followed by Boxer (n = 2), German Shepherd (n = 2), Hungarian Vizla (n = 2) and Springer Spaniel (n = 2). Mn concentrations and PCVs in each group are summarised in Figure 1 and Table 2. Manganese concentrations were significantly different between the four groups ($P = 0.0001$), being higher in healthy dogs compared to: anaemic dogs with CE ($P = 0.0056$), dogs with IDA ($P = 0.0001$), and non-anaemic ill controls ($P < 0.0001$). No differences were observed between Mn concentrations in anaemic dogs with CE, dogs with IDA and non-anaemic ill controls. Mn concentrations were also higher in overall non-anaemic compared to anaemic dogs ($P = 0.0078$), with an overall moderate positive correlation between PCV and Mn concentration ($r_s = 0.6252$, $P < 0.0001$).

Table 1. Problem list/diagnoses of a cohort of non-anaemic ill dogs (n = 9).

Diagnosis	Patients (n)
Chronic cystitis	2
Chronic intermittent diarrhoea	2
Acute gastroenteritis	1
Cervical carcinoma, prostatic mass	1
Hepatosplenic nodules, gastric mass, chronic kidney disease	1
Septic peritonitis of unknown origin	1
Sinonasal aspergillosis	1

Table 2. Descriptive statistics of manganese concentrations and packed cell values distribution within four cohorts.

Cohort	Mn (nmol/L)		PCV (l/l)	
	Median	Range	Median	Range
Anaemic CE	366	219-1817	0.27	0.13-0.32
IDA	292	170-710	0.20	0.13-0.30
Non-anaemic ill	608	303-839	0.46	0.42-0.51
Healthy	1006	893-1240	0.53	0.45-0.64

Footnote: CE – chronic enteropathy; IDA – iron-deficiency anaemia; Mn – manganese; PCV – packed cell value.

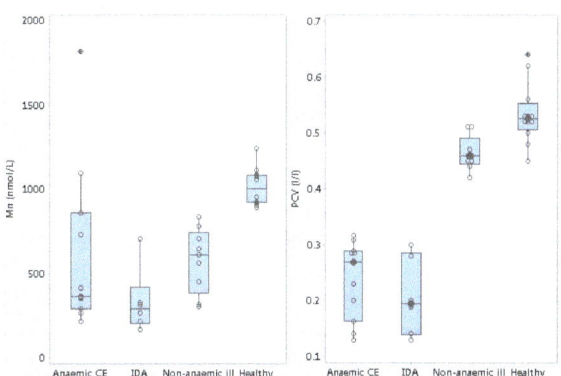

Fig. 1. Box and whisker plots and individual values depicting manganese (Mn) concentrations (left) and packed cell values (PCV, right) distribution within four cohorts. (CE): Chronic enteropathy; (IDA): Iron-deficiency anaemia.

However, when analysing healthy dogs alone, there was no correlation between PCV and Mn ($r_s = -11.35$, $P = 0.7329$). Moreover, when comparing PCV overall amongst groups, the difference obtained ($P < 0.0001$) was attributed only to the comparison between each of the anaemic groups (dogs with CE or ID), with each of the non-anaemic ill or healthy control groups, and no difference was seen in between the latter two cohorts on post-test Dunn's multiple comparisons test.

Discussion

Anaemia in canine CE was frequent within the population studied. The obtained prevalence of 20.6% was higher than previously reported, as was the overall number of patients assessed, totalling 160, compared with 22 and 77 in other studies (Craven et al., 2004; Marchetti et al., 2010). This prevalence is similar to that of 24% obtained in a meta-analysis in human IBD (Filmann et al., 2014). This confirms that anaemia is a common clinicopathological abnormality in canine CE and may be contributing towards overall morbidity.

The results obtained in this study showed no evidence that ID is associated with increased whole blood Mn concentrations. Moreover, anaemic dogs with CE or IDA, as well as non-anaemic ill dogs, had lower Mn concentrations when compared to healthy controls. This does not support the hypothesis that Mn neurotoxicity contributes to the clinical sign of lethargy in these cases.

There are many potential factors which may explain this result. As the majority of circulating Mn is within erythrocytes, it is possible that anaemia may be a confounding factor, although no correlation between Mn and PCV was found in the healthy controls (Pleban and Pearson, 1979).

Measurement of whole blood Mn is recommended to reflect whole body manganese (Clegg et al., 1986). Whole blood Mn is less variable within an individual, when compared to plasma, better reflecting Mn in a single sample (Baker et al., 2015). A higher risk of inaccuracy is seen with serum measurements, combined with wider variation of reference ranges (Baruthio et al., 1988). Even if no macroscopic haemolysis is present, there can be a considerable amount of Mn that is released from the red blood cells into the serum or plasma if not separated, leading to potential erroneous interpretations. In addition, to be reliable, serum or plasma analysis requires very sensitive assays, since Mn concentration is approximately 10-30 times lower than within erythrocytes (Versieck et al., 1974).

Moreover, other studies have used whole blood samples to assess Mn status in ID and were able to confirm increased Mn concentrations in anaemic samples (Meltzer et al., 2010; Kim and Lee, 2011; Smith et al., 2013).

Whole blood manganese is obtained from dietary intake. These clinical cases were on a range of diets, which would likely have widely different Mn content, as previously documented on a comparison of several commercial diets (Gagne et al., 2013). Hyporexia is a common finding in any illness, and one of the main clinical signs of canine CE (Gianella et al., 2017), therefore reduced dietary intake is a potential confounding factor for both the non-anaemic ill and CE groups. The healthy control group dogs were all fed a standard complete diet with a Mn content of 25.1mg/kg on a dry matter basis, which is within the minimum and maximum amounts (5.8mg/kg and 170mg/kg, respectively) recommended for adult dogs, by the European Pet Food Industry Federation (Zentek, 2016). It is possible that this standardised diet may explain the higher concentrations seen in the healthy group in this study.

Inflammation seen in canine CE might stimulate hepcidin, a peptide produced in the liver, controlling iron homeostasis by inhibiting iron transport (Brasse-Lagnel et al., 2011). This hormone downregulates DMT1 and also binds to the iron and Mn exporter ferroportin 1, leading to its internalisation and degradation, resulting in iron (and likely Mn) entrapment and decreased transport across the basolateral membrane (Seo and Wessling-Resnick, 2015). Hepcidin has been shown to be upregulated in human IBD, resulting in ACD due to relative ID (Bergamaschi et al., 2013). As a further variable, Vitamin D is an important suppressor of hepcidin, and dogs with severe CE have been shown to have reduced vitamin D concentrations (Gow et al., 2011; Bacchetta et al., 2014). Moreover, in inflammatory conditions, the action of metal transporters can be disrupted, independently of hepcidin (Guida et al., 2015). In human IBD, active disease was seen to correlate with decreased mucosal DMT1 expression (Wu et al., 2015). Conversely, in a study of human IBD, where 14/19 patients were anaemic while in histological remission, upregulation of DMT1 was confirmed, and negatively correlated with haemoglobin, possibly explained by absolute ID overriding the effects of ACD (Sukumaran et al., 2014). Investigation of DMT1 expression in enterocytes in canine CE would help define this effect. In addition, is unknown how the presence of other iron and Mn transporters, namely ZIP8 and ZIP14, might influence overall canine Mn homeostasis (Shawki et al., 2015). Given that dogs with gastrointestinal disease (CE, lymphoma, and non-specified) were present within the absolute IDA and non-anaemic ill groups (n = 3 in each group), is possible that impaired Mn absorption in these patients has accounted for the lower concentrations observed, alongside the anaemic CE group.

Finally, the liver is responsible for removing most of the Mn absorbed through the gastrointestinal tract from the portal circulation, excreting it via the biliary system and allowing only around 2% of the absorbed Mn to reach the systemic circulation (Papavasiliou et al., 1966; Klaassen, 1974). This system is very efficient and dogs fed large quantities of Mn over many weeks demonstrated no significant increase in whole blood manganese concentrations, yet had increased hepatic concentrations, thought to be due to trafficking through the liver for excretion in bile (Reiman and Minot,

1920). Therefore, it is possible that despite increased Mn delivery in the portal vasculature, the canine liver is more efficient at Mn extraction, leading to no systemic increase. Dogs with hepatic dysfunction and portosystemic shunting have altered Mn homeostasis, leading to Mn accumulation (Kilpatrick *et al.*, 2014). Consequently, further research would be needed to assess if ID could play a role in exacerbating increased Mn concentrations in dogs with established liver pathology, as reported in human chronic liver disease (Malecki *et al.*, 1999).

This study carries several limitations. Although Mn levels were prospectively measured, the population was retrospectively assessed, thereby leading to lack of standardisation within and between groups. The number of dogs in each group was also small, which could have led to subsequent type II error regarding the absence of difference between anaemic and non-anaemic ill dogs. Iron status analysis was only available for eight subjects, precluding further conclusions. In addition, diet was not standardised, which could have affected results (Lopez-Alonso *et al.*, 2007).

This study demonstrates that anaemia is common in dogs with chronic enteropathy. However, anaemic dogs with chronic enteropathy and/or iron-deficiency anaemia do not have increased whole blood manganese concentrations, compared to non-anaemic ill or healthy cohorts. More investigation is warranted to understand the complex interplay of canine anaemia, iron deficiency and inflammatory disease, namely chronic enteropathy, in manganese concentrations.

Acknowledgments

Manganese analyses were reported by Antony Catchpole, Scottish Trace Element & Micronutrient Diagnostic & Research Laboratory, North Glasgow Biochemistry Department, NHS Great Glasgow and Clyde, United Kingdom.

No external funds were used for this study.

Conflict of interest

The authors declare that there is no conflict of interest.

References

Allenspach, K., Culverwell, C. and Chan, D. 2016. Long-term outcome in dogs with chronic enteropathies: 203 cases. Vet. Rec. 178(15), 368.

Allenspach, K., Wieland, B., Grone, A. and Gaschen, F. 2007. Chronic enteropathies in dogs: evaluation of risk factors for negative outcome. J. Vet. Intern. Med. 21(4), 700-708.

Au, C., Benedetto, A. and Aschner, M. 2008. Manganese transport in eukaryotes: the role of DMT1. Neurotoxicology 29(4), 569-576.

Bacchetta, J., Zaritsky, J.J., Sea, J.L., Chun, R.F., Lisse, T.S., Zavala, K., Nayak, A., Wesseling-Perry, K., Westerman, M., Hollis, B.W., Salusky, I.B. and Hewison, M. 2014. Suppression of iron-regulatory hepcidin by vitamin D. J. Am. Soc. Nephrol. 25(3), 564-572.

Bager, P. 2014. Fatigue and acute/chronic anaemia. Dan. Med. J. 61(4), B4824.

Baker, M.G., Simpson, C.D., Sheppard, L., Stover, B., Morton, J., Cocker, J. and Seixas, N. 2015. Variance components of short-term biomarkers of manganese exposure in an inception cohort of welding trainees. J. Trace Elem. Med. Biol. 29, 123-129.

Baruthio, F., Guillard, O., Arnaud, J., Pierre, F. and Zawislak, R. 1988. Determination of manganese in biological materials by electrothermal atomic absorption spectrometry: a review. Clin. Chem. 34(2), 227-234.

Bergamaschi, G., Di Sabatino, A., Albertini, R., Costanzo, F., Guerci, M., Masotti, M., Pasini, A., Massari, A., Campostrini, N., Corbella, M., Girelli, D. and Corazza, G.R. 2013. Serum hepcidin in inflammatory bowel diseases: biological and clinical significance. Inflamm. Bowel Dis. 19(10), 2166-2172.

Brasse-Lagnel, C., Karim, Z., Letteron, P., Bekri, S., Bado, A. and Beaumont, C. 2011. Intestinal DMT1 cotransporter is down-regulated by hepcidin via proteasome internalization and degradation. Gastroenterology 140(4), 1261-1271 e1261.

Brna, P., Gordon, K., Dooley, J.M. and Price, V. 2011. Manganese toxicity in a child with iron deficiency and polycythemia. J. Child Neurol. 26(7), 891-894.

Burkhard, P.R., Delavelle, J., Du Pasquier, R. and Spahr, L. 2003. Chronic parkinsonism associated with cirrhosis: a distinct subset of acquired hepatocerebral degeneration. Arch. Neurol. 60(4), 521-528.

Cerquetella, M., Spaterna, A., Laus, F., Tesei, B., Rossi, G., Antonelli, E., Villanacci, V. and Bassotti, G. 2010. Inflammatory bowel disease in the dog: differences and similarities with humans. World J. Gastroenterol. 16(9), 1050-1056.

Chervier, C., Cadore, J.L., Rodriguez-Pineiro, M.I., Deputte, B.L. and Chabanne, L. 2012. Causes of anaemia other than acute blood loss and their clinical significance in dogs. J. Small Anim. Pract. 53(4), 223-227.

Clegg, M.S., Lonnerdal, B., Hurley, L.S. and Keen, C.L. 1986. Analysis of whole blood manganese by flameless atomic absorption spectrophotometry and its use as an indicator of manganese status in animals. Anal. Biochem. 157(1), 12-18.

Craven, M., Simpson, J.W., Ridyard, A.E. and Chandler, M.L. 2004. Canine inflammatory bowel disease: retrospective analysis of diagnosis and outcome in 80 cases (1995-2002). J. Small Anim. Pract. 45(7), 336-342.

Dodd, C.A. and Filipov, N.M. 2011. Manganese potentiates LPS-induced heme-oxygenase 1 in microglia but not dopaminergic cells: role in controlling microglial hydrogen peroxide and inflammatory cytokine output. Neurotoxicology 32(6), 683-692.

El Muhtaseb, M.S., Duncan, A., Talwar, D.K., O'Reilly, D.S., McKee, R.F., Anderson, J.H. and Finlay, I.G. 2007. Assessment of dietary intake and trace element status in patients with ileal pouch-anal anastomosis. Dis. Colon. Rectum. 50(10), 1553-1557.

Erikson, K.M. and Aschner, M. 2006. Increased manganese uptake by primary astrocyte cultures with altered iron status is mediated primarily by divalent metal transporter. Neurotoxicology 27(1), 125-130.

Filmann, N., Rey, J., Schneeweiss, S., Ardizzone, S., Bager, P., Bergamaschi, G., Koutroubakis, I., Lindgren, S., Morena Fde, L., Moum, B., Vavricka, S.R., Schroder, O., Herrmann, E. and Blumenstein, I. 2014. Prevalence of anemia in inflammatory bowel diseases in european countries: a systematic review and individual patient data meta-analysis. Inflamm. Bowel Dis. 20(5), 936-945.

Forton, D.M., Patel, N., Prince, M., Oatridge, A., Hamilton, G., Goldblatt, J., Allsop, J.M., Hajnal, J.V., Thomas, H.C., Bassendine, M., Jones, D.E. and Taylor-Robinson, S.D. 2004. Fatigue and primary biliary cirrhosis: association of globus pallidus magnetisation transfer ratio measurements with fatigue severity and blood manganese levels. Gut 53(4), 587-592.

Gagne, J.W., Wakshlag, J.J., Center, S.A., Rutzke, M.A. and Glahn, R.P. 2013. Evaluation of calcium, phosphorus, and selected trace mineral status in commercially available dry foods formulated for dogs. J. Am. Vet. Med. Assoc. 243(5), 658-666.

Gianella, P., Lotti, U., Bellino, C., Bresciani, F., Cagnasso, A., Fracassi, F., D'Angelo, A. and Pietra, M. 2017. Clinicopathologic and prognostic factors in short- and long-term surviving dogs with protein-losing enteropathy. Schweiz. Arch. Tierheilkd. 159(3), 163-169.

Gow, A.G., Else, R., Evans, H., Berry, J.L., Herrtage, M.E. and Mellanby, R.J. 2011. Hypovitaminosis D in dogs with inflammatory bowel disease and hypoalbuminaemia. J. Small Anim. Pract. 52(8), 411-418.

Guida, C., Altamura, S., Klein, F.A., Galy, B., Boutros, M., Ulmer, A.J., Hentze, M.W. and Muckenthaler, M.U. 2015. A novel inflammatory pathway mediating rapid hepcidin-independent hypoferremia. Blood 125(14), 2265-2275.

Herrera-deGuise, C., Casellas, F., Robles, V., Navarro, E. and Borruel, N. 2016. Iron Deficiency in the Absence of Anemia Impairs the Perception of Health-Related Quality of Life of Patients with Inflammatory Bowel Disease. Inflamm. Bowel Dis. 22(6), 1450-1455.

Kilpatrick, S., Jacinto, A., Foale, R.D., Tappin, S.W., Burton, C., Frowde, P.E., Elwood, C.M., Powell, R., Duncan, A., Mellanby, R.J. and Gow, A.G. 2014. Whole blood manganese concentrations in dogs with primary hepatitis. J. Small Anim. Pract. 55(5), 241-246.

Kim, Y. and Lee, B.K. 2011. Iron deficiency increases blood manganese level in the Korean general population according to KNHANES 2008. Neurotoxicology 32(2), 247-254.

Klaassen, C.D. 1974. Biliary excretion of manganese in rats, rabbits, and dogs. Toxicol. Appl. Pharmacol. 29(3), 458-468.

Kwik-Uribe, C.L., Golubt, M.S. and Keen, C.L. 1999. Behavioral consequences of marginal iron deficiency during development in a murine model. Neurotoxicol. Teratol. 21(6), 661-672.

Lopez-Alonso, M., Miranda, M., Garcia-Partida, P., Mendez, A., Castillo, C. and Benedito, J.L. 2007. Toxic and trace metal concentrations in liver and kidney of dogs: influence of diet, sex, age, and pathological lesions. Biol. Trace Elem. Res. 116(2), 185-202.

Ma, X., Zhao, K., Wei, L., Song, P., Liu, G., Han, H. and Wang, C. 2013. Altered plasma concentrations of trace elements in ulcerative colitis patients before and after surgery. Biol. Trace Elem. Res. 153(1-3), 100-104.

Malecki, E.A., Devenyi, A.G., Barron, T.F., Mosher, T.J., Eslinger, P., Flaherty-Craig, C.V. and Rossaro, L. 1999. Iron and manganese homeostasis in chronic liver disease: relationship to pallidal T1-weighted magnetic resonance signal hyperintensity. Neurotoxicology 20(4), 647-652.

Marchetti, V., Lubas, G., Lombardo, A., Corazza, M., Guidi, G. and Cardini, G. 2010. Evaluation of erythrocytes, platelets, and serum iron profile in dogs with chronic enteropathy. Vet. Med. Int. 2010. Article ID 716040, doi:10.4061/2010/716040.

Meltzer, H.M., Brantsaeter, A.L., Borch-Iohnsen, B., Ellingsen, D.G., Alexander, J., Thomassen, Y., Stigum, H. and Ydersbond, T.A. 2010. Low iron stores are related to higher blood concentrations of manganese, cobalt and cadmium in non-smoking, Norwegian women in the HUNT 2 study. Environ. Res. 110(5), 497-504.

Papavasiliou, P.S., Miller, S.T. and Cotzias, G.C. 1966. Role of liver in regulating distribution and excretion of manganese. Am. J. Physiol. 211(1), 211-216.

Pleban, P.A. and Pearson, K.H. 1979. Determination of manganese in whole blood and serum. Clin. Chem. 25(11), 1915-1918.

Racette, B.A., Searles Nielsen, S., Criswell, S.R., Sheppard, L., Seixas, N., Warden, M.N. and

Checkoway, H. 2017. Dose-dependent progression of parkinsonism in manganese-exposed welders. Neurology 88(4), 344-351.

Reiman, C.K. and Minot, A.S. 1920. Absorption and elimination of manganese ingested as oxides and silicates. J. Biol. Chem. 45(1), 133-143.

Seo, Y.A. and Wessling-Resnick, M. 2015. Ferroportin deficiency impairs manganese metabolism in flatiron mice. FASEB J. 29(7), 2726-2733.

Shawki, A., Anthony, S.R., Nose, Y., Engevik, M.A., Niespodzany, E.J., Barrientos, T., Ohrvik, H., Worrell, R.T., Thiele, D.J. and Mackenzie, B. 2015. Intestinal DMT1 is critical for iron absorption in the mouse but is not required for the absorption of copper or manganese. Am. J. Physiol. Gastrointest. Liver Physiol. 309(8), G635-647.

Smith, E.A., Newland, P., Bestwick, K.G. and Ahmed, N. 2013. Increased whole blood manganese concentrations observed in children with iron deficiency anaemia. J. Trace Elem. Med. Biol. 27(1), 65-69.

Smith, M.R., Fernandes, J., Go, Y.M. and Jones, D.P. 2017. Redox dynamics of manganese as a mitochondrial life-death switch. Biochem. Biophys. Res. Commun. 482(3), 388-398.

Sukumaran, A., James, J., Janardhan, H.P., Amaladas, A., Suresh, L.M., Danda, D., Jeyeseelan, V., Ramakrishna, B.S. and Jacob, M. 2014. Expression of iron-related proteins in the duodenum is up-regulated in patients with chronic inflammatory disorders. Br. J. Nutr. 111(6), 1059-1068.

Torisu, S., Washizu, M., Hasegawa, D. and Orima, H. 2008. Measurement of brain trace elements in a dog with a portosystemic shunt: relation between hyperintensity on T1-weighted magnetic resonance images in lentiform nuclei and brain trace elements. J. Vet. Med. Sci. 70(12), 1391-1393.

Versieck, J., Barbier, F., Speecke, A. and Hoste, J. 1974. Manganese, copper, and zinc concentrations in serum and packed blood cells during acute hepatitis, chronic hepatitis, and posthepatitic cirrhosis. Clin. Chem. 20(9), 1141-1145.

Whineray, E., Inder, W.J., Roche, D., Dobbs, B.R. and Frizelle, F.A. 2000. Comparison of micronutrients in patients having had panproctocolectomy and either ileal pouch anal anastomosis or Brooke ileostomy for chronic ulcerative colitis (UC). Colorectal. Dis. 2(6), 351-354.

Wu, W., Song, Y., He, C., Liu, C., Wu, R., Fang, L., Cong, Y., Miao, Y. and Liu, Z. 2015. Divalent metal-ion transporter 1 is decreased in intestinal epithelial cells and contributes to the anemia in inflammatory bowel disease. Sci. Rep. 5, 16344. doi: 10.1038/srep16344.

Yin, Z., Aschner, J.L., dos Santos, A.P. and Aschner, M. 2008. Mitochondrial-dependent manganese neurotoxicity in rat primary astrocyte cultures. Brain Res. 1203, 1-11.

Yokoyama, N., Ohta, H., Mizukawa, H., Kagawa, Y., Nakayama, S., Sasaki, N., Morishita, K., Nakamura, K., Ikenaka, Y., Ishizuka, M. and Takiguchi, M. 2016. Plasma essential trace element concentrations in dogs with chronic enteropathy. In the Proceedings of the 2016 American College of Veterinary Internal Medicine Forum, pp: 1415.

Zentek, J. 2016. Nutritional guidelines for complete and complementary pet food for cats and dogs. FEDIAF - European Pet Food Industry Federation.

29

Medical infrared imaging and orthostatic analysis to determine lameness in the pelvic limbs of dogs

Erika Fernanda V. Garcia[1], Catherine A. Loughin[1,*], Dominic J. Marino[1], Joseph Sackman[1], Scott E. Umbaugh[2], Jiyuan Fu[2], Samrut Subedi[2], Martin L. Lesser[3], Meredith Akerman[3] and João Eduardo W. Schossler[4]

[1]*Department of Surgery, Long Island Veterinary Specialists, 163 South Service Road, Plainview, NY 11803, USA*
[2]*Computer Vision and Image Processing Laboratory, Electrical and Computer Engineering Department, Southern Illinois University at Edwardsville, Edwardsville, IL 62026-1801, USA*
[3]*North Shore - LIJ Health System Feinstein Institute for Medical Research, Biostatistics Unit, Manhasset, NY 11030, USA*
[4]*Universidade Federal de Santa Maria, Santa Maria, Brazil*

Abstract

Subtle lameness makes it difficult to ascertain which is the affected limb. A study was conducted to investigate a change in the thermal pattern and temperature of the thermal image of the paw print in a lame pelvic limb compared to a non-lame pelvic limb of dogs confirmed by orthostatic analysis. Fourteen client owned dogs with a unilateral pelvic limb lameness and 14 healthy employee dogs were examined and the pelvic limbs radiographed. Thermal images of the paw print were taken after each dog was kept in a static position on a foam mat for 30 seconds. Average temperatures and thermographic patterns were analyzed. Analysis was performed in a static position. The asymmetry index for each stance variable and optimal cutoff point for the peak vertical force and thermal image temperatures were calculated. Image pattern analysis revealed 88% success in differentiating the lame group, and 100% in identifying the same thermal pattern in the healthy group. The mean of the peak vertical force revealed a 10.0% difference between the left and right pelvic limb in healthy dogs and a 72.4% between the lame and non-lame limb in the lame dog group. Asymmetry index analysis revealed 5% in the healthy group and 36.2% in the lame group. The optimal cutoff point for the peak vertical force to determine lameness was 41.77% (AUC = 0.93) and for MII 0.943% (AUC = 0.72). The results of this study highlight the change in the thermal pattern of the paw print in the lame pelvic limb compared to a non-lame pelvic limb in the lame group and the healthy group. Medical infrared imaging of the paw prints can be utilized to screen for the lame limb in dogs.

Keywords: Cruciate, Infrared imaging, Lameness, Orthostatic analysis.

Introduction

Examination of the gait is the first diagnostic step in the evaluation of a patient with a lameness (Griffon, 2008), and relies on the assessment of asymmetry (Budsberg *et al.*, 1993; Fanchon and Grandjean, 2007). Watching a dog walk is subjective, and it can be difficult to differentiate left versus right sided lameness if asymmetry is subtle (Fanchon and Grandjean, 2007; Voss *et al.*, 2007).

Force plate analysis has been used for a wide range of kinetic applications in veterinary medicine, and its use has been proven as a valuable tool in gait analysis (Anderson, 1994; Voss *et al.*, 2007; Gillette and Angle, 2008). This analysis provides a noninvasive, objective and quantitative evaluation of the forces occurring between the paw and the ground during the stance phase of the stride (Anderson, 1994), as well as the pressure distributions of the paw in a standing position (orthostatic pattern) (Barbosa *et al.*, 2011). However, the complicated logistics, high cost of the equipment,

and laborious interpretation makes this method typically inaccessible in most clinics for small animals. Medical infrared imaging (MII) has proven to be a sensitive method for detecting changes in superficial temperature of the skin (Turner, 2001). This non-contact, non-invasive diagnostic technique measures heat emitted from a body surface as infrared radiation (Van hoogmoed and Snyder, 2002). The infrared image is a color map of warm colors representing areas of elevated temperature (e.g. associated with inflammation, increased circulation or metabolic rate), and cool colors representing areas of decreased tissue temperature or perfusion (e.g. vascular shunt, infarction or change in autonomic nervous system) (Eddy *et al.*, 2001; Turner, 2001; Van hoogmoed and Snyder, 2002). The change in superficial heat detected by the infrared camera is related to sympathetic nerve control of skin blood flow and the increase and decrease of postganglionic pressure that regulates microdermal blood flow.

*Corresponding Author: Catherine A. Loughin. Department of Surgery, Long Island Veterinary Specialists, 163 South Service Road, Plainview, NY 11803, USA. Email: cloughin@livs.org

Medical infrared imaging has been reported mostly for use in large animals, such as llamas, cattle, and horses to aid in the diagnosis of infectious (Colak *et al.*, 2008; Rainwater-Lovett *et al.*, 2009), reproductive (Purohit *et al.*, 1985), orthopedic (Purohit and McCoy, 1980; Eddy *et al.*, 2001), and neurologic conditions (Purohit *et al.*, 1980; Purohit, 2008). Recently, studies in small animals have been published evaluating normal thermal patterns in limbs of healthy dogs (Loughin and Marino, 2007), differentiation of cranial cruciate ligament deficient stifles from normal in dogs (Infernuso *et al.*, 2010), assessing for intervertebral disc disease in chondrodystrophic dogs (Grossbard *et al.*, 2014), assessing for elbow dysplasia in dogs (McGowan *et al.*, 2015), and to assist in detection of hyperthyroidism in cats (Waddell *et al.*, 2015). Another study in cats (Vainionpaa *et al.*, 2013) revealed that MII of the paw prints can detect a change in weight bearing. In this study, the author observed a change in the paw print thermal image, suggesting a painful process in the limb of the cat. Palpation of the cat and a questionnaire filled out by the owner were used for comparison to the images, but no other diagnostics were performed to support the suspicion of a pain or diagnose a specific disease process.

The purpose of this study was to investigate a change in the thermal pattern and temperature of the thermal image of the paw print in a lame pelvic limb compared to a non-lame pelvic limb in dogs with cranial cruciate ligament rupture. We also evaluated the thermal images of the paw prints of non-lame pelvic limbs of healthy dogs for comparison purposes, and used orthostatic analysis to objectify the data. We hypothesized that MII could be used to detect changes in the thermal pattern and temperatures of the thermal image of paw prints in dogs with a documented lameness as compared to the non-lame limb and the limbs of healthy dogs.

Materials and Methods

Criteria for case selection

Client-owned dogs (>18 kg) that presented between January through July 2013 for unilateral pelvic limb lameness due to cranial cruciate ligament rupture (CCLR) were included in this study. The diagnosis of unilateral CCLR was determined by clinical history, orthopedic examination, and radiographic evaluation (radiographs of the pelvis, bilateral stifles and hocks were reviewed) and was confirmed by exploratory surgery of the stifle.

Thermal imaging was performed before induction of anesthesia for surgery. A board-certified surgeon assessed the lameness and classified it with a clinical lameness grade (Table 1) (Witte and Scott, 2011). Written consent from the owner was acquired for each dog included in the study. Dogs were excluded if another orthopedic or neurologic condition was diagnosed.

Table 1. Lameness grade at a walk and trot.

Grade	Description
0 (None)	No lameness is observed at a walk or trot
1 (Mild)	Lameness is present, but may only be consistently apparent at a trot
2 (Mild to moderate)	Mild lameness is obviously present at a walk and is worse at a trot
3 (Moderate)	Obvious lameness is present at both gaits
4 (Moderate to severe)	Obvious lameness is present at both gaits and may be intermittently non-weight bearing
5 (Severe)	Lameness is non-weight bearing most or all of the time

Control group

Healthy employee-owned dogs with absence of orthopedic and neurologic disease assessed via physical examination and radiographic evaluation of the hips, stifles and tarsus were selected. Written consent from the owner was acquired for each control dog in the study. Dogs were excluded from the study if an orthopedic or neurologic condition was diagnosed.

Infrared Imaging

All the thermal images were obtained in the same room with an ambient temperature of 21°C that is controlled by a centralized climate control system. The dogs were housed in runs at the same temperature. All thermal images were obtained before sedation or general anesthesia. A portable infrared camera (Med 2000 IRIS, Meditherm Inc., Fort Meyers, FL) with a silicone microbolometer with a spectral range between 7 and 14 µm, resolution 160x120 pixels with a focal plane array amorphous, and an emissivity setting of one (e = 1) was used. The camera was connected to a laptop computer for real-time data analysis. The dogs were positioned symmetrically as possible on a foam mat in a static standing position. The dog was kept in this position for 30 seconds, while the handler remained beside the dog to facilitate positioning. If the dog moved the limbs before 30 seconds, the dog was again positioned. After the 30 seconds, the dog was allowed to walk forward, and the thermographer captured images of the paw prints left by the pelvic limbs on the foam mat. To capture these images, the camera was held approximately 1.5m directly over the mat.

Each image was saved within the software program (WINTES 2, Compix Inc., Lake Oswego, OR) for further evaluation and review. The program was preset for a temperature range of 8°C with a 16-shade color map. The color map indicated warmer temperatures as white and red and cooler temperatures as blue and black. Each image was focused and saved by the operator of the computer. After each image was saved, the temperature scale was adjusted so that the color range of the image was balanced. The program saved the final image with the specific 8°C temperature range for each image as a tiff file.

Force plate orthostatic analysis

Orthostatic analysis was performed in the same room as MII. Two permanently mounted force plates (AMTI-model# OR6-7-1000, 18.25x20x3.25 in, Advanced Mechanical Technology Inc, Watertown, MA) placed lengthwise on a platform and connected to a computer equipped with a software program (Acquire version 7.33V, Advanced Mechanical Technology Inc, Watertown, MA) designed for data collection and storage were used.

The force plates were embedded in a carpeted runway 1.16 meters long and 0.45 meters wide. The dog was placed in a standing, static position as symmetrically and naturally as possible so that each pelvic limb was on one of the force plates. The dog remained in this position for 5 seconds for data collection. A minimum of three valid trials for each dog was used to obtain mean peak vertical force (PVF) values. Peak vertical forces were expressed in percent of body weight (%BW). The asymmetry index (ASI) for each gait variable for each dog was calculated by use of the following equation (Fanchon and Grandjean, 2007):

$$(|XR - XL| / [|XR + XL| \times 0.5]) \times 100$$

Where XR is the mean of a given gait variable for static peak force ($100 \times N/N$) of the right pelvic limb and the XL is the mean of a given gait variable for static peak force ($100 \times N/N$) of the left pelvic limb. According to this method, an ASI of 0% indicates perfect gait symmetry for the measured variable, whereas positive or negative values indicate right or left hind limb asymmetry, respectively (Voss *et al.*, 2007).

Imaging Pattern Analysis

An image processing software program (CVIPtools, Computer Vision and Image Processing Laboratory, Department of Electrical and Computer Engineering, School of Engineering, Southern Illinois University, Edwardsville, IL) that included a collection of computer vision and image processing routines was used to analyze images.

Ten sets of experiments were performed with the thermal images. The left and right side were not separated. Four color normalization methods were used along with the original RGB images. Three data normalization were used on the feature data, soft-max, standard normal density as well as the original raw feature data.

The experiments were performed with the Computer Vision and Image Processing – Feature extraction and Pattern Classification (CVIP-FEPC), with each set having 2047 permutations, and using Nearest Neighbor (NN) and Train/Test Set as the classification methods; histogram, spectral and texture features with a pixel distance of six. The testing method used was the leave-one-out method.

Statistical analysis

For each of the analyses, standard logistic regression (PROC LOGISTIC, SAS Institute Inc., Cary, NC) was used, where the predictor value was either absolute percent difference in peak force (using orthostatic analysis) or absolute percent difference in thermal images, and the outcome variable was whether or not the dog was lame.

Absolute percent difference was calculated as follows:
% difference = ((absolute value ((Right – Left) / ((Right + Left)/2)))*100)/2

An optimal rule was defined as the rule corresponding to the point on the receiver operating characteristic (ROC) curve closest to (0,1) (i.e. closest to 100% sensitivity and 0% false positive rate). The area under the ROC curve (AUC) was calculated separately for each predictor variable. The ROC comparisons were performed using a contrast matrix to take differences of the areas under the empirical ROC curves (DeLong *et al.*, 1988).

A result was considered statistical significant at the $p<0.05$ level of significance. All analyses were performed using SAS version 9.3. The mean peak vertical force and asymmetry indexes were also calculated to compare the healthy and lame groups.

Results

Fourteen lame dogs (9 female spayed, 1 female intact and 4 males neutered) with confirmed CCLR were included in the study. Nine dogs had a lameness associated with the left pelvic limb and five dogs in the right pelvic limb. Breeds represented were 5 mixed-breed dogs, 3 Pit Bulls, 2 Labrador Retrievers; and 1 each Golden Retriever, Boxer, Portuguese Water Dog and Shetland Sheepdog. The mean age was 4.7 years old (range 1 to 9 years, median 4.7 years) and mean body weight was 29.5 kg (range 19.9 to 43.5 kg, median 28.9 kg). Six dogs had grade 4 lameness, two dogs had grade 3, three dogs had grade 2, and three dogs had grade 1. The normal dogs consisted of fourteen dogs (8 female spayed and 6 male neutered), 6 were mixed breed dogs, 2 Boxers, and 1 each Pit Bull, Doberman, Australian Cattle Dog, Greyhound, German Shepherd Dog and Labradoodle. The mean age was 4.9 years old (range 0.8 to 9.7 years, median 4 years) and mean body weight was 28.3 kg (range 18.8 to 41.7 kg, median 26.9 kg). The paw print image temperatures were separated into the following groups: healthy dogs (right limb versus left limb), lame dogs (lame limb versus non-lame limb), lame limb (lame dog) versus normal limbs (healthy dogs) and non-lame limb (lame dog) versus normal limb (healthy dogs). In the lame dog group, the temperature difference between the paw print thermal image of the lame limb versus the non-lame limb revealed a difference in temperature of 0.5°C (Table 2).

Table 2. Average, ± SD, minimum and maximum of temperatures (°C) of the paw print obtained in healthy (left and right pelvic limb) and lame dogs (lame limb and non-lame pelvic limb).

Dog	Limb	Mean ± SD	Avg min	Avg max
Healthy	Left limb	21.67 ± 1.3	20.5	22.8
Dogs	Right limb	21.82 ± 1.3	20.7	23.1
Lame	Lame limb	21.08 ± 1.2	20.5	21.7
Dogs	Non-lame limb	21.61 ± 1.2	20.6	23.0

In the healthy dog group, the temperature difference between the right and left limb was 0.1°C. Image pattern analysis revealed an 88% success rate in differentiating the paw print thermal image in the lame pelvic limb versus the non-lame limb (lame group). For the paw print thermal image of the right pelvic limb versus the left pelvic limb (healthy group) the success rate was 100%. Fig. 1 (lame group) and Fig. 2 (healthy group) show these image pattern differences.

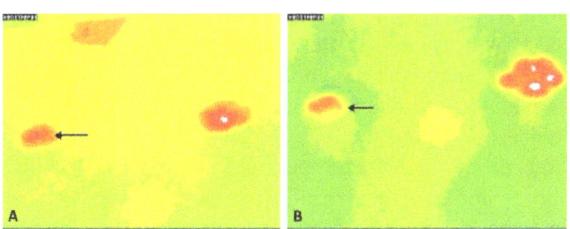

Fig. 1. (A): Thermal image of the paw print in a dog with grade 2 lameness (black arrow). **(B):** Thermal image of the paw print in a dog with grade 4 lameness (black arrow). Note the difference in the temperature in the paw print of the lame limb between figures 1A and 1B.

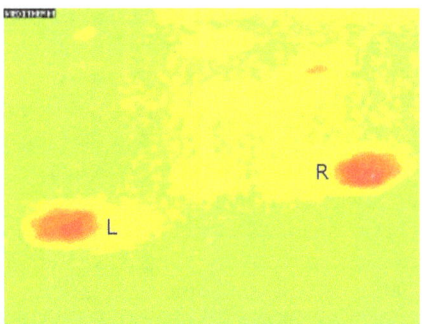

Fig. 2. Thermal image of the paw prints in a healthy dog (L= left, R=right side).

The mean of the peak vertical force (100*N/N) showed a 10.0% difference between left (20.9 ± 2.1) and right (18.1 ±2.9) limb in the healthy dogs. In the lame dogs, the difference between the lame limb (5.4 ± 6.4) and the non-lame limb (30.0 ± 5.0) was 72.4%. Asymmetric index analysis showed that there are significant differences between the healthy group (5%) and the lame group (36.2%) ratings (Table 3).

Table 3. Ground reaction forces (mean ± SD), average (avg) of the percentage (%) difference of the peak vertical force (PVF) in static position of the healthy and lame dogs and asymmetry index (ASI) of the healthy and lame dogs.

	Healthy Dogs mean		Lame Dogs mean	
	Left limb	Right limb	Lame limb	Non-lame limb
PVF (100*N/N)	20.94±2.1	18.05±2.9	5.44±6.4	30.01±5.0
Avg % difference*	10.0 %		72.4 %	
ASI (%)	5%		36.2%	

*(Avg % difference): The average of all trials for each patient was calculated and then the percentage difference between the left and right was calculated.

Based on the ROC curve using percent difference in peak force (Fig. 3), the optimal cutoff point was determined to be 41.8% with an AUC = 0.93. Using this cutoff point for percent difference in peak force, the sensitivity = 78.6% and the specificity = 100.0%.

Based on the ROC curve using percent difference in thermal imaging (Fig. 4), the optimal cutoff point was determined to be 0.943% with an AUC = 0.72. Using this cutoff point for percent difference in peak force, the sensitivity = 64.3% and the specificity = 78.6%.

The AUC for orthostatic analysis was significantly greater than for thermal imaging (difference = 0.21, $p<0.032$). Figure 5 shows the ROC curves for comparison.

Discussion

The present study evaluated the use of MII to detect lameness in dogs by the change in the thermal pattern and lower temperature of the paw prints. Image pattern analysis was successful in differentiating the paw print thermal image of the lame limb versus the non-lame limb in lame dogs.

The only other comparative study (Vainionpaa *et al.*, 2013), revealed an uneven thermal pattern in the images of cat paw prints associated with differences in weight bearing, but did not use any objective data analysis to support their findings. In this study, lameness was detected by the temperature difference observed in the paw print thermal image of the dog, and confirmed with force plate orthostatic analysis.

This information in conjunction with a physical examination and gait assessment may be able to assist with confirmation of a lame limb in situations where the lameness is subtle or subclinical, but further studies with larger groups of dogs with a subtle or subclinical lameness would need to be done to confirm this. Further diagnostics such as anatomical MII, radiographs, computed tomography or magnetic resonance imaging could then be performed to assess for a more specific diagnosis.

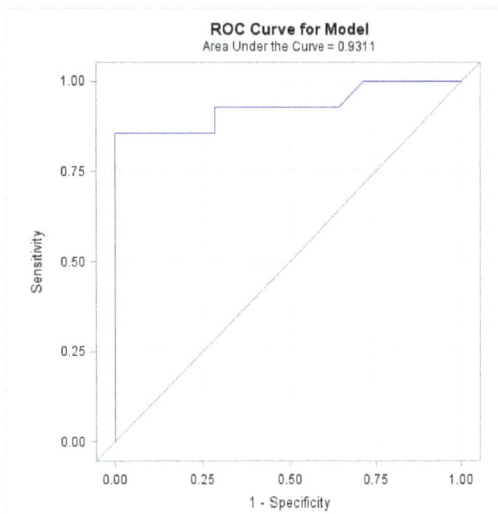

Fig. 3. ROC curve for percent difference in peak force.

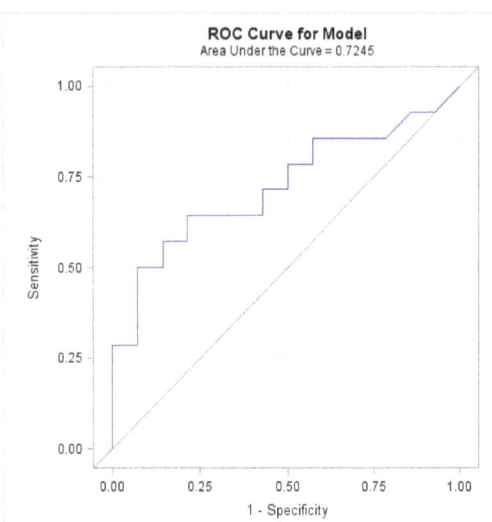

Fig. 4. ROC curve for percent difference in MII.

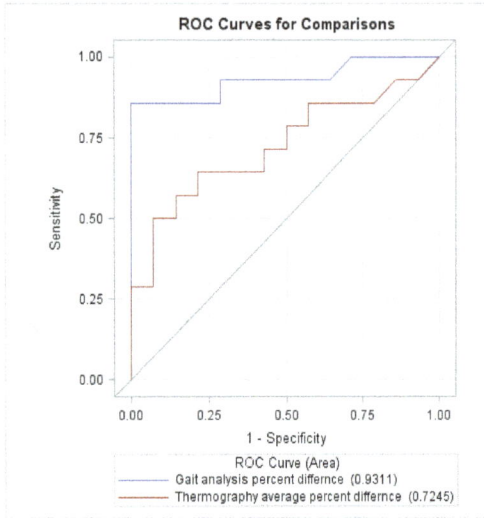

Fig. 5. ROC curves for comparison.

Temperature analysis revealed an increase of 0.5°C between the paw prints of the lame dogs lame limb versus the non-lame limb, and in the healthy dogs the difference was 0.1°C between the right and left limbs.

Studies in healthy humans, horses, and dogs have shown symmetry between right and left sides with temperature differences a fracture of a degree centigrade (Uematsu *et al.*, 1988; Loughin and Marino, 2007; Purohit, 2008; Westermann *et al.*, 2013). Studies of clinical disease have shown that a difference greater than 1°C of temperature between two of the same anatomic regions indicate an abnormality such as inflammation (Purohit *et al.*, 1985; Turner, 1991, 2001; Eddy *et al.*, 2001). The comparison of this data with the thermal paw print image would not be possible because it comes from different surfaces. However, when reviewing the data from the imaging pattern analysis and the orthostatic analysis between healthy and lame dogs, the data supports differences in weight bearing in lame versus non-lame limbs in lame dogs and similarities in data between the non-lame limbs. In this case, we argue that the difference of 0.5°C in the temperature of the paw print between the pelvic limbs is actually significant.

When evaluating the data for the lame pelvic limb in dogs the value of the temperature difference is less than the temperature in healthy dogs, the significance becomes stronger when we observe the thermal pattern differences, where the color distribution is remarkably different. The ability to differentiate between lame and healthy dogs using force plate orthostatic analysis increases with the severity of the lameness (Voss *et al.*, 2007), which is supported by the AUC of 0.93 for the percent difference in the peak force. The optimal cutoff for the peak force was abnormally high due to 2 dogs with a higher percent difference in peak force. This could be explained by the difficulty in positioning some of the dogs on the force plates and keeping them in place for a measurement. Dogs move and many of them will lean toward the handler. Kinetic gait analysis studies have analyzed variation due to handlers, acclimation and day-to-day variations (Rumph *et al.*, 1997, 1999), which supports this falsely elevated number.

Similar observations were made with the thermal images where it was noted that the higher the grade of lameness, the greater the color change (cooler color pattern), and the paw print became smaller. The AUC of 0.72 was not as high as for peak force, but is still considered supportive of MII of the paw prints as a viable option to help determine lameness. In the study with cats, irregular heat patterns were observed in paw prints by the change in weight bearing of cats that showed signs of discomfort during palpation; however, they showed no significant lameness (Vainionpaa *et al.*, 2013). Taking both studies into consideration, it is possible that MII could be useful in screening cases of subtle lameness to determine the affected limb, but since we only had 3 dogs with a subtle lameness in this study further investigation would be necessary.

In this study, the temperature of the paw print was observed on a foam mat. The thermal pattern was detected from the transfer of heat by conduction (Eddy et al., 2001; Turner, 2001) from the paw to the foam mat, and the camera detected the print by radiation emission from the mat.

Emissivity of the object is the ability to absorb and emit infrared radiation (Eddy et al., 2001; Turner, 2001). This is an important concept in thermal imaging, because the ability of a material to reflect or emit heat must be considered in the interpretation of an image. The thermal camera generates images based on the amount of heat generated rather than reflected; meaning, they actually detect differences in temperatures of the target and surroundings (Eddy et al., 2001). The foam mat was chosen because the thermal conductivity was high, besides being inexpensive and easily accessible.

There was no significant asymmetry in the paw print observed by temperature and imaging pattern analysis in healthy dogs. All species studied thus far have provided remarkable bilateral symmetrical patterns of infrared emission (Purohit and McCoy, 1980; Loughin and Marino, 2007; Purohit, 2008). The high degree of right-to-left symmetry is a valuable asset in the diagnosis of a unilateral problem associated with various inflammatory disorders (Loughin and Marino, 2007; Purohit, 2008). In gait analysis, the assessment of the asymmetry index is a good method to evaluate lameness, because it is based on right versus left comparisons with modification of the balance of the dog (Fanchon and Grandjean, 2007). In this study, the orthostatic analysis revealed 5% asymmetry in the healthy dogs, which is not significant. These results are consistent with another study (Budsberg et al., 1993), in which the author found in the vertical symmetry indices a deviation of < 8 % from perfect for all variables tested, reflecting near perfect symmetry in the vertical axis.

The clinical lameness score is used routinely in veterinary medicine as part of the orthopedic examination. Mild lameness cannot always be detected when the dog walks but may become evident at a trot (Witte and Scott, 2011). In the present study, data from the lameness score was helpful and, although not the objective of this study, it was possible to compare the degree of lameness with the changes in size and temperature of the thermal image of the paw print of the dogs. Future studies with a larger number of animals may produce more accurate results.

The limitation of the present study was the ability to keep the dog in a standing position for 30 seconds, especially the dogs with lameness. The time was arbitrarily determined, but during the course of the study it was observed that it might be possible to obtain images in less time. Another limitation was the low number of dogs, decreasing the statistical power. This was most likely due to the strict selection criteria of no orthopedic or neurologic deficits in the pelvic limbs. Many clinical patients have contralateral cruciate tears or hip dysplasia, which made them ineligible for this study. It may be beneficial to conduct additional studies with different weights, breeds of dogs, and contralateral disease to assess the changes in thermal patterns.

Based on the results obtained, we concluded that there was a change in the thermal pattern of the paw print in the lame pelvic limb compared to non-lame pelvic limb in lame and limbs of healthy dogs. Medical infrared imaging could be useful as a screening method, allowing the targeting of a disease or injury to a specific limb or region of interest. Further investigations are required to specify variations of the paw print in different orthopedic conditions.

Acknowledgments

This paper was supported in part by CNPq, Conselho Nacional de Desenvolvimento Científico e Tecnológico - Brazil. The authors thank Dr. Peter Leando for technical assistance.

Conflict of interest

The authors declare that there is no conflict of interest.

References

Anderson, M.A. 1994. Force plate analysis: a non-invasive tool for gait evaluation. Comp. Cont. Ed. Pract. Vet. 16, 857-867.

Barbosa, A.L.T., Schossler, J.E.W., Bolli, C.M., Lemos, L.F.C. and Medeiros, C. 2011. Test and standardize of force plate in orthostatic pattern in dogs. Arq. Bras. Med. Vet. Zootec. 63, 559-566.

Budsberg, S.C., Jevens, D.J., Brown, J., Foutz, T.L., DeCamp, C.E. and Reece, L. 1993. Evaluation of limb symmetry indices, using ground reaction forces in healthy dogs. Am. J. Vet. Res. 54, 1569-1574.

Colak, A., Polat, B., Okumus, Z., Kaya, M., Yanmaz, L.E. and Hayirli, A. 2008. Short communication: early detection of mastitis using infrared thermography in dairy cows. J Dairy Sci. 91:4244-4248.

DeLong, E.R., DeLong, D.M. and Clarke-Pearson, D.L. 1988. Comparing the areas under two or more correlated receiver operating characteristic curves: a nonparametric approach. Biometrics 44, 837-845.

Eddy, A.L., Van hoogmoed, L.M. and Snyder, J.R. 2001. The role of thermography in the management of equine lameness. Vet. J. 162, 172-181.

Fanchon, L. and Grandjean, D. 2007. Accuracy of asymmetry indices of ground reaction forces for diagnosis of hind limb lameness in dogs. Am. J. Vet. Res. 68, 1089-1094.

Gillette, R.L. and Angle, T.C. 2008. Recent developments in canine locomotor analysis: a review. Vet. J. 178, 165-176.

Griffon, D.J. 2008. Canine gait analysis: a decade of computer assisted technology. Vet. J. 178, 159-160.

Grossbard, B.P., Loughin, C.A., Marino, D.J., Marino, L.J., Sackman, J., Umbaugh, S.E., Solt, P.S., Afruz, J., Leando, P., Lesser, M.L. and Akerman, M. 2014. Medical infrared imaging (thermography) of type I thoracolumbar disk disease in chondrodystrophic dogs. Vet. Surg. 43, 869-876.

Infernuso, T., Loughin, C.A., Marino, D.J., Umbaugh, S.E. and Solt, P.S. 2010. Thermal imaging of normal and cranial cruciate ligament-deficient stifles in dogs. Vet. Surg. 39, 410-417.

Loughin, C.A. and Marino, D.J. 2007. Evaluation of thermographic imaging of the limbs of healthy dogs. Am. J. Vet. Res. 68, 1064-1069.

McGowan, L., Loughin, C.A., Marino, D.J., Umbaugh, S.E., Liu, P., Amini, M., Solt, P., Lesser, M.L. and Akerman, M. 2015. Medical Infrared Imaging of Normal and Dysplastic Elbows in Dogs. Vet. Surg. 44, 874-882.

Purohit, R.C. 2008. Use of thermography in veterinary medicine. In: Lee HMN CJ, ed. Rehabilitation Medicine and Thermography. Wilsonville, OR: Impress Publications, pp: 129-144.

Purohit, R.C., Hudson, R.S., Riddell, M.G., Carson, R.L., Wolfe, D.F. and Walker, D.F. 1985. Thermography of the bovine scrotum. Am. J. Vet. Res. 46, 2388-2392.

Purohit, R.C. and McCoy, M.D. 1980. Thermography in the diagnosis of inflammatory processes in the horse. Am. J. Vet. Res. 41, 1167-1174.

Purohit, R.C., McCoy, M.D. and Bergfeld, W.A. 3rd. 1980. Thermographic diagnosis of Horner's syndrome in the horse. Am. J. Vet. Res. 41, 1180-1182.

Rainwater-Lovett, K., Pacheco, J.M., Packer, C. and Rodriguez, L.L. 2009. Detection of foot-and-mouth disease virus infected cattle using infrared thermography. Vet. J. 180, 317-324.

Rumph, P.F., Steiss, J.E. and Montgomery, R.D. 1997. Effects of selection and habituation on vertical ground reaction force in greyhounds. Am. J. Vet. Res. 58, 1206-1208.

Rumph, P.F., Steiss, J.E. and West, M.S. 1999. Interday variation in vertical ground reaction force in clinically normal Greyhounds at the trot. Am. J. Vet. Res. 60, 679-683.

Turner, T.A. 1991. Thermography as an aid to the clinical lameness evaluation. Vet. Clin. North Am. Equine Pract. 7, 311-338.

Turner, T.A. 2001. Diagnostic thermography. Vet. Clin. North Am. Equine Pract. 17, 95-113.

Uematsu, S., Edwin, D.H., Jankel, W.R., Kozikowski, J. and Trattner, M. 1988. Quantification of thermal asymmetry. Part 1: Normal values and reproducibility. J. Neurosurg. 69, 552-555.

Vainionpaa, M.H., Raekallio, M.R., Junnila, J.J., Hielm-Björkman, A.K., Snellman, M.P. and Vainio, O.M. 2013. A comparison of thermographic imaging, physical examination and modified questionnaire as an instrument to assess painful conditions in cats. J. Feline Med. Surg. 15, 124-131.

Van hoogmoed, L.M. and Snyder, J.R. 2002. Use of infrared thermography to detect injections and palmar digital neurectomy in horses. Vet. J. 164, 129-141.

Voss, K., Imhof, J., Kaestner, S. and Montavon, P.M. 2007. Force plate gait analysis at the walk and trot in dogs with low-grade hindlimb lameness. Vet. Comp. Orthop. Traumatol. 20, 299-304.

Waddell, R.E., Marino, D.J., Loughin, C.A., Tumulty, J.W., Dewey, C.W. and Sackman, J. 2015. Medical infrared thermal imaging of cats with hyperthyroidism. Am. J. Vet. Res. 76, 53-59.

Westermann, S., Buchner, H.H., Schramel, J.P., Tichy, A. and Stanek, C. 2013. Effects of infrared camera angle and distance on measurement and reproducibility of thermographically determined temperatures of the distolateral aspects of the forelimbs in horses. J. Am. Vet. Med. Assoc. 242, 388-395.

Witte, P. and Scott, H. 2011. Investigation of lameness in dogs: 2. hindlimb. In Practice 33, 58-66.

30

Long-term follow-up of surgical resection alone for primary intracranial rostrotentorial tumors in dogs: 29 cases (2002-2013)

Anna Suñol[1], Joan Mascort[1], Cristina Font[1,2], Alicia Rami Bastante[3], Martí Pumarola[4] and Alejandro Lujan Feliu-Pascual[1,5,*]

[1]*Hospital Ars Veterinaria, carrer Cavallers nº37, 08034, Barcelona, Spain*
[2]*Hospital Canis Girona. Carrer Can Pau Birol, 38. 17006 Girona, Spain*
[3]*Neuroscience Institute of Barcelona. Universitat Autònoma de Barcelona, edifici M1, campus de Bellaterra E-98193, Cerdanyola del Vallès, Spain*
[4]*Department of Animal Medicine and Surgery, Veterinary Faculty, Universitat Autonoma de Barcelona, 08193 Bellaterra (Cerdanyola del Vallès), Barcelona, Spain*
[5]*AÚNA Especialidades Veterinarias, Calle Algepser 22-1, 46980 Paterna, Valencia, Spain*

Abstract

Intracranial neoplasia is frequently encountered in dogs. After a presumptive diagnosis of intracranial neoplasia is established based on history, clinical signs and advanced imaging characteristics, the decision to treat and which treatment to choose must be considered. The objective of this study is to report survival times (ST) for dogs with intracranial meningiomas and gliomas treated with surgical resection alone (SRA), to identify potential prognostic factors affecting survival, and to compare the results with the available literature. Medical records of 29 dogs with histopathologic confirmation of intracranial meningiomas and gliomas treated with SRA were retrospectively reviewed. For each dog, signalment, clinical signs, imaging findings, type of surgery, treatment, histological evaluation, and ST were obtained. Twenty-nine dogs with a histological diagnosis who survived >7 days after surgery were included. There were 15 (52%) meningiomas and 14 (48%) gliomas. All tumors had a rostrotentorial location. At the time of the statistical analysis, only two dogs were alive. Median ST for meningiomas was 422 days (mean, 731 days; range, 10-2735 days). Median ST for gliomas was 66 days (mean, 117 days; range, 10-730 days). Kaplan-Meier analysis indicated that ST was significantly longer for meningiomas than for gliomas ($P<0.05$). A negative correlation between the presence of a midline shift and ST ($P=0.037$) and ventricular compression and ST ($P=0.038$) was observed for meningiomas. For gliomas, there were no significant associations between ST and any of the variables evaluated. In conclusion, the results of this study suggest that, for dogs that survived >7 days postoperatively, SRA might be an appropriate treatment, particularly for meningiomas, when radiation therapy is not readily available. Also, the presence of midline shift and ventricular compression might be negative prognostic factors for dogs with meningiomas.

Keywords: Dog, Glioma, Intracranial tumor, Meningioma, Survival time.

Introduction

Intracranial neoplasia is frequently encountered in dogs (Song *et al.*, 2013) and represent a major cause of morbidity and mortality (Dickinson, 2014). Meningiomas are the most commonly reported primary intracranial neoplasm in this species, followed by glial tumors, including astrocytomas, oligodendrogliomas, and oligoastrocytomas (Snyder *et al.*, 2006; Sessums and Mariani, 2009; Song *et al.*, 2013). After a presumptive diagnosis of intracranial neoplasia is established based on history, clinical signs and advanced imaging characteristics, the decision to treat and which treatment to choose must be considered. The therapeutic modalities most commonly available for veterinary patients with intracranial neoplasia include palliative care, surgery, chemotherapy and radiation therapy, all of which can be used either alone or in combination (Dickinson, 2014). Definitive diagnosis of intracranial tumors is based on histopathologic examination, (Dickinson, 2014) typically following the World Health Organization (WHO) classification system published in 2007 (Louis *et al.*, 2007).

Palliative care for intracranial tumors often involves glucocorticoids targeting peritumoral edema together with antiepileptic drugs to control seizures, (Dickinson, 2014) which is the most common presenting complaint for intracranial tumors in dogs (Bagley *et al.*, 1999; Snyder *et al.*, 2006).

Mean survival time (ST) reported for dogs with rostrotentorial meningiomas that received only palliative treatment ranged from 54 to 195 days, (Turrel *et al.*, 1984; Foster *et al.*, 1988; Bilderback *et al.*, 2006)

***Corresponding Author:** Alejandro Lujan Feliu-Pascual. Hospital Ars Veterinaria, Carrer Cardedeu nº3, 08023, Barcelona, Spain. Email: alejandrolujan@colvet.es* whereas a median ST of 45 days was reported for gliomas (Adams *et al.*, 2005).

Efficacy of surgical cytoreduction of intracranial tumors is highly operator and equipment dependent (Dickinson, 2014). Most published information is related to more easily accessible canine and feline meningiomas, with only anecdotal data for other tumor types such as gliomas (Dickinson, 2014). Surgical excision alone for canine meningiomas resulted in median ST of 180-210 days (Kostolich and Dulisch, 1987; Niebauer and Dayrell-Hart, 1991; Axlund *et al.*, 2002; Bilderback *et al.*, 2006; Rossmeisl, 2014). Neurosurgical treatment using devices such as intracranial endoscopy or ultrasonic surgical aspirator, which either improve intraoperative visualization or facilitate tumor excision, have been associated with longer median ST after surgical resection for intracranial meningiomas, with ST ranging from 1260 to 2100 days. (Greco *et al.*, 2006; Klopp and Rao, 2009; Rossmeisl, 2014).

Currently, no meaningful conclusions can be made from published data relating to surgery of intraaxial tumors (Dickinson, 2014) and, to the best of the authors' knowledge, a retrospective or prospective paper looking for ST for gliomas treated with surgical resection alone (SRA) has not been previously reported.

There is little information available about the efficacy of chemotherapeutic agents for canine intracranial neoplasia. Most data relate to the use of nitrosurea-based alkylating agents, such as lomustine (CCNU) and carmustine, or the ribunucleotide reductase inhibitor hydroxyurea (Dickinson, 2014). Anecdotal published data show apparent survival benefits and occasional responses with survival of many months in some cases (Jung *et al.*, 2006; Tamura *et al.*, 2007).

However, a large retrospective study suggested no benefit from lomustine chemotherapy compared to palliative care (93 days versus 60 days) for brain masses diagnosed via computed tomography and without a histologic diagnosis (Van Meervenne and Verhoeven, 2014).

Radiation therapy has become a mainstay of treatment for intracranial neoplasia in both human and veterinary patients, either as a primary or adjunctive treatment (Dickinson, 2014). Radiotherapy has demonstrated to improve ST in presumptive and confirmed meningiomas, with ST ranging from 240 to 577 days (Turrel *et al.*, 1984; Evans *et al.*, 1993; Axlund *et al.*, 2002; Bley *et al.*, 2005; Griffin *et al.*, 2014; Rossmeisl, 2014). Radiation therapy has been reported to be beneficial when compared to SRA for the treatment of meningiomas (Axlund *et al.*, 2002).

A study including 12 dogs with gliomas treated with radiotherapy only, showed a median ST of 255 days (Adams *et al.*, 2005). In this same study, the combination of surgery and radiotherapy increased the median ST to 300 days (Adams *et al.*, 2005). A large prospective study analyzing the outcome, ST, and complications of the different treatment modalities in veterinary medicine is lacking. Consequently, the information necessary to choose a particular treatment is mainly based on published clinical studies with a limited number of cases with variable treatment modalities and follow-up, and the personal experience of the neurologist/neurosurgeon (Dickinson, 2014).

Until a large prospective study is designed, conducted and published, our aim was to report the long-term survival in a cohort of dogs with primary brain tumors (meningiomas and gliomas), where standard surgical resection was the main treatment modality due to the limited availability of radiotherapy, and to compare our results with previously published studies.

We also aimed to assess potential prognostic factors pertaining to signalment, magnetic resonance imaging (MRI) characteristics or type of tumor associated with ST. We hypothesized that ST for meningiomas treated with SRA would be longer than previously reported and that ST for gliomas following SRA would be longer than the ST reported with palliative care across previous publications.

We also hypothesized that the tumor type and some specific MRI characteristics, such as the presence of a midline shift, peritumoral edema and ventricular compression, would have a negative influence on ST.

Materials and Methods

Case selection criteria

Medical records of dogs examined at our hospital from April 2002 to December 2013 were retrospectively reviewed. All dogs with a histopathologic diagnosis of primary intracranial tumor following surgical resection were included.

Medical records review

Information obtained from the medical records included signalment, type and duration of clinical signs, tumor location, MRI findings, type of surgery, duration of hospitalization, WHO histopathological classification, date of recurrence of clinical signs, and date and cause of death. If not available in the medical records, referring veterinarians and clients were contacted by telephone in order to obtain follow-up information.

Procedures and follow-up

For each dog, hematology, serum biochemistry profile, and systemic tumor staging (including 3-view thoracic radiographs and abdominal ultrasound) were performed to rule out potential underlying or concurrent diseases in preparation for surgery. Additional ancillary testing was performed as indicated.

For all dogs, a tentative diagnosis of intracranial neoplasia was obtained following 0.25 T MRI of the brain (Esaote VetMR Grande, Genoa, Italy) and cerebrospinal fluid analysis, both performed under general anesthesia.

A second year neurology resident and a board-certified neurologist examined all MR images. For each MRI study, tumor type (suspected meningioma versus glioma), neuroanatomical location (frontal, parietal, temporal), and size of the presumptive brain tumor, as well as any secondary changes observed, including the presence of a midline shift, peritumoral edema and compression of the ventricular system, were recorded. The percentage of midline shift was calculated on transverse T2-weighted (T2W) fast spin echo images. The midline shift was measured as the distance of maximum shift from the midline using commercial software (Osirix version 4.1.2 DICOM viewer, Pixmeo SARL, Bernex, Switzerland) as previously reported (Beltran et al., 2014).

This value was multiplied by 100 and divided by the distance from the midline to the convexity surface at the same level to calculate the percentage of midline shift (Beltran et al., 2014). Peritumoral edema was classified as present or absent based on T2W images. If present, it was graded as peritumoral if it extended ≤10 mm beyond the tumor margin on T2W images or as diffuse if it extended for >10 mm beyond the tumor margin (Sturges et al., 2008).

Ventricular system compression was evaluated in dorsal T1 post contrast images at the level of corpus callosum. If there were any abnormality in the symmetry, location or size of the ventricles that was attributed to direct tumor compression or surrounding edema, it was classified as present. If there were no abnormality it was classified as absent (Fig. 1).

Animals were anesthetized for surgery using standard hospital protocols. Preanesthetic medications included a combination of methadone (0.2-0.4 mg/kg SC/IM, Metasedin, Laboratorio Esteve) and acepromazine (0.05-0.1mg/kg SC/IM, Equipromacina, Fatro Iberica SA). Anesthesia was induced with thiopental (3.0–6.6 mg/kg, IV, Tiobarbital, Braun) or propofol (4.0–6.0 mg/kg, IV, Propofol Hospira, Hospira SL) and diazepam (0.5 mg/kg IV, Valium, Roche Farma SA) and maintained with isoflurane and oxygen (1–2% Isoflo, Laboratorio Esteve). All animals received perioperative antibiotics (cefazolin, 25 mg/kg, IV, every 90 min, Cefazolin Normon, Laboratorios Normon SA).

Two board-certified neurologists performed all surgical resections using magnifying loupes and a non-vibrating surgical aspirator (Ferguson suction tube, Instrumevet, Barcelona, Spain). Surgical approaches and operative techniques were performed according to the nature and location of the lesion in order to remove the maximal volume of tumor observed macroscopically.

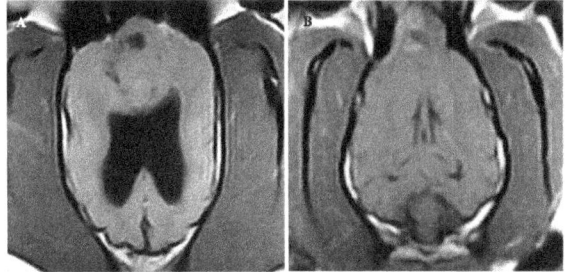

Fig. 1. T1W post contrast dorsal images at the level of corpus callosum. **(A):** Ventricular compression considered as present. **(B):** Ventricular compression considered as absent.

Once the tumor was located, surgical resection was performed as follows: for meningiomas, once a clear dissection plane was identified, blunt separation and removal of the macroscopic neoplastic tissue was achieved with nerve hooks, flat curettes, and bipolar cautery.

For gliomas, since no clear dissection plane was evident, a biopsy was obtained using curettes and the remaining tumor was removed using a non-vibrating surgical aspirator (Ferguson suction tube, Instrumevet, Barcelona, Spain) until removal was considered macroscopically complete. Hemorrhage was controlled via bipolar electrocautery and application of hemostatic sponges, when appropriate. Intraoperative mannitol was administered prior to dural opening when advanced imaging suggested increased intracranial pressure. The dura mater was not sutured but hemostatic sponges were placed tightly over the craniectomy defect. The bone flap was only replaced in dogs that underwent transfrontal craniotomy. Soft tissues were closed routinely.

While in recovery, dogs were positioned with the head above the level of the heart until alert and responsive, and were closely monitored for seizure activity, decreased mentation, or hypoventilation.

For the histopathological study, a biopsy sample was obtained during the surgical procedure and fixed in 10% formalin. A board-certified pathologist evaluated all tumors.

Animals were recovered in the intensive care unit for administration of supportive care, broad-spectrum antibiotics, and opioid analgesia (methadone at 0.2-0.4 mg/kg SC (Metasedin, Laboratorio Esteve), or fentanyl continuous rate infusion at 3–6 µg/kg/h IV (Fentanest, Kern pharma) until discharge. After surgery, treatment included oral anticonvulsants and glucocorticoids for epileptic seizure control and peritumoral edema reduction, respectively. Regular monitoring of anticonvulsant blood level was conducted as indicated. Median hospital stay was recorded and the first postoperative control was performed at our hospital within the first week after surgery.

For ST analysis, recurrence of clinical signs and date and cause of death were obtained from the medical records, or from the referring veterinarian or client via telephone conversation.

Statistical analyses

For the purpose of the statistical analyses, dogs were classified into two groups depending on the histopathological results. Group I included all dogs diagnosed with meningiomas and group II included all dogs with gliomas.

Survival time was defined as the time from surgery until the date of death. Dogs that died within 7 days of surgery from complications directly related to the surgical procedure and those with incomplete medical records were excluded from the survival analysis. Dogs that died of causes unrelated to tumor progression were censored. For dogs that were still alive at the time of data analysis, the corresponding number of days between surgery and time where data was collected was considered.

The Kaplan-Meier product limit method was used to calculate median ST by means of a commercially available statistical analysis software (Statistical Package for the Social Sciences v.20 (SPSS Inc., Chicago, IL)(SPSS)). The effect of age, sex, and type of tumor (meningioma versus glioma) on ST was evaluated.

Categorical data was evaluated using Fisher's exact test. Shapiro-Wilk test confirmed the majority of the continuous variables were not normally distributed; therefore, a non-parametric test (Kruskal-Wallis) was used. In addition, for each MRI study the effects of the severity of the midline shift, perilesional edema, and ventricular compression on the ST were evaluated. Severity of the midline shift and its potential correlation with ST was evaluated for each group separately by means of Pearson's correlations. An ANOVA test was used to evaluate the association between perilesional edema and ST, and the effect of ventricular compression on ST was evaluated using a t-test. Significance level was set at P value ≤ 0.05.

Results

During the study period, SRA was performed on 35 dogs with intracranial tumors. Four dogs (3 with a meningioma and 1 with a glioma) were excluded from the study because they died within 7 days following surgical resection. Two of them died secondary to middle cerebral artery thrombosis occurring 4 and 12 hours after surgery. Post-mortem examination was performed in both cases. The other 2 dogs were euthanized due to postoperative aspiration pneumonia, and intraoperative hypotension and cardiorespiratory failure, respectively. Two additional dogs were excluded because of incomplete medical records. Therefore, 29 dogs with a histopathologically confirmed primary intracranial neoplasia survived >7

days following surgical resection and were included in the study. There were 15 (52%) meningiomas (group I) and 14 (48%) gliomas (group II).

In group I, 6 (40%) dogs were male (4 intact, 2 neutered) and 9 (60%) were female (3 intact, 6 spayed). Median age at initial presentation was 11 years (mean, 10.3 years; range, 5-14.6 years). Seven dogs were purebreds and 8 were mixed breeds. Only German shepherd dogs were represented by >1 dog (n=2). In Group II, 8 (57%) dogs were male (5 intact, 3 neutered) and 6 (43%) were female (1 intact, 5 spayed). Median age at initial presentation was 8.8 years (mean, 8.6 years; range, 6-12.5 years). Eight dogs in group II were purebreds and 6 were mixed breeds. Breeds represented by >1 dog included Golden Retriever (n=4) and Boxer (n=2). Clinical signs reflected the neuroanatomic location of the tumor in all dogs. The most common clinical signs were seizures and behavioral changes, present in 24 of 29 dogs. Contralateral motor and sensory deficits were noted in 3 of 29 dogs. Two dogs also showed clinical signs consistent with central vestibular disease including obtundation, head tilt, tetraparesis and spontaneous nystagmus. The duration of clinical signs prior to diagnosis varied widely, ranging from 1 day to 1 year (mean, 54 days).

Three types of surgical approaches were used to resect the 29 intracranial masses visualized on MRI including transfrontal (20 dogs), frontoparietal (5 dogs), and parietotemporal (4 dogs) approaches. Median hospital stay for all surviving dogs was 3 days (range, 2–6 days). All dogs but two had one surgery performed. Two dogs with meningiomas underwent more than one surgery. One of these two dogs was still alive 2735 days (7.5 years) after the first surgery, with a total of three surgeries performed. A second surgery was performed 1440 days after first one, and a third surgery 450 days after the second surgical procedure. This dog had a Grade I psammomatous meningioma, with little histopathological change between the first and second biopsies. The other dog had a histopathological confirmation of transitional meningioma, and died 1740 days (4.7 years) after the first surgery having had a second surgery performed 1224 days after the first tumor resection. In addition, two dogs were censored because they died from causes unrelated to tumor progression. One dog, which had a meningioma, died 768 days after surgery due to renal failure. One dog with an oligodendroglioma died 15 days after surgery after developing a pericardial effusion apparently unrelated to the tumor. Post-mortem examination was performed and no underlying etiology for the pericardial effusion was found.

A board-certified pathologist evaluated all tumors and classified them according to the WHO classification system (Louis *et al.*, 2007). There were 15 (52%) meningiomas and 14 (48%) gliomas.

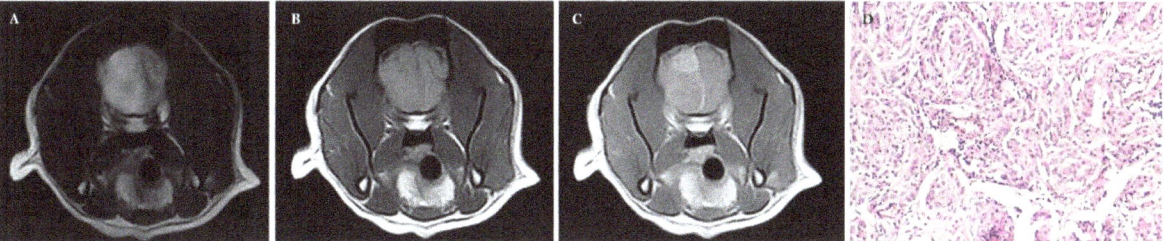

Fig. 2. Grade I canine frontal lobe transitional meningioma. Transverse T2W, T1W and T1W post contrast (T1+C) magnetic resonance image at the level of frontal lobe. **(A):** T2W: The tumor shows hyperintensity respect the grey matter and peritumoral edema. **(B):** T1W: the tumor shows isointensity respect the grey matter. **(C):** T1W+C: the tumor enhanced homogenously and there is also meningeal enhancement. Also noted the midline shift present in all three sequences. **(D):** Transverse T1WHematoxylin and eosin stain showing whorls of spindle-shaped cells. Original magnification 40x.

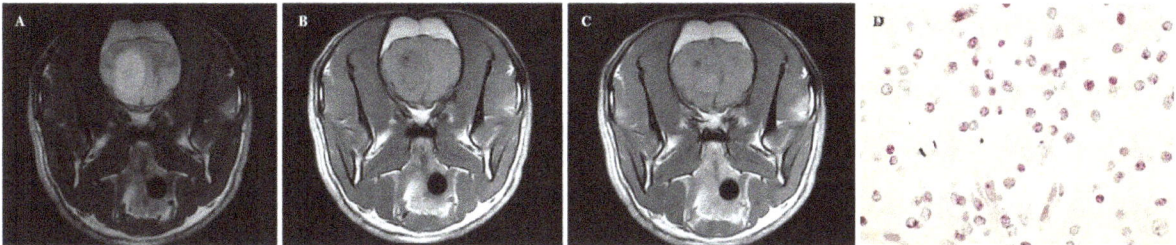

Fig. 3. Grade III canine frontal lobe oligodendroglioma. Transverse T2W, T1W and T1W post contrast (T1W+C) magnetic resonance image at the level of the frontal lobes. **(A):** T2W: Well-defined T2-hyperintensity lesion respect the grey matter. **(B):** T1W: The lesion shows heterogeneously T1-hypointensity respect the grey matter. **(C):** T1W+C: Mild enhancement in the medial ventral part of the lesion. Also noted the midline shift present in all three sequences. **(D):** Hematoxylin and eosin stain showing the honeycomb pattern characteristic of these tumors. Original magnification 400x.

All tumors had a rostrotentorial location. Meningioma subtypes represented included transitional (7), psammomatous (1), fibroblastic (1), meningothelial (1), atypical (2), and anaplastic (3). According to the WHO classification system (Louis *et al.*, 2007), there were 10 Grade I meningiomas, 2 Grade II meningiomas, and 3 Grade III meningiomas (Fig. 2). The gliomas resected included oligodendrogliomas (8), astrocytomas (4), and anaplastic gliomas (2). There was 1 Grade I glioma, 5 Grade II gliomas, and 8 Grade III gliomas (Fig. 3).

Median ST for dogs with meningiomas was 422 days (mean, 731 days; range, 10-2735 days). Median ST for dogs with gliomas was 66 days (mean, 117 days; range, 10-730 days). Kaplan-Meier survival analysis indicated that ST for dogs with meningiomas treated with SRA was statistically longer than ST for dogs with gliomas treated with SRA (F= 0.024; *P*<0.05) (Fig. 4).

In the meningioma group, 6/15 (40%) had ≥ 20% of midline shift displacement, whereas 5/14 (36%) gliomas showed this feature. A negative correlation between the presence of a midline shift and ST was observed for meningiomas (*P*=0.037). In the meningioma group, 14/15 (93%) had ≤10% of edema, with only 1 dog meningioma having >10% of edema. In the glioma group, 4/14 (28.6%) had >10% of edema, 9/14 (64.3%) had <10% of edema, and 1/14 (7.1%) had no observable edema on MRI. No significant association between the presence of peritumoral edema

and ST was observed for either type of tumor. Ten of 15 (66.7%) meningiomas had ventricular compression in comparison with 9/14 cases (64.3%) in the glioma group. A statistically significant negative association between the presence of ventricular compression and ST was observed for meningiomas (*P*=0.038). For gliomas, there were no significant associations between any of the MRI variables and ST. Among all data collected, only tumor histopathology (meningioma vs. glioma) (Fig. 3), and the presence of a midline shift and ventricular compression in meningiomas had a significant influence on ST.

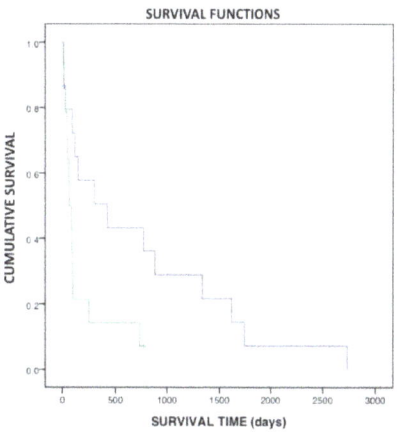

Fig. 4. Kaplan-Meier survival curve. Median survival times in dogs with intracranial primary tumors treated with SRA for meningiomas (blue) compared with gliomas (green).

Discussion

The results of the present study suggest that in dogs with intracranial rostrotentorial meningiomas, SRA might result in ST longer than previously reported. In our study, dogs with meningiomas treated with SRA had a median ST of 422 days, which compares favorably to previously published median ST after standard surgical resection, which have typically ranged from 180 to 210 days (Kostolich *et al.*, 1987; Niebauer *et al.*, 1991; Axlund *et al.*, 2002; Bilderback *et al.*, 2006; Rossmeisl, 2014). In addition, we report ST for 14 gliomas treated with SRA, with a median survival of 66 days, which is slightly longer than previously reported with palliative treatment (Adams *et al.*, 2005). Of the secondary changes evaluated on MRI, the presence of a midline shift and ventricular compression were significantly associated with a lower ST in dogs with meningiomas treated with SRA, suggesting a negative prognostic implication. For the glioma group, we did not observe any associations between MRI characteristics and ST.

All the tumors included in our study had a rostrotentorial location, which might have influenced the decision to operate as well as the long-term ST. In general, rostrontentorial tumors have been reported to have a better prognosis than infratentorial neoplasms (Dickinson, 2014). Focusing on meningiomas, the available literature has reported median ST of 180-210 days after SRA (Kostolich *et al.*, 1987; Niebauer *et al.*, 1991; Axlund *et al.*, 2002; Bilderback *et al.*, 2006; Rossmeisl, 2014). However, dogs with meningiomas treated with SRA in this study achieved a longer median ST (median, 422 days; mean, 731 days). Similar to previous studies, (Axlund *et al.*, 2002; Klopp *et al.*, 2009) dogs that died within 7 days after surgery were not included in the ST analyses. However, not all previously published studies followed the same criteria, making comparisons between studies challenging. Most of the reports available described surgical resection of olfactory bulb or frontal lobe meningiomas, similar to our study. One of the first reports describing intracranial surgery in dogs (Kostolich *et al.*, 1987) included 4 olfactory meningiomas treated with surgery with a median ST of 135 days, with all dogs surviving beyond the first 7 days after surgery. The longest median ST described for dogs with meningiomas treated with SRA was 210 days, based on 18 cases (Axlund *et al.*, 2002). This report excluded from the survival analyses those dogs that died within the first 7 days following surgical resection, similar to the method that was followed in the present study. The most recent report describing SRA for the treatment of canine brain tumors (Bilderback *et al.*, 2006) reported a median ST of 201 days. However, this study comprised a small number of cases and only included 5 meningiomas. Moreover, one of these 5

dogs died during the third day after surgery. With the data available it was difficult to obtain the exact ST for the remaining 4 patients, although a median ST of 204 days was inferred from the data provided. Overall, our study achieved a longer median ST for dogs with meningiomas surviving >7 days after SRA, in comparison to previous studies that used similar criteria to calculate ST (Axlund *et al.*, 2002). In our study the two cases with meningioma that had more than one surgery have had a slightly positive influence in our ST. If these animals had been included only for the first procedure, the median ST for meningiomas would also have been 422 days, with a mean of 611 days.

History and signalment from the dogs included in this study were similar to previous studies, including a majority of older dogs, consistent with the previously reported average age at presentation of 9.5-11 years (Bagley *et al.*, 1999; Axlund *et al.*, 2002; Song *et al.*, 2013; Dickinson, 2014). Also, both genders appeared equally represented, which matches the lack of a sex predisposition described in the literature (Dickinson, 2014). It has been suggested that meningiomas are overrepresented in Golden Retrievers, Boxers, and Miniature Schnauzers, and that astrocytomas and oligodendrogliomas are overrepresented in brachycephalic breeds (Dickinson, 2014). In our study, we did not observe a clear breed predisposition in the meningioma group, but there were 4 gliomas diagnosed in Golden Retrievers and 3 in brachycephalic dogs (2 Boxers, 1 French Bulldog). Seizures were the most common initial complaint in our study with 24 of 29 dogs initially examined for this reason. This is also consistent with previous publications (Bagley *et al.*, 1999; Snyder *et al.*, 2006) and it is not surprising considering the rostrontentorial origin of all tumors included in the present study. Of the signalment variables analyzed in this study (age, sex, and type of tumor), only tumor type was found to have a significant influence on ST, with meningiomas having longer ST than gliomas.

In humans, meningiomas are histologically categorized as Grade I, II, and III according to the 2007 WHO classification (Louis *et al.*, 2007). Grade I meningiomas include psammomatous, transitional, meningothelial and fibroblastic subtypes. Grade II meningiomas include atypical and choroid subtypes. Grade III meningiomas include anaplastic and papillary subtypes and are considered to be the most aggressive (Louis *et al.*, 2007). WHO classification of meningiomas in domestic animals does not include categorization of subtypes into different grades (Koestner *et al.*, 1999) therefore, the use of the human classification has been suggested (Sturges *et al.*, 2008; Mandara *et al.*, 2009). Due to the limited sample size of our study, we were unable to evaluate any associations between meningiomas subtypes/grades and survival.

However, most of the meningiomas included in this study were classified as Grade I, which could have positively impacted median ST, since Grade I meningiomas are typically considered "benign" (Sturges *et al.*, 2008). Ideally, future larger studies would investigate a potential relationship between meningioma subtype/grade and ST, which might add useful information for prognostic purposes.

The recurrence rate of intracranial meningiomas in humans is 9-12% with grossly complete excision and may be as high as 40% with incomplete excision (Spagnuolo *et al.*, 2003) Meningioma recurrence depends on extension of resection, location and histological grade of the tumor (Schiffer *et al.*, 2005). In our study, the main cause of death was the progression of neurological signs, behavioral changes, and uncontrolled seizures, allegedly related to tumor re-growth, scar tissue formation or brain herniation trough craniectomy defect. In most cases a follow-up MRI to confirm tumor recurrence could not be performed, but the clinical signs and the neurological exam suggested recurrence. Hence, euthanasia due to suspected progression of clinical signs was the most common cause of death in our patients.

Fewer studies document ST for canine gliomas. In humans, gliomas are categorized as Grade I, II, III, and IV according to their histopathologic features and the 2007 WHO classification system, with Grade IV gliomas being the most aggressive type (Louis *et al.*, 2007).

Grade I include: subependymal giant cell astrocytoma and pilocytic astrocytoma. Grade II include: pilomyxoid astrocytoma, diffuse astrocytoma, pleomorphic xanthoastrocytoma, oligodendroglioma and oligoastrocytoma. Grade III include: anaplastic astrocytoma, anaplastic oligodendroglioma and anaplastic oligoastrocytoma. Grade IV, the most aggressive type, include: glioblastoma, giant cell glioblastoma and gliosarcoma (Louis *et al.*, 2007).

To the authors' knowledge, this is the first study reporting ST in canine gliomas treated with SRA showing a median ST of 66 days (mean 117 days). Interestingly, one dog with an anaplastic glioma survived for 2 years after surgery before dying of uncontrolled seizures.

In human medicine, it has been suggested that repeated surgery with maximal extend of resection should be standard of care for recurrent low-grade gliomas (Uppstrom *et al.*, 2016).

In the present study, ST for gliomas appeared slightly longer than the ST that had been previously reported following palliative care (Adams *et al.*, 2005), but considerably shorter than the ST previously reported following radiotherapy or following surgery and radiotherapy (Adams *et al.*, 2005). Furthermore, this type of surgery allows the possibility of a histopathological confirmation and the use of alternatives or adjunctive future therapies, such as radiation therapy or chemotherapy.

There are important factors to consider when comparing the results of ST for meningiomas and gliomas. The different nature and growth patterns of both types of tumors (extra- versus intra-axial) is the most likely factor influencing the differences in ST observed after SRA. Gliomas, being intra-axial tumors, may be more difficult to access because they often have deeper locations than meningiomas; moreover, gliomas may also be more challenging to resect because they typically lack a clear plane of dissection (Niebauer *et al.*, 1991; Rossmeisl, 2014). Another important factor to consider is that most meningiomas included in this study were Grade I, whereas most gliomas were Grade III. Therefore, it is likely that in the present study meningiomas showed a less aggressive biological behavior than gliomas.

Regarding the MRI secondary changes evaluated in this study (midline shift, ventricular compression and peritumoral edema), there was a correlation between the presence of a midline shift and ventricular compression and ST for meningiomas. A study investigated the MRI characteristics of histological confirmed meningiomas and concluded that it was not possible to predict the meningioma subtype or grade based on MRI features, emphasizing the need for histopathology for an antemortem diagnostic confirmation (Sturges *et al.*, 2008). Another study evaluated potential prognostic factors associated with ST in brain tumors and found no significant correlation between the edema observed on MRI and ST, (Rossmeisl *et al.*, 2013) which was also observed in the present study.

At our institution, radiation therapy is always recommended following surgical resection of intracranial tumors; however, radiotherapy was not available in our country during the study period, and owners elected to not pursue this treatment modality due to the logistic difficulties and the expenses that would be associated with pursuing radiotherapy in a different country.

There were several limitations and strengths to our study. Limitations included the retrospective nature of the study, along with a limited sample size. As in all retrospective studies, multiple variables existed that could not be controlled, which might have influenced our results. At the time of the surgery, information regarding whether the excision was considered to be complete or incomplete was not included in the medical records. Thus, it was not possible to correlate if the completeness or not of the surgical resection might have had an influence on recurrence or ST. Euthanasia due to recurrence or progression of clinical signs was the most common cause of death. In most of these cases, tumor recurrence was suspected, but a repeat MRI or a postmortem histopathological examination were not performed, which is another limitation of the study.

Our decision to exclude the patients that did not survive pass >7 days after surgery was intended to eliminate the direct influence of postsurgical complications on the ST, as well as to be able to compare the results with previously published studies that calculated ST following the same approach (Axlund et al., 2002).

One of the strengths of this study is that all biopsies were obtained during the initial surgical resection. Other previous clinical studies, in particular during the treatment of gliomas, rely on suspected gliomas by MRI characteristics or biopsy or postmortem samples obtained following radiation or chemotherapy, which might change the nature or histopathological grade of those tumors (Brearley et al., 1999; Spugnini et al., 2000; Adams et al., 2005).

Moreover, radiation therapy itself has been reported to induce the formation of brain tumors in people (Salvati et al., 2003; Umansky et al., 2008; Ecemis et al., 2013) and dogs (Luján Feliu-Pascual et al., 2009).

Our study also provides ST data after SRA for a group of 14 dogs with gliomas. There is very limited information available on ST after SRA for histopathologically confirmed canine gliomas. As such, the results from the present study add extra data to the scant information currently available, and provide additional evidence that neurologists can use when choosing treatment options for presumptive glial tumors.

The results of this study suggest that SRA might be an appropriate treatment, particularly for meningiomas, when radiation therapy is not readily available. Also, the presence of midline shift and ventricular compression might be negative prognostic factors for dogs with meningiomas.

For canine gliomas, this is the first clinical study reporting ST using SRA. Results shows longer survival time with surgery compared to previously reported palliative treatment for glioma. Also, no MRI characteristics appeared to be associated with ST in this group of dogs with gliomas.

Studies that investigate the ST associated with the different therapies available to treat brain tumors, such as the one presented here, provide veterinary neurologists with additional evidence to aid in the decision-making process and to estimate the most likely prognosis for each one of these patients.

Acknowledgments

No third-party funding or support was received in connection with this study or the writing or publication of the manuscript.

Conflict of interest

The authors declare that there is no conflict of interest.

References

Adams, V.J., Platt, S.R., Garosi, L.S., Murphy, S. and Abramson, C.J. 2005. Survival analysis of canine gliomas and meningiomas treated with corticosteroids hypofractionated radiotherapy or surgery and radiotherapy. Proceedings of the Symposium BSAVA, April 7 to 10, Birmingham, UK.

Axlund, T.W., McGlasson, M.L. and Smith, A.N. 2002. Surgery alone or in combination with radiation therapy for treatment of intracranial meningiomas in dogs: 31 cases (1989-2002). J. Am. Vet. Med. Assoc. 221, 1597-1600.

Bagley, R.S., Gavin, P.R., Moore, M.P., SIlver, G.M., Harrington, M.L. and Connors, R.L. 1999. Clinical signs associated with brain tumors in dogs: 97 cases (1992-1997). J. Am. Vet. Med. Assoc. 215, 818-819.

Beltran, E., Platt, S.R., McConnell, J.F., Dennis, R., Keys, D.A. and De Risio, L. 2014. Prognostic value of early magnetic resonance imaging in dogs after traumatic brain injury: 50 cases. J. Vet. Intern. Med. 28, 1256-1262.

Bilderback, A., Faissler, D., Sato, A.F., Keating, J.H. and Mc Donnell, J.J. 2006. Transfrontal craniectomy, radiation therapy, and/or chemotherapy in the treatment of canine meningiomas. Proceedings of the American College of Veterinary Internal Medicine Symposium, May 31 to June 3, Louisville, USA, pp: 784.

Bley, C.R., Sumova, A., Roos, M. and Kaser-Hotz, B. 2005. Irradiation of brain tumors in dogs with neurologic disease. J. Vet. Intern. Med. 19, 849-854.

Brearley, M.J., Jeffery, N.D., Phillips, S.M. and Dennis, R. 1999. Hypofractionated radiation therapy of brain masses in dogs: a retrospective analysis of survival of 83 cases (1991-1996). J. Vet. Intern. Med. 13, 408-412.

Dickinson, P.J. 2014. Advances in diagnostic and treatment modalities for intracranial tumors. J. Vet. Intern. Med. 28, 1165-1185.

Ecemis, G.C., Atmaca, A. and Meydan, D. 2013. Radiation-associated secondary brain tumors after conventional radiotherapy and radiosurgery. Expert. Rev. Neurother. 13, 557-565.

Evans, S.M., Dayrell-Hart, B., Powlis, W., Christy, G. and VanWinkle, T. 1993. Radiation therapy of canine brain masses. J. Vet. Intern. Med. 7, 216-219.

Foster, E.S., Carrillo, J.M. and Patnaik, A.K. 1988. Clinical signs of tumors affecting the rostral cerebrum in 43 dogs. J. Vet. Intern. Med. 2, 71-74.

Greco, J.J., Aiken, S.A. and Berg, J.M. 2006. Evaluation of intracranial meningioma resection with a surgical aspirator in dogs:17 cases (1996–2004). J. Am. Vet. Med. Assoc. 229, 394-400.

Griffin, L.R., Nolan, M.W., Selmic, L.E., Randall, E., Custis, J. and LaRue, S. 2014. Stereotactic Radiation Therapy for Treatment of Canine Intracranial Meningiomas. Vet. Comp. Oncol. 14, 158-170.

Jung, D.-I., Kim, H.-J., Park, C., Kim, J.-W., Kang, B.-T., Lim, C.-Y., Park, E.H., Sur, J.H., Seo, M.G., Hahm, D.H. and Park, H.M. 2006. Long-term chemotherapy with lomustine of intracranial meningioma occurring in a miniature schnauzer. J. Vet. Med. Sci. 68, 383-386.

Klopp, L.S. and Rao, S. 2009. Endoscopic-assisted intracranial tumor removal in dogs and cats: long-term outcome of 39 cases. J. Vet. Intern. Med. 23, 108-115.

Koestner, A., Bilzer, T., Fatzer, R., Schulman, F.Y. and Van Winkle, T.J. 1999. World Health Organization histological classification of tumors of the nervous system of domestic animals, in: World Health Organization histological classification of tumors of the nervous system of domestic animals. Second. DC, pp: 27-29.

Kostolich, M. and Dulisch, M.L. 1987. A surgical approach to the canine olfactory bulb for meningioma removal. Vet. Surg. 16, 273-277.

Louis, D.N., Ohgaki, H., Wiestler, O.D., Cavenee, W.K., Burger, P.C., Jouvet, A., Scheithauer, B.W. and Kleihues, P. 2007. The 2007 WHO Classification of Tumours of the Central Nervous System. Acta Neuropathol. 114, 97-109.

Luján Feliu-Pascual, A., Dennis, R., Murphy, S., De Risio, L. and Matasiek, K. 2009. Cerebral necrosis following hypofractionated radiotherapy for canine intracranial tumors: a magnetic resonance imaging and pathological study. In: Proceedings of the 22nd Symposium ESVN- ECVN, September 24 to 26, 2009. Bologna, Italy, pp: 43.

Mandara, M.T., Pavone, S., Brunetti, B. and Mandrioli, L. 2009. A comparative study of canine and feline meningioma classification based on the WHO histological classification system in humans. In: Proceedings of the 22nd Symposium ESVN-ECVN, September 24 to 26, 2009. Bologna, Italy, pp: 41.

Niebauer, G.W. and Dayrell-Hart, B.L. 1991. Evaluation of craniotomy in dogs and cats. J. Am. Vet. Med. Assoc. 198, 89-95.

Rossmeisl, J.H. 2014. New treatment modalities for brain tumors in dogs and cats. Vet. Clin. North Am. Small Anim. Pract. 44, 1013-1038.

Rossmeisl, J.H., Jones, J.C., Zimmerman, K.L. and Robertson, J.L. 2013. Survival time following hospital discharge in dogs with palliatively treated primary brain tumors. J. Am. Vet. Med. Assoc, 242,
193-198.

Salvati, M., Frati, A., Russo, N., Caroli, E., Polli, F.M., Minniti, G. and Delfini, R. 2003. Radiation-induced gliomas: report of 10 cases and review of the literature. Surg. Neurol. 60, 60-67.

Schiffer, D., Ghimenti, C. and Fiano, V. 2005. Absence of histological signs of tumor progression in recurrences of completely resected meningiomas. J. Neurooncol. 73, 125-130.

Sessums, K. and Mariani, C. 2009. Intracranial meningioma in dogs and cats: a comparative review. Compend. Contin. Educ. Vet. 31(7), 330-339.

Snyder, J.M., Shofer, F.S., Van Winkle, T.J. and Massicotte, C. 2006. Canine intracranial primary neoplasia: 173 cases (1986-2003). J. Vet. Intern. Med. 20, 669-675.

Song, R.B., Vite, C.H., Bradley, C.W. and Cross, J.R. 2013. Postmortem evaluation of 435 cases of intracranial neoplasia in dogs and relationship of neoplasm with breed, age, and body weight. J. Vet. Intern. Med. 27, 1143-1152.

Spagnuolo, E., Calvo, A., Erman, A. and Tarigo, A. 2003. Recurrent meningiomas with progressive aggressiveness and posterior extracranial extension. Neurocirugia (Astur). 14, 409-416.

Spugnini, E.P., Thrall, D.E., Price, G.S., Sharp, N.J., Munana, K. and Page, R.L. 2000. Primary irradiation of canine intracranial masses. Vet. Radiol. Ultrasound. 41, 377-380.

Sturges, B.K., Dickinson, P.J., Bollen, A.W., Koblik, P.D., Kass, P.H., Kortz, G.D., Vernau, K.M., Knipe, M.F., Lecouteur, R.A. and Higgins, R.J. 2008. Magnetic resonance imaging and histological classification of intracranial meningiomas in 112 dogs. J. Vet. Intern. Med. 22, 586-595.

Tamura, S., Tamura, Y., Ohoka, A., Hasegawa, T. and Uchida, K. 2007. A canine case of skull base meningioma treated with hydroxyurea. J. Vet. Med. Sci. 69, 1313-1315.

Turrel, J.M., Fike, J.R., LeCouteur, R.A., Pflugfelder, C.M. and Borcich, J.K. 1984. Radiotherapy of brain tumors in dogs. J. Am. Vet. Med. Assoc. 184, 82-86.

Umansky, F., Shoshan, Y., Rosenthal, G. and Fraifeld, S. 2008. Radiation-induced meningioma, Neurosurg. Focus. 24, E7.

Uppstrom, T.J., Singh, R., Hadjigeorgiou, G.F., Magge, R. and Ramakrishna, R. 2016. Repeat surgery for recurrent low-grade gliomas should be standard of care. Clin. Neurol. Neurosurg. 151, 18-23.

Van Meervenne, S. and Verhoeven, P.S. 2014. Comparison between symptomatic treatment and lomustine supplementation in 71 dogs with intracranial, space-occupying lesions. Vet. Comp. Oncol. 12, 66-77.

31

Tear ferning in normal dogs and dogs with keratoconjunctivitis sicca

David Williams* and Heather Hewitt

Department of Veterinary Medicine, University of Cambridge, Madingley Road, Cambridge CB3 0ES, UK

Abstract

This study evaluates tear ferning as an ancillary technique for the evaluation of the canine tear film in normal eyes and eyes affected by keratoconjunctivitis sicca (KCS). Thirty dogs with KCS and 50 control dogs with normal tear film were evaluated with a full ophthalmoscopic examination and a Schirmer tear test type 1 (STT) determined before tear samples were obtained from the medial canthus with a microhaematocrit capillary tube. 10ul of tear was placed on a microscope slide and the time to first formation of a fern of crystallised tear solute was determined. The appearance of the ferning pattern was graded and correlated with the STT value. All eyes with KCS had abnormal ferning patterns while 39 out of the 50 normal dogs (78%) had so-called 'normal' ferning patterns. The mean STT for dogs showing 'normal' ferning patterns was 20.6mm/min for the left eye and 21.3mm/min for the right eye. STT values for eyes with 'abnormal' ferning patterns were 10.9mm/min and 12.4mm/min, these differing from the normal eyes with STT above 15mm/min significantly. These findings suggest that tear ferning could be a valuable technique for assessment of the tear film in dogs with KCS.
Keywords: Dog, Dry eye, Ferning, Keratoconjunctivitis sicca, Tear.

Introduction

The phenomenon of crystal formation in a fern-like pattern in drying solutions of body fluids has been recognised for several years. First described in human cervical mucus in the context of cervical smear (Papanicolau, 1946), ferning has been reported in other fluids from saliva (Guida *et al.*, 1993), serum (Reece *et al.*, 1984), nasal mucus (Ullery *et al.*, 1959) as well as tears (Rolando, 1984).

In 1986 Rolando and colleagues devised a grading system for tear ferning (Rolando *et al.*, 1986), dividing the ferning into one of four grades depending on the extent and pattern of the ferns. Rolando's four grades are detailed in Table 1.

One paper has demonstrated that tear ferning occurs in tears from dogs but only in the context of evaluating tear formation in canine eyes rendered tear deficient experimentally and treated with nerve growth factor (Coassin *et al.*, 2005).

Silva and colleagues have documented tear ferning in 30 horses (Silva *et al.*, 2016) and sought to quantify the ferning pattern with a computerised stereology tool. No detailed study of tear ferning in normal dogs and dogs with naturally occurring keratoconjunctivitis sicca has to date been published and thus it is our aim here to provide such a report.

Keratoconjunctivitis sicca (KCS) is a common ophthalmic disease in the dog (Williams, 2008) in which the Schirmer tear test (STT) is the standard diagnostic test (Gelatt *et al.*, 1975).

Table 1. Classification of human tear ferning patterns (Rolando *et al.*, 1986).

Tear fern grade	Description of ferning pattern
I	Uniform arborisation in the entire field of observation without spaces among the ferns, with single ferns big and close branching
II	Ferning phenomenon still abundant but the single ferns are smaller and with lower frequency of branching compared with type I. Empty spaces begin to appear among the ferns
III	Arborization of mucus is partially present. Single ferns are little and incompletely formed with no or rare branching. Large spaces without ferning are present in the field, including conglomerates of mucus without any sign of organization
IV	Ferning phenomenon is absent. The specimen collected does not show any organization and the mucus appears in clusters and threads, which represent possibly contaminated and degenerated mucus mixed with exfoliated cells

A number of other criteria are important in determining the ocular pathology in KCS from Rose Bengal staining, tear osmolality and tear ferning, these being considered central to a diagnosis of KCS in human patients to a greater degree than in veterinary ophthalmology (Van Bijsterveld, 1990).

---
*Corresponding Author: David Williams. Department of Veterinary Medicine, University of Cambridge, Madingley Road, Cambridge CB3 0ES, UK. Email: *dlw33@cam.ac.uk*

The use of tests such as tear ferning is not essential to a diagnosis of canine KCS but can assist in the evaluation of dogs with the condition, especially in animals with qualitative rather than quantitative tear film deficiency, in which STT may be normal but ocular surface pathology occurs through mucin or tear lipid deficiency with consequent increased tear evaporation.

We have shown in this study that animals with KCS and STT values below 10mm/min tended to have abnormal ferning patterns (types III or IV) while animals with STT above 10mm/min tended to have normal tear ferning patterns (types I or II) and demonstrated that tear ferning can be a valuable additional assessment of the properties of the tear film to supplement but not replace the Schimer tear test.

Materials and Methods

Eighty dogs examined at the Queen's Veterinary School Hospital, University of Cambridge were involved in the study described herein. Animals included 30 with KCS and 50 included as normal control animals. Dogs with KCS were evaluated prior to treatment with tear replacement medication or topical cyclosporine. The control animals were matched to the clinical cases as closely as possible for age, gender and breed but this was not always possible. All animals underwent a full ophthalmic evaluation using direct and indirect ophthalmoscopy and slit lamp biomicroscopy before undergoing a Schirmer tear test 1. After these examinations tear fluid was obtained as previously described (Norn, 1988). Over 10 µl of tear fluid was obtained from the medial canthus with a glass capillary tube (Fig. 1).

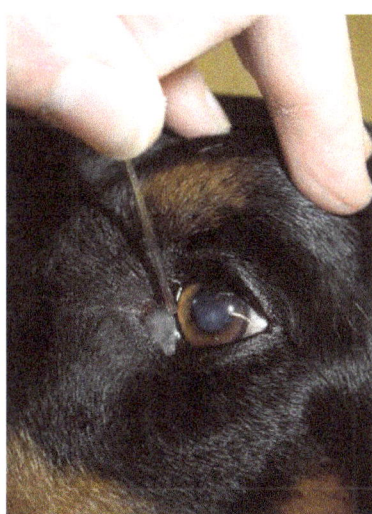

Fig. 1. Sampling of tear fluid from the medial canthus in a dog with mild KCS.

The order of sampling, i.e. using left or right eye first was randomised using an online random number table (http://stattrek.com/statistics/random-number-generator.aspx). An aliquot of 10µl of the fluid thus

acquired was drawn up using a Gilson pipette and applied to a clean microscope slide kept at 20±2oC and 30±2% humidity. The slide was viewed by phase contrast microscopy at x40 magnification until all tear fluid had evaporated. The time taken to the earliest fern formation was determined and the final form of the tear fern was photographed after 5 minutes, by which time the slide was dry in all cases. The temperature and humidity at the point of sample taking and drop evaluation was determined using a LCD Digital Temperature Humidity 88 Meter Thermometer (DTYHTC8, White Industries, Reading UK).

A Fishers exact test was performed on the data to compare the ferning patterns of dogs with normal tear production and KCS (STT<10mm/min). A student t test was used to compare time to fern formation for dogs with different ferning patterns after Levene's test for equality of variance was performed. Data from right and left eyes was compared using a paired samples T test. Data analysis of fern type and time to fern formation was performed separately for the left and right eyes to avoid the conundrum of over-estimating the population size by using the data from both eyes together (Newcombe and Duff, 1987).

Results

The signalment of the dogs in this study in summarised in Table 2.

Table 2. Signalment of animals in KCS and control groups.

	KCS group	Control group
Number of animals	30	50
Mean age of animals	12.2±3.4 years	11.4±2.2 years
Percentage of KCS-predisposed breeds	50	56
Mean STT value for both eyes	6.2±3.5mm/min	16.2±5.6mm/min

KCS patients were predominantly breeds predisposed to the condition (English Cocker spaniel 7 cases, West Highland white terrier 4 cases, Cavalier King Charles spaniel 2 cases, Yorkshire terrier 2 cases, Lhasa Apso 1 case) and a similar proportion of control animals were chosen from the same breeds to avoid inter-breed differences providing uncontrolled variation. The four types of tear ferning, as delineated by Rolando *et al.* (1986) are shown in Figure 2.

All 30 of the dogs with KCS had ferning patterns of types 3 and 4 while 39 out of the 50 normal dogs (78%) had ferning patterns of types 1 and 2. The mean STT for dogs showing normal (types 1 and 2) ferning patterns was 20.6mm/min for the left eye and 21.3mm/min for the right eye, these two populations of STT values not being statistically different.

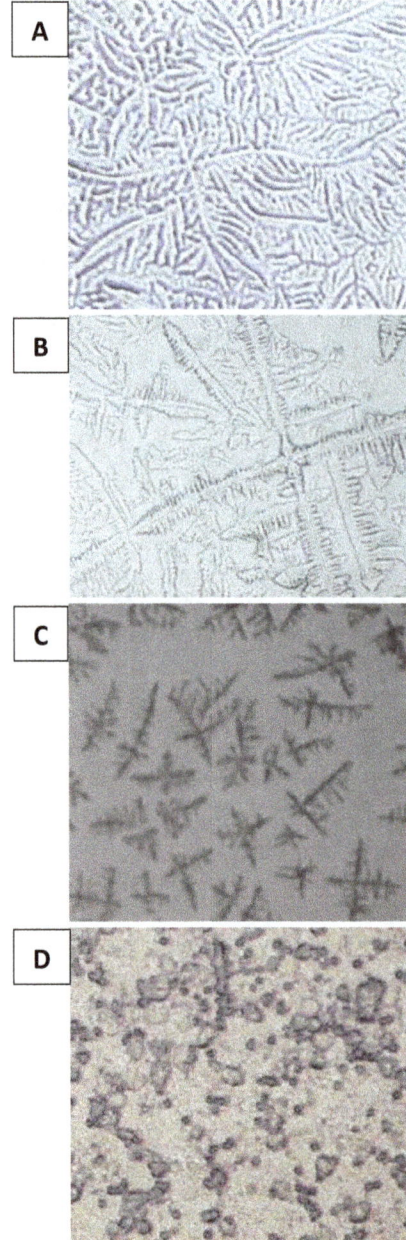

Fig. 2. The four grades of tear ferning taken at 20x magnification. **(A)**: Tear ferning grade 1. **(B)**: Tear ferning grade 2. **(C)**: Tear ferning grade 3. **(D)**: Tear ferning grade 4.

STT values for eyes with abnormal ferning patterns (types 3 and 4) were 10.9mm/min (type 3) and 12.4mm/min (type 4) for the left eye and 11.3mm/min (type 3) and 11.9mm/min (type 4) for the right, these not being significantly different between left and right eye but differing from the normal eyes with STT above 10mm/min significantly with p values of 0.001 and 0.002 respectively. Time to drying of the tear sample was 3.2±1.2 minutes for eyes with STT above 15mm/min and 1.8±1.6 minutes for eyes with STT below 15mm/min (p<0.05).

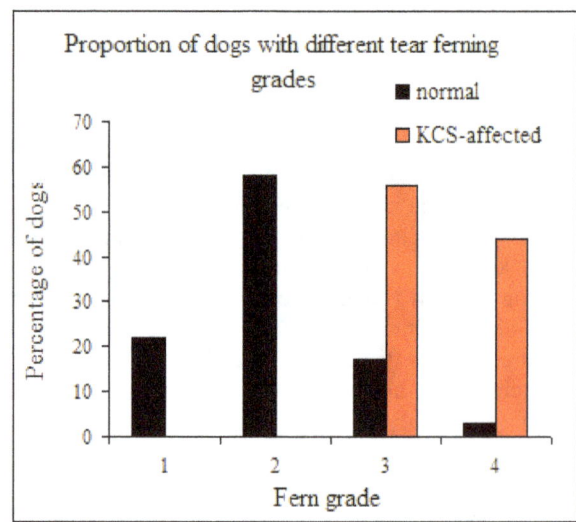

Fig. 3. Proportion of normal and KCS-affected dogs with differing grades of tear film ferning.

Figure 3 shows the percentage of dogs with the four different types of tear ferning in dogs with and without signs of keratoconjunctivitis sicca.

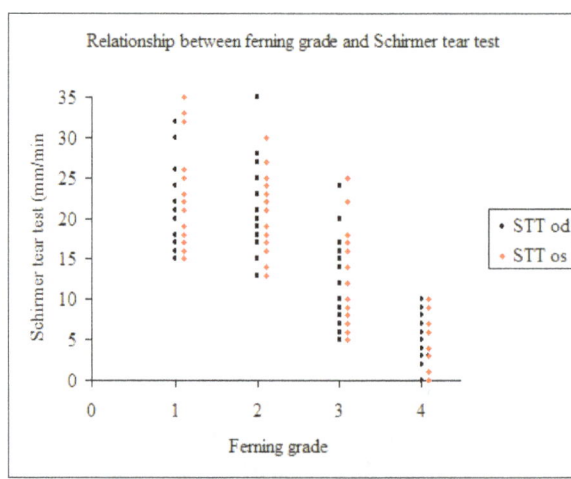

Fig. 4. Graphical representation of the relationship between ferning grade and Schirmer tear test.

Figure 4 shows the correlation between tear ferning pattern and STT value in the dogs evaluated. Mean STT for eyes with ferning types 1, 2 3 and 4 were 22.5±5.9mm/min, 20.6±5.0mm/min, 11.5±5.6mm/min and 5.2±3.2mm/min respectively.

Time to initiation of fern formation was 310±63 seconds in dogs with STT greater than 10mm/min and no ophthalmic signs of ocular surface dysfunction and 125±86 seconds in dogs with STT lower than 10mm/min and signs of ocular surface pathology such as mucoid discharge, keratitis or ocular surface pigmentation.

Discussion

Tear ferning has proved to be a useful tool in the evaluation of the ocular surface in human ophthalmology, in the diagnosis of keratoconjunctivitis sicca and cicatrising keratoconjunctivitis as well as predicting tolerance of the human eye to contact lenses. Here we have shown that tear ferning can be a valuable tool in veterinary ophthalmology too. All tear samples from dogs with keratoconjunctivitis sicca have shown abnormal ferning patterns while a number of animals with apparently normal tear production have shown abnormal ferning patterns. The molecular basis of tear ferning is still somewhat unclear. It may be that mucus is the key to fern production. Mucus lowers tear surface tension facilitating spreading of the tear drop. Tabbara and Okumoto were the first to recognise that tear ferning does not occur in human patients with mucus deficiency (Tabbara and Okumoto, 1982). Norn reported more extensive ferning in human patients with keratitis and bacterial conjunctivitis where mucus production is increased (Norn, 1987), however he also showed that ferning does not relate to the presence of mucus in the tear film on the ocular surface and that tear ferns do not stain with alcian blue and rose bengal, molecules interacting with mucus components (Norn, 1994). Kogbe et al. (1991) showed that a biopolymer is necessary for fern formation but that this need not be mucus.

It is widely accepted that electrolytes are essential for ferning in biological fluids. Ferning occurs in cervical mucus when organic matter is removed but Zondek (1959) found that dialysed cervical mucus, with electrolytes removed, will not form a ferning pattern until electrolytes are replenished. Indeed the same researcher reported demonstrating ferning in solutions of sodium chloride (Zondek, 1959) but that finding has not been repeated by other workers. Increased osmolarity in tear samples from human patients with keratoconjunctivitis sicca may explain the different ferning patterns in those cases and Rolando specifically investigated the effect of hyperosmolarity on tear ferning in samples from human patients, finding that experimental increases in tear osmolarity by adding sodium chloride to the inferior conjunctival sac caused deterioration in grade of tear ferning.

In vitro dilution of tear samples with sodium chloride changed the ferning pattern from grades I and II to grades III and IV but adding glucose to increase the osmolarity did not have the same effect (Rolando, 1988); clearly it is not osmolarity alone which is the important factor but perhaps electrolyte concentration which is more critical to the ferning phenomenon. Protein concentration may be an important factor. Body fluids with a high protein concentration do not exhibit a ferning pattern unless diluted with electrolyte solutions (Zondek and Rozin, 1954). Electrophoretic assessment of tear protein profile and correlation with tear ferning suggested that there is an association with protein concentration (Kogbe and Liolet, 1987). The same research group also showed that tear proteins have an important effect on tear ferning by lowering surface tension of the drop in the same manner that mucus does (Kogbe et al., 1991). In one *in vitro* experiment stark tear crystal skeletons formed by mixing electrolyte solutions only turn to classic fern patterns when protein is added, but only in a limited range of salt-to-protein ratios. Since electrolyte concentrations in tears from patients with KCS are increased and tear protein concentrations are decreased (Kogbe et al., 1991), this critical ratio for tear fern formation may be the central factor in fern formation. But the very constituents of the electrolyte mix may be critical. The ratio of monovalent sodium and potassium ions to divalent calcium and magnesium ions may also be important, this being suggested by the study conducted by Kogbe et al. (1991). Sequestration of divalent cations with EDTA inhibits fern formation. The truth is that tear ferning is probably influenced by several interacting moieties in the tear film, as suggested by Golding and Brennan (1989), rather than any one in isolation.

A critical paper is that of Pearce and Tomlinson (2000) who used scanning electron microscopy and energy dispersive X-ray analysis to analyse the chemical composition of human tear ferns. Sodium, potassium and chloride were all detected within the fern structure as was sulphur, indicative of the presence of mucin and/or protein, but this latter element was only found at the periphery of the dried tear-film drop. Earlier analysis by X-ray fluoresecence also detected sodium, potassium, chlorine, calcium and sulphur (Golding et al., 1994) but electron microscopy by the same group showed crystalline fern patterns surrounded by globular structures, presumed to be of protein and/or mucin composition. A hypothesis to explain the generation of tear film ferning might thus suggest that as the tear drop dries with water evaporating the electrolyte solution reaches maximal solute concentration and that the proteins are deposited at the drop margin. As evaporation proceeds the solubility limit of electrolytes is reached and ferning proceeds. Given that the protein and mucins have already been deposited at the drop boundary the ferning proceeds unhindered (Pearce and Tomlinson, 2000). The shift in the ratio of electrolytes and macromolecule in eyes with keratoconjunctivitis thus may be the key factor inhibiting fern formation. This hypothesis, however, has been generated with studies of human tear film ferning and it still has to be shown that the equivalent is occurring in the companion animal species.

Collecting tears can be difficult, especially in dogs with a pathologically lower tear production. The animal in

Figure 1 for instance had a mucoid discharge in the medial canthus associated with an STT value of 9mm/min in that eye. It might be argued that this should be wiped away before collecting a lacrimal sample and this might well be a valuable topic for further study of this technique. In that particular dog the capillary tube was held a millimeter away from the mucus itself to avoid the discharge abnormally affecting the ferning result. As with all tests, familiarity with sampling improves the ease with which one can obtain samples for the tear ferning test. Given the results we have obtained in this study we would recommend that tear ferning be used as an evaluative technique in all cases of canine KCS and would encourage other ophthalmologists to share their experience with this new technique.

Conclusion

This study has shown that tear ferning occurs with canine tear samples and that the pattern of ferning correlates with tear production as measured by the Schirmer tear test. The correlation is not exact, with some apparently normal tear films yielding abnormal ferning patterns. It may be that tear ferning yields additional information on tear film health not provided by the Schirmer tear test and that tear ferning can be a valuable technique in the evaluation of ocular surface pathology in the dog.

Conflict of interest

The authors declare that they have no competing interests.

References

Coassin, M., Lambiase, A., Costa, N., De Gregario, A., Squelleta, R., Sachetti, M., Aloe, L. and Bonini, S. 2005. Efficacy of nerve growth factor treatment in dogs affected by dry eye. Graefes Archiv. Clin. Exp. Ophthalmol. 243, 151-155.

Gelatt, K.N., Peiffer, R.L. Jr., Erickson, J.L. and Gum, G.G. 1975. Evaluation of tear formation in the dog, using a modification of the Schirmer tear test. J. Am. Vet. Med. Assoc. 166, 368-370.

Golding, T.R. and Brennan, N.A. 1989. The basis of tear ferning. Clin. Exp. Optom. 72, 102-112.

Golding, T.R., Baker, A.T., Rechberger, J. and Brennan, N.A. 1994. X-ray and scanning electron microscopic analysis of the structural composition of tear ferns. Cornea 13, 58-66.

Guida, M., Barbato, M., Bruno, P., Lauro, G. and Lampariello, C. 1993. Salivary ferning and the menstrual cycle in women. Clin. Exp. Obstet. Gynecol. 20, 48-54.

Kogbe, O. and Liolet, S. 1987. An interesting use of the study of tear ferning patterns in contactology. Ophthalmologica 194, 150-153.

Kogbe, O., Liotet, S. and Tiffany, J.M. 1991. Factors responsible for tear ferning. Cornea 10, 433-444.

Newcombe, R.G. and Duff, G.R. 1987. Eyes or patients? Traps for the unwary in the statistical analysis of ophthalmological studies. Brit. J. Ophthalmol. 71, 645-646.

Norn, M. 1987. Ferning in conjunctival-cytologic preparations. Crystallisation in stained semiquantitative pipette samples of conjunctival fluid. Acta Ophthalmol. 65, 118-122.

Norn, M. 1988. Quantitative tear ferning. Methodologic and experimental investigations. Acta Ophthalmol. 66, 201-205.

Norn, M. 1994. Quantitative tear ferning. Clinical investigations. Acta Ophthalmol. 72, 369-372.

Papanicolau, G. 1946. A general survey of the vaginal smear and its use in research and diagnosis. Am. J. Obstet. Gynecol. 11, 30-37.

Pearce, E.I. and Tomlinson, A. 2000. Spatial location studies on the chemical composition of human tear ferns. Ophthal. Physiol. Opt. 20, 306-313.

Reece, E.A., Chervenak, F.A., Moya, F.R. and Hobbins, J.C. 1984. Amniotic fluid arborization: effect of blood, meconium, and pH alterations. Obstet. Gynecol. 64, 248-250.

Rolando, M. 1984. Tear mucus ferning test in normal and keratoconjunctivitis sicca eyes. Chib. Int. J. Ophthalmol. 2, 32-41.

Rolando, M. 1988. Tear mucus crystallization in children with cystic fibrosis. Ophthalmologica 197, 202-206.

Rolando, M., Baldi, F. and Calabria, G. 1986. The effect of hyperosmolarity on tear mucus ferning. Fortsch. Ophthalmol. 83, 644-646.

Silva, L.R., Gouveia, A.F., de Fátima, C.J., Oliveira, L.B., Reis, J.L. Jr., Ferreira, R.F., Pimentel, C.M. and Galera, P.D. 2016. Tear ferning test in horses and its correlation with ocular surface evaluation. Vet. Ophthalmol. 19, 117-123.

Tabbara, K.F. and Okumoto, M. 1982. Ocular ferning test. A qualitative test for mucus deficiency. Ophthalmology 89, 712-714.

Ullery, J.C., Livingstone, N. and Aboushabanah, E.H. 1959. The mucous fern phenomenon in the cervical and nasal smears; a review and current concept of arborization. Obstet. Gynecol. Surv. 14, 1-25.

Van Bijsterveld, O.P. 1990. Diagnosis and differential diagnosis of keratoconjunctivitis sicca associated with tear gland degeneration. Clin. Exp. Rheumatol. 8(Suppl. 5), 3-6.

Williams, D.L. 2008. Immunopathogenesis of keratoconjunctivitis sicca in the dog. Vet. Clin. N. Am. Sm. Anim. Pract. 38, 251-268.

Zondek, B. 1959. Arborization of cervical and nasal mucus and saliva. Obstet. Gynecol. 13, 477-481.

Zondek, B. and Rozin, S. 1954. Cervical mucus arborisation. Its use in the determination of corpus luteum function. Obstet. Gynecol. 3, 463-470.

32

A rare case of pituitary chromophobe carcinoma in a dog: clinical, tomographic and histopathological findings

M. Longo[1,2]*, D. Binanti[3], P.G. Zagarella[2], F. Iocca[2], D. De Zani[1], G. Ravasio[1], M. Di Giancamillo[1] and D.D. Zani[1]

[1]*Dipartimento di Medicina Veterinaria (DIMEVET), Università degli Studi di Milano, Az.Polo Veterinario di Lodi, Lodi, Italy*
[2]*Centro Traumatologico Ortopedico Veterinario, Arenzano (GE), Italy*
[3]*AbLab, Veterinary Diagnostic Laboratory, Sarzana (SP), Italy*

Abstract

A 9 year old male mixed-breed dog was presented for progressive aggressiveness towards the owner. The neurological evaluation was consistent with a forebrain syndrome. Magnetic Resonance Imaging (MRI) of the brain revealed enlargement of the third ventricle and presence of a large spheroidal neoplasm in the sellar/parasellar region suggestive of a pituitary macroadenoma. On the owner request, the dog was euthanized. Histopathological examination revealed the presence of a pituitary chromophobe carcinoma. To the author's knowledge, pituitary carcinomas have been rarely described in dogs, especially the chromophobe subtype.

Keywords: Brain, Chromophobe carcinoma, Histology, Pituitary neoplasm, Tumour.

Introduction

Pituitary tumors are considered the most common intracranial neoplasms in dogs, making up 25% of secondary intracranial neoplasms in middle-aged and geriatric patients (O'Brien and Coates, 2010). However, in people they only account for 10-12% of all intracranial tumors (Oruçkaptan *et al.*, 2000). The classification of these neoplasms is based on their size and in humans there is a 10 mm cut off that differentiates between pituitary micro and macroadenomas, with giant pituitary adenomas having a diameter of 50 mm (Fracassi *et al.*, 2014). In dogs sellar/parasellar pituitary neoplasms typically refer to micro and macroadenomas and the terminology enlarged and non-enlarged has only recently been introduced, considering that even large adenomas can measure less than 10 mm in diameter (Fracassi *et al.*, 2014).

Clinical signs are mainly related to the serial hormonal dysfunction that leads to Pituitary Dependent Hypercortisolism (PDH) and/or the mass effect on the adjacent brain tissues. This is more significant in the case of large neoplasms. The malignancy of a pituitary lesion is reserved in humans for pituitary tumors that show invasiveness towards the adjacent structures and even local or distant metastatic behaviour (Pollard *et al.*, 2010; Kopczak *et al.*, 2014). In veterinary literature there are few reports concerning pituitary adenocarcinomas, especially the chromophobe subtype (Shimada *et al.*, 1996; Sato *et al.*, 2001) and a recent review of 33 cases showed a 6% prevalence of adenocarcinomas, confirmed by imaging results and subsequent histopathology (Pollard *et al.*, 2010). The present report describes clinical, tomographic, and histopathological features of a pituitary chromophobe carcinoma in a dog.

Case Details

A 9-year-old, male mixed-breed dog was referred for progressive aggressiveness towards its owner. At the clinical examination, the patient presented normothermic, polypnoic (>50 apm), and tachycardic (>140 bpm). Neurological evaluation revealed mental depression, normal gait, and normal postural reaction consistent with a forebrain syndrome. Due to the aggressiveness of the patient, a complete neurological examination was not performed. The diagnostic procedure included blood analysis with leukocyte formula, chest x-rays, abdominal ultrasound (with no relevant findings detected), and brain Magnetic Resonance Imaging (MRI). MRI scans were performed with a low field MRI unit (0,2 T) model Vet-MR® (Esaote S.p.A. Genova, Italy) and 4 mm thick T1-weighted pre and post paramagnetic contrast administration, T2-weighted and FLAIR sequences. At the end of the MRI exam, a total body CT scan was carried out employing a 16-slice CT unit model Brightspeed® (General Electric Healthcare, Milan, Italy), with a pitch of 1, a slice thickness of 1.25 mm, 120 kV and 200 mA.

MRI revealed a moderate ventricular asymmetry, discrete left deviation of the *falx cerebri*, enlargement of the third ventricle and the presence of a large (18x20x15 mm) spheroidal mass in the sellar/parasellar region characterized by isointense on T1 weighted images (Fig. 1a,f) and increased signal on T2 weighted (Fig. 1b,e) and FLAIR (Fig. 1c). In the dorso-lateral portion of the mass, a circular lesion (6 mm diameter)

*****Corresponding Author:** Maurizio Longo. Dipartimento di Medicina Veterinaria (DIMEVET), Università degli Studi di Milano, Az. Polo Veterinario di Lodi, via dell'Università n.6, Lodi, Italy. E-mail: *maurizio.longo@unimi.it* characterized by intense and homogeneous signal hyperintensity on T2 weighted images was detected (Fig. 1e). After gadolinium-based contrast medium was administered intravenously (0.2 ml/kg), the mass showed heterogeneous intense enhancement (Fig. 1d). A pituitary enlarged adenoma/macroadenoma (invasive adenoma/adenocarcinoma) characterized by the presence of a necrotic/cystic lesion was suspected. Craniopharyngioma was also considered and included as a less likely MRI differential diagnosis. At the CT examination, no metastasis was observed in the chest and abdomen. Moreover, no adrenal hyperplasia was detected, confirming the normal blood tests and the non-secreting nature of the pituitary lesion. Due to the invasive nature of the lesion and the aggressive

behavior of the patient the owner elected not to pursue further treatment. The animal was euthanized and the brain was fixed in 10% buffered formalin and submitted for histopathology examination, after written informed consent was obtained from the owner. Samples were processed routinely, embedded in paraffin wax, and sections were stained with hematoxylin and eosin. Pituitary gland was completely effaced by a wide, infiltrative, unencapsulated, not well circumscribed, densely cellular neoplasm composed of polygonal cells arranged in nests and packets supported by a fine fibrovascular stroma with numerous small hyperemic vessels (Fig. 2a). Neoplastic cells had variably distinct cell borders, intermediate N/C ratio, moderate amount of eosinophilic cytoplasm occasionally finely granular

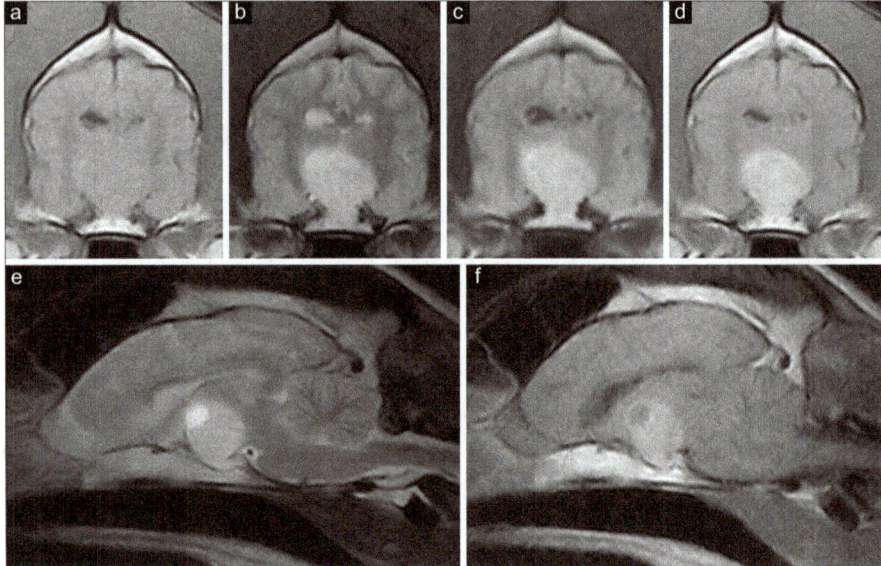

Fig. 1. Transverse (a,b,c,d) and Sagittal (e,f) MRI images of the brain showing a large spheroideal mass in the sellar/parasellar region. The mass was characterized by isointense signal on T1-weighted images (a) and high signal on T2-weighted (b and e) and FLAIR (c) sequences. A circular lesion hypointense on T1-weighted (f) and hyperintense on T2-weighted images was observed in the dorso-lateral aspect of the mass. After contrast medium administration, the mass showed a heterogeneous intense enhancement. Note the ventricular asimmetry and the moderate deviation of the falx cerebri on the transverse images of the brain (a,b,c,d).

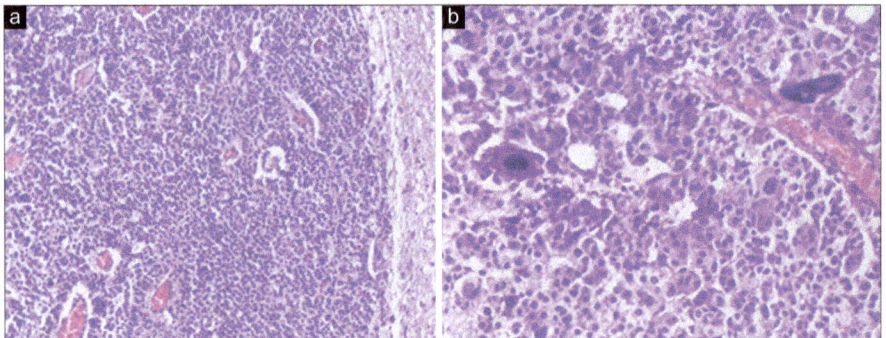

Fig. 2. Histological findings of the pituitary gland. (a) Histological examination showed a wide, infiltrative, unencapsulated, not well circumscribed, densely cellular neoplasm composed of polygonal cells arranged in nests and packets supported by a fine fibrovascular stroma with numerous small hyperemic vessels. (b) Details of the neoplastic cells with severe anisokaryosis, anisocytosis and karyomegaly.

(Fig. 2a,b). Nuclei were round to ovalar, with one or two magenta nucleoli. Mitosis ranged from 0 to 1 per HPF (2 mitosis in 10 HPF). Severe anisokaryosis, anisocytosis and karyomegaly were evident with rare binucleated cells (Fig. 2b). The neoplasm had infiltrative growth throughout the adjacent brain parenchyma, with invasion of the third ventricle. A focal marginal residual area of pituitary parenchyma was evident. The other portion of evaluated brain was characterized by mild gliosis and satellitosis. No other neoplastic cerebral lesions were detected. Histological findings supported the diagnosis of pituitary chromophobe carcinoma.

Discussion

Pituitary carcinomas have been rarely observed in old dogs; moreover, cases of pituitary neoplasm with intense cellular pleomorphism and elevate mitotic index in absence of metastatic lesions are extremely rare. These neoplasms can cause serious functional disorders due to the destruction of the pars distalis of the neurohypophysis. Even though different therapeutical approaches have been described in literature, including trans-sphenoidal surgery and adjuvant therapies like radiotherapy (Oruçkaptan et al., 2000; Hanson et al., 2005; Fracassi et al., 2014), little evidence, concerning large pituitary tumors, of surgical outcome have been described in literature. In the present case the owner decided to euthanize the patient and histopathology revealed the infiltrative nature of the neoplasm towards the adjacent brain tissue.

Cranipharyngioma was considered as a less likely MRI differential diagnosis due to the rounded shape of the neoplasm in continuity with the hypophysis and its sellar/parasellar location peculiar for pituitary tumours. In fact craniopharyngiomas have been rarely reported in dogs (Hawkins et al., 1985; Eckersley et al., 1991) and cats (Nagata et al., 2005), with a more suprasellar and pharyngeal localization, sometimes adjacent to the dura (Hawkins et al., 1985).

Due to the absence of clinical findings compatible with hormonal imbalance or hormonal problem the neoplasm was considered a not-hormonally active tumor, and immunohistochemistry for pituitary hormones was therefore not performed.

In case of not-hormonally active neoplasm, the histological finding is the only strictly clarified method to classify the tumor. Previously a similar neoplasm was reported (Hawkins et al., 1985), based only on histological findings.

The images in the paper show severe anisokaryosis and anisocytosis typical of malignant chromophobe neoplasm. Neoplastic cells were polygonal with a small to moderate amount of eosinophilic to faintly-basophilic finely granular cytoplasm and a large, oval nucleus compatible with chromophobic cells.

In humans the distinction between invasive adenoma and pituitary adenocarcinoma is based on the finding of intracranial or systemic metastasis. It is believed that adenocarcinomas originate from malignant transformation of pre-existing adenomas after a variable latency period. In the presented case, despite the absence of systemic and intracranial metastasis, the infiltrating growth pattern and the presence of neoplastic cells that reach and surround the third ventricle, together with the intense cellular pleomorphism support the diagnosis to a rare malignant form of the neoplasm.

References

Eckersley, G.N., Geel, J.K. and Kriek, N.P. 1991. A craniopharyngioma in a seven-year-old dog. J. S. Afr. Vet. Assoc. 62, 65-67.

Fracassi, F., Mandrioli, L., Shehdula, D., Diana, A., Grinwis, G.C. and Meij, B.P. 2014. Complete Surgical Removal of a Very Enlarged Pituitary Corticotroph Adenoma in a Dog. J. Am. Anim. Hosp. Assoc. 50, 192-197.

Hanson, J.M., van't, H.M., Voorhout, G., Teske, E., Kooistra, H.S. and Meij, B.P. 2005. Efficacy of Transsphenoidal Hypophysectomy in Treatment of Dogs with Pituitary-Dependent Hyperadrenocorticism. J. Vet. Intern. Med. 19, 687-694.

Hawkins, K.L., Diters, R.W. and McGrath, J.T. 1985. Craniopharyngioma in a dog. J. Comp. Pathol. 95, 469-474.

Kopczak, A., Renner, U. and Karl Stalla, G. 2014. Advances in understanding pituitary tumors. F1000Prime Rep. 6, 5. http://doi.org/10.12703/P6-5.

Nagata, T., Nakayama, H., Uchida, K., Uetsuka, K., Yasoshima, A., Yasunaga, S., Masuda, K., Tsujimoto, H., Kuwajima, E., Nishimura, R., Sasaki, N. and Doi, K. 2005. Two cases of feline malignant craniopharyngioma. Vet. Pathol. 42, 663-665.

O'Brien, D.P. and Coates, J.R. 2010. Brain disease. In Textbook of Veterinary Internal Medicine Expert Consult, Eds. Ettinger, S.J. and Feldman E.C. St. Louis, Missouri, USA: Elsevier Saunders, pp: 1445.

Oruçkaptan, H.H., Senmevsim, O., Ozcan, O.E. and Ozgen, T. 2000. Pituitary Adenomas: Results of 684 Surgically Treated Patients and Review of the Literature. Surg. Neurol. 53, 211-219.

Pollard, R.E., Reilly, C.M., Uerling, M.R., Wood, F.D. and Feldman, E.C. 2010. Cross-Sectional Imaging Characteristics of Pituitary Adenomas, Invasive Adenomas and Adenocarcinomas in Dogs: 33 Cases (1988 –2006). J. Vet. Intern. Med. 24, 160-165.

Sato, J., Sato, R., Kinai, M., Tomizawa, N., Osawa, T., Nakada, K., Yano, A., Goryo, M. and Naito, Y.

2001. Pituitary Chromophobe Carcinoma with a Low Level of Serum Gonadotropin and Aspermatogenesis in a Dog. J. Vet. Med. Sci. 63, 183-185.

Shimada, A., Hara, K., Umemura, T., Kagota, K., Yamaga, Y., Ozaki, K. and Narama, I. 1996. Non-functional Pituitary Chromophobe Adenoma in a Calf. J. Comp. Pathol. 115, 89-93.

33

Congenital deformity of the distal extremities in three dogs

F. Di Dona[1,*], G. Della Valle[1], L. Meomartino[2], F. Lamagna[1] and G. Fatone[1]

[1]*Department of Veterinary Medicine and Animal Productions, University of Napoli "Federico II", Italy*
[2]*Interdepartmental Center of Veterinary Radiology, University of Napoli "Federico II", Italy*

Abstract
Congenital limb deformities are very rare conditions and the knowledge about etiology, pathogenesis, clinical presentation and treatment is still poor. Moreover, many defects are still not reported in veterinary literature. This report documents clinical and radiographic findings in three dogs with congenital deformity involving the distal extremities. Case 1 was affected with bilateral aphalangia of the pedes, case 2 presented a combination of brachydactyly and syndactyly, whereas in case 3 a unilateral ectrodactyly was observed. To the authors' knowledge, brachydactyly, as well as aphalangia, are very uncommon anomalies and have been rarely documented. Moreover, association between syndactyly and brachydactyly has still not been reported.
Keywords: Aphalangia, Brachydactyly, Congenital deformity, Dog, Syndactyly.

Introduction

Congenital skeletal deformities, also referred as dysostoses, are defects arising from errors during development and characterized by abnormal growth of individual bones or part of bones (Noden and de Lahunta, 1985). Causes can be hereditary, or intrinsic (abnormal developmental process), and environmental, or extrinsic (interference with a normal developmental process), and result in failure of a mesenchymal bone model to form, failure of anlagen to properly transform into cartilage, or failure to convert cartilage into bone (Towle and Breur, 2004).
In dogs, limb formation is a complex process that occurs between the 3rd and 5th week of gestation and that includes limb bud formation, limb elongation, digit formation, and bone and joint formation (Evans, 1993). The morphologic developmental aberrations and genes responsible for these aberrations have still not been identified in canine and feline dysostoses. Differently, several environmental factors have also been implicated in development of dysostoses and may include: drugs, maternal diseases, faulty maternal diet, modified-live vaccines, radiations, and trauma to the mother, embryo, or placenta (Towle and Breur, 2004). Although a wide number of dysostoses have been previously reported in domestic animals (Towle *et al.*, 2007; Barrand and Cornillie, 2008; Lockwood *et al.*, 2009; Pisoni *et al.*, 2012; Macrì *et al.*, 2014; Di Dona *et al.*, 2016), comparing to human literature, in veterinary medicine, a complete description of congenital skeletal malformations is still lacking (Temtamy and Aglan, 2008). Moreover, a clear classification of the possible anomalies detectable does not exist.

Congenital anomalies of the distal extremities include: aphalangia (A = without; Phàlanx = phalanx), absence of a digit or of one or more phalanges (Macrì *et al.*, 2012); polydactyly (Polys = many; Dactylos = digit), increase number of digits (Jezyk, 1985); oligodactyly (Oligos = few), decreased number of digits (Clark *et al.*, 2001); adactyly, absence of one or more digits (Barrand and Cornillie, 2008); brachydactyly (Brachus = short), reduced size of digits (Hoskins, 1995); syndactyly (Syn = together), adjacent digits are fused and can be classified as simple or complex, incomplete or complete, and uncomplicated or complicated (Towle and Breur, 2004); ectrodactyly (Ektroma = abortion), is congenital digital cleft formation extending between the metacarpal bones (Towle and Breur, 2004).
The current knowledge about congenital limb deformity in dogs and cats is very poor, and many congenital defects are still not described. In order to improve the knowledge about congenital limb anomalies in dogs, the aim of this report is to describe the clinical and radiographic findings in three dogs affected by dysostoses of the distal extremities.

Case details

Case 1
A 2-year-old, male miniature poodle was referred for left hind limb lameness. The dog had a story of a previous lameness occurred when he was 4-month-old due to an abnormal digits development that determined a severe skin lesion; the owner referred that the dog's activity was restricted previously, but no improvement on the gait was noticed. Successively the dog was submitted to amputation of the most distal portions of the III and IV digits. The owner was not able to provide any radiographic images prior the surgery.

*****Corresponding Author:** Francesco Di Dona. Department of Veterinary Medicine and Animal Productions, University of Napoli "Federico II". Via Federico Delpino, 1 – 80138 Napoli, Italy. Email: *francesco.didona@unina.it*

Inspection of the feet revealed a malformation of both pedes characterized by the absence of all digits and the underdevelopment of the metatarsal pad. Palpation of the distal end of the left foot showed discomfort and eliciting pain, while on the right side the dog was unresponsive. The physical examination was within normal limits and did not reveal any additional abnormality. On radiographic examination, all of the digits had missing of some phalangeal bones: in the right foot, there was the absence of one row of phalangeal bones (II or III row) and the distal row was characterized by "V" shaped phalangeal bones; in the left foot, II and V digits presented a single "V" shaped phalangeal bone, whereas the III and IV digits presented just portion of the base, probably as consequence of the amputation (Fig. 1).

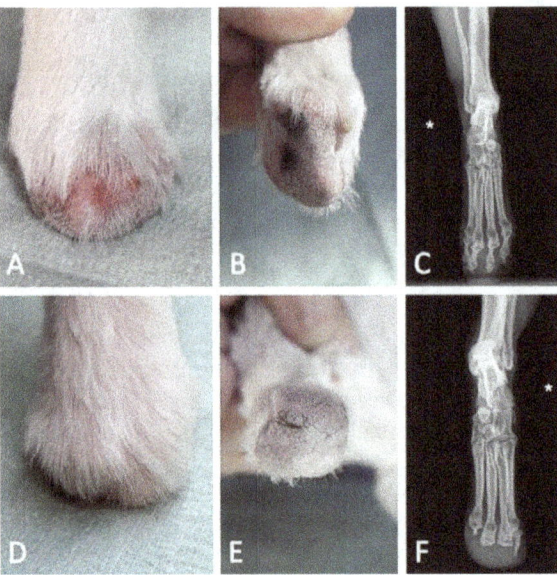

Fig. 1. Case 1: 2-year-old male miniature poodle. (A,B): Dorsal and plantar view of the right pes showing the absence of all the digits and all digital pads. (C): Dorso-plantar radiographic projection of the right pes [* = lateral side] showing the absence of all second phalangeal bones (brachymesophalangy). (D,E): Dorsal and plantar view of the left pes showing the absence of all the digits and all digital pads. (F): Dorso-plantar radiographic projection of the left pes showing the absence of the first and second phalangeal bones of the II and V digits, whereas the two intermediate digits present just a sketch.

Clinical and radiographic findings showed bilateral partial aphalangia. The dog was managed by using orthopedic braces for protecting the pads.
The dog adapted to the use of protections and no evidence of skin lesion or lameness were detected after 2 months.
Case 2
A 3-month-old female English setter was referred with lameness and paw malformation to the left front limb. On clinical examination, the IV and V digits of the left

paw were shorter than normal. Moreover, the left shoulder joint showed local soft tissue swelling and flexion-extension maneuvers elicited pain. The physical examination was within normal limits and did not reveal any additional abnormality. On radiographic examination, the IV and V digits of the left paw had short metacarpi (i.e. only the bases were visible), both hypoplastic first phalanx and second phalanx of the V digit fused with the first phalangeal bone of the IV digit. The V digit was the most affected and just the III phalangeal bone was clearly identifiable, whereas the I phalangeal bone appeared as an isolated sketch, shorter and thinner than normal (Fig. 2).

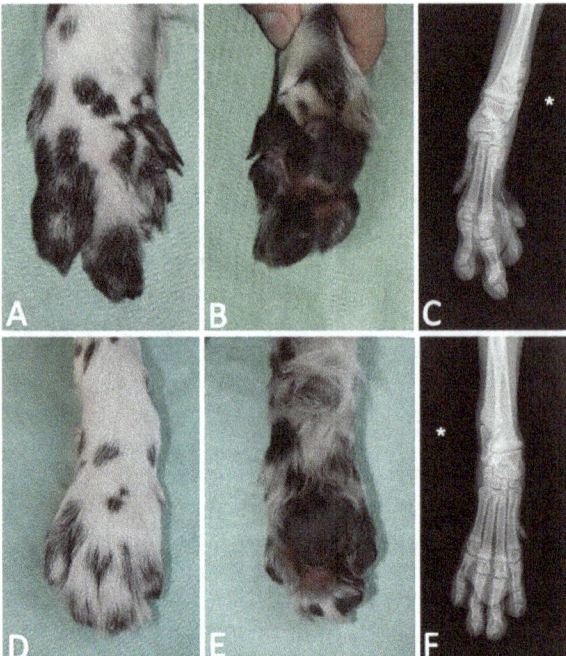

Fig. 2. Case 2: 3-month-old female English setter. (A,B): Dorsal and plantar view of the left manus showing an abnormal development and the evident shortening of the most lateral digits, however all the pads are present. (C): Dorso-plantar radiographic projection of the left manus [* = lateral side] showing short (or partially developed) IV and V metacarpal bones, hypoplastic phalanges of the V digit (just the III phalangeal bone was clearly identifiable, whereas the I phalangeal bone appeared as an isolated sketch, shorter and thinner than normal), synostosis between the I phalangeal bone of the IV digit and the II phalangeal bone of the V digit. (D,E,F): Dorsal and plantar view and dorso-plantar radiographic projection of the right manus showing a normal development.

Radiographic examination of the left shoulder joint revealed a severe deformity of the proximal humeral epiphysis characterized by an irregularly flattening and hypoplasia of the head; the shaft of the humerus showed a more pronounced sigmoid-shape and shortness compared to the contralateral. Moreover, the infraglenoid tubercle and the caudal end of the glenoid cavity of the scapula were hypoplastic and sclerotic (Fig. 3).

Clinical and radiographic findings showed a partial brachydactyly and syndactyly, in association to avascular necrosis of the humeral head. No treatment was considered at time for managing the congenital deformity. Unfortunately, after the first evaluation, the follow up was lost.

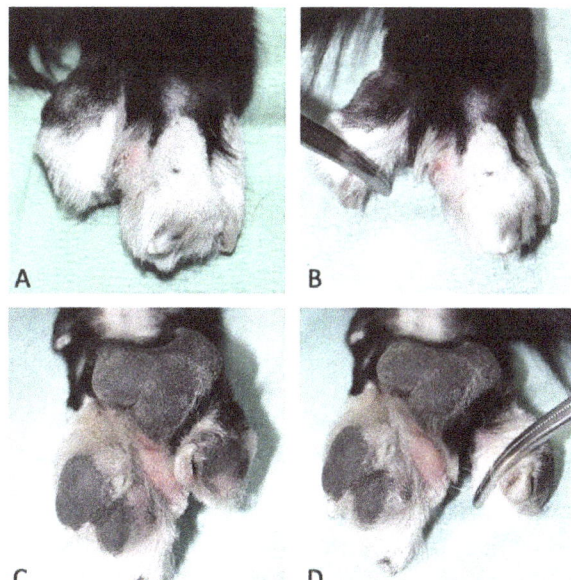

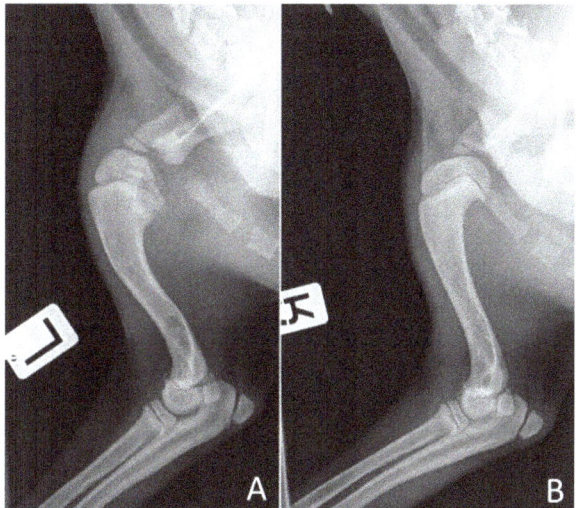

Fig. 3. Case 2: 3-month-old female English setter. (A): Lateral radiographic projection of the left shoulder joint. There is a severe deformity characterized by collapse and flattening of the proximal humeral epiphysis, as well as a more pronounced sigmoid-shape and shortness of the shaft of the humerus. Moreover, the infraglenoid tubercle and the caudal end of the glenoid cavity of the scapula were hypoplastic and sclerotic. (B): Lateral radiographic projection of the right shoulder joint. The anatomy is preserved and no abnormalities are detectable.

Fig. 4. Case 3: 3-year-old male Border collie. Dorsal (A,B) and palmar (C,D) macroscopic view of the right manus. Note the complete absence of the IV digit, visible in all the pictures, and the cutaneous syndactyly between the II and III digits, visible in pictures C and D.

Case 3

A 3-years-old, male border collie was referred for the presence of an abnormal right front paw not associated to any lameness. Physical examination of the involved limb revealed a deformity of the paw characterized by the absence of the IV digit and the fusion of the II and the III digits which determined a "cleft hand aspect" (Fig. 4).

The physical examination was otherwise within normal limits and did not reveal any additional congenital anomaly. Dorso-palmar radiographic view of both manus were taken. On the right side, there was the absence of the IV digit distal to the base of the metacarpal bone, that, however, was thinner than normal, and the V digit showed a varus deviation. On the left side, the clinical unaffected paw, the radiographic examination revealed, as an incidental finding, a varus deviation of the last two phalangeal bones of the V digit (Fig. 5).

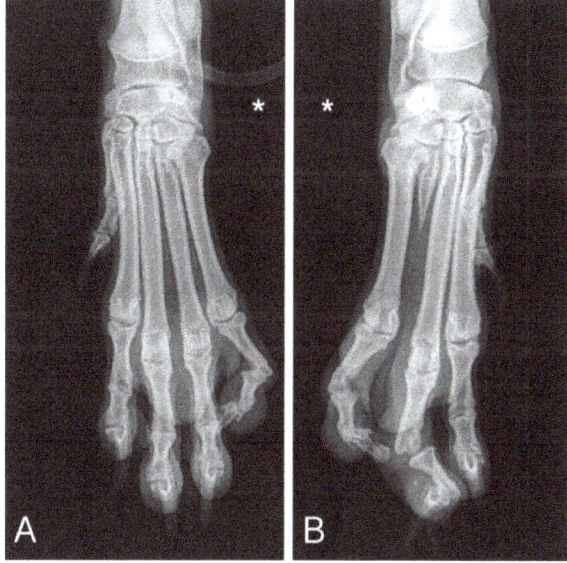

Fig. 5. Case 3: 3-year-old male Border collie. (A): Dorso-palmar radiographic projection of the left manus [* = lateral side] showing a normal development of all the digits and a varus deviation of the last two phalangeal bones of the V digit. (B): Dorso-palmar radiographic projection of the right manus showing the absence of the IV digits with a residual sketch of the relative metacarpal on the right side, as well as varus deviation of the last two phalangeal bones of the III and V digits.

Clinical and radiographic findings showed unilateral ectrodactyly. No treatment was instituted at time because the dog had no evidence of discomfort.

Discussion

The definition of limb malformations is quite complex since the lack of a uniform and consistent nomenclature. Nomina Embryologica Veterinaria (2006) represents the gold standard about the identification and classification of congenital anomalies in animals, but as previously indicated by Cornillie *et al.* (2004), it needs to be expanded and ambiguous definition should be agreed upon. Many terms used in human literature for the identification of specific dysostoses are still not mentioned in the official list. Moreover many affections can be distinctly identified and named, whereas many others cannot be easily classified and in such cases more than one term can be used for describing the same anomaly (Ogino, 2007).

Case 1 was clinically characterized by the involvement of both hind paws with the absence/shortening of all the digits, the global hypoplasia of the extremity and the cutaneous fusion; whereas, on radiographic examination, the lesions characterized by the absence of many phalanges bilaterally. In our opinion, the clinical presentation can be identified by using the term adactyly; however the radiographic findings led us to identify the affection with the term of partial aphalangy. Case 2 was, clinically and radiographically, characterized by the involvement of the left front paw with the abnormal shortening of the IV and V digits. According to the definitions previously introduced, this congenital anomaly can be classified as brachydactyly on the basis of the clinical presentation, whereas, on radiographic examination, a combination of more anomalies including brachydactyly and syndactyly can be appreciated. The concurrent shoulder affection on the same side of the congenital defect could support a common origin of both lesions; however, a different and independent origin cannot be excluded.

Case 3 was clinically characterized by a V-shaped cleft situated in the centre of the right paw, the absence of the IV digit and cutaneous fusion of the II and III digits. Radiographically, the defects were less severe because clearly involved exclusively the IV digit that showed just a sketch of its proximal metacarpal. According to the definitions previously introduced, this affection can be classified as ectrodactyly based on the clinical presentation, but can be identified as oligodactyly, partial adactyly or aphalangy based on radiographic aspect.

The use of some terms is still controversial and probably this can influence the modality of description and classification of many congenital anomalies. For example, the term brachydactyly has not been used frequently in animals and currently, in literature, there are few reports dealing with this anomaly. Towle and Breur (2004) in a review about dysostoses of the canine and feline appendicular skeleton provided a concise guide to the clinical signs, diagnosis, treatment, prognosis, and heritability for each reported appendicular dysostosis; however, they did not report any mention to brachydactyly. On the other hand, in two guides on canine and feline congenital defects, where a schematic list of abnormalities is provided, the term brachydactyly is reported and defined as "reduced size and function of outer toes", but the authors did not provide any reference about this congenital anomaly (Hoskins and Taboada, 1992; Hoskins, 1995). To our knowledge, in literature, this lesion has been documented in the dog exclusively by Hudson and Money (1995), reporting a case affected by abnormal shortening of the II and V digits bilaterally, identifying the affection as abnormal development of the metacarpal bones. Although the authors named the affection as brachymetacarpalia (Hudson and Money, 1995). In our opinion, and according to the human literature, it can be considered a particular form of brachydactyly (Schwabe and Mundlos, 2004).

Descriptions of adactily and aphalangy have been recently reported in both dogs and cats (Macrì *et al.*, 2011, 2012). These papers added contribution to the literature but different widely from the cases described here. Adactyly is defined partial when there is the absence of one to four digits and their metacarpals or metatarsals; whereas partial aphalangy refers to the absence of one or more phalanges from one to four digits (Macrì *et al.*, 2012). According to this classification, case 1 was clearly affected by a bilateral partial aphalangy of both pedes. Whereas case 3 could be classified as aphalangy and not as adactyly because the metacarpal bone was present, even though only in part.

Ectrodactyly has been frequently reported and probably it is the most common malformation involving the manus in dogs (Pratschke, 1996; Barrand, 2004; Carvallo *et al.*, 2011). However, there are various types of ectrodactyly and some defects can differ much from others (Ogino, 2007). Some reports defined ectrodactyly as congenital digital cleft formation extending between the metacarpal bones, associated with hypoplasia or absence of one or more bones in the adjacent area of the distal portion of the limb, and characterized by severely hypoplastic or missing carpal bones (Carrig *et al.*, 1981; Towle and Breur, 2004).

The affection of the dog in case 3, showing clinically the typical "cleft-hand aspect" and the absence of one central digit, was classified as ectrodactyly, even though the carpus did not show any morphological alteration.

The knowledge about etiology, pathogenesis, presentation, and treatment of congenital skeletal defects in the dog is still weak. In the Online Mendelian Inheritance in Animals database (OMIA; http://omia.angis.org.au), which offers the most recent references about inheritable disorders in several animal species, has listed only the terms brachydactyly and ectrodactyly of all the aforementioned terms; but no specific reference about the genetic influence is reported in dogs. However, some authors investigated the inheritance of brachydactyly and allied abnormalities in rabbits, defining the types of deformities, the inheritance, and the embryological changes, concluding that this disorder is "a recessive mutant which reduces the size and function of the outside toes on the front and sometimes the hind feet" (Greene and Saxton, 1939; Green, 1957).

There is no general or specific treatment to manage a dog with a congenital limb deformity. The treatment must be planned based on the type and severity of the malformation, as well as if the lesion is separated or more structures are involved. Surgical management of ectrodactyly has been described in dogs; the main goal of the surgery is to provide metacarpal synostosis and recover the function of the manus (Innes *et al.*, 2001; Harasen, 2010; Pisoni *et al.*, 2014).

Differently, there is no mention in literature to the management of the other digital anomalies in dogs. In human medicine, the main goal of surgery is to improve child's ability to grasp and pinch. Surgery may also have an esthetic role making the child's hand look more typical. Possible options include skin separation in case of a combination with syndactyly, phalangeal transfer and bone lengthening. Prognosis for the brachydactylies, and terminal transverse defects in general, is strongly dependent on the nature of the lesion, and may vary from excellent to severely influencing hand function. If the limb defect is part of a syndrome, prognosis often depends on the nature of the associated anomalies (Temtamy and Aglan, 2008). In dogs, the surgical management of terminal transverse defects of the distal extremities is not considered in most of the cases, because the affection can be compatible with a normal life, as experienced in the cases presented here. Conservative management with the use of protective braces can avoid the secondary lesions that can be associated to the underdevelopment of the toes and the digital pads in particular.

This report enriches the available literature about congenital limb deformities, describing the features of rarely reported lesions and discussing about how difficult it is to know the correct identification and classification. We would like to underline the need for a standard resource of unequivocal and well-defined nomenclature. In our opinion many dysostoses are either not diagnosed or not reported and large-scale studies are necessary to understand the real prevalence of these affections in companion animals.

Conflict of interest
The authors declare that there is no conflict of interest.

References

Barrand, K.R. 2004. Ectrodactyly in a West Highland white terrier. J. Small Anim. Pract. 45, 315-318.

Barrand, K.R. and Cornillie, P. 2008. Bilateral hindlimb adactyly in an adult cat. J. Small Anim. Pract. 49, 252-253.

Carrig, C.B., Wortman, J.A., Morris, E.L., Blevins, W.E., Root, C.R., Hanlon, G.F. and Suter, P.F. 1981. Ectrodactyly (split-hand deformity) in the dog. Vet. Radiol. Ultrasound 22, 123-144.

Carvallo, F.R., Domínguez, A.S. and Morales, P.C. 2011. Bilateral ectrodactyly and spinal deformation in a mixed-breed dog. Can. Vet. J. 52, 47-49.

Clark, R.M., Marker, P.C., Roessler, E., Dutra, A., Schimenti, J.C., Muenke, M. and Kingsley, D.M. 2001. Reciprocal mouse and human limb phenotypes caused by gain- and loss-of-function mutations affecting Lmbr1. Genetics 159, 715-726.

Cornillie, P., Van Lancker, S. and Simoens, P. 2004. Two cases of Brachymelia in cats. Anat. Histol. Embryo. 33, 115-118.

Di Dona, F., Murino, C., Della Valle, G. and Fatone G. 2016. Bilateral tibial agenesis and syndactyly in a cat. Vet. Comp. Orthop. Traumatol. 29, 277-282.

Evans, H.E. 1993. Prenatal development. In Miller's anatomy of the dog, Ed., Miller, M.E.: W.B. Saunders, Philadelphia, pp: 32-97.

Green, E.L. 1957. Mutant stocks of cats and dogs offered for research. J. Hered. 48, 56-58.

Greene, H.S.N. and Saxton, J.A. 1939. Hereditary brachydactylia and allied abnormalities in the rabbit. J. Exp. Med. 69, 301-314.

Harasen, G. 2010. Surgical management of ectrodactyly in a Siberian husky. Can. Vet. J. 51, 421-424.

Hoskins, J.D. and Taboada, J. 1992. Congenital defects of the dog. Compend. Contin. Educ. Vet. 14, 873-897.

Hoskins, J.D. 1995. Congenital defects of cats. Compend. Contin. Educ. Vet. 17, 385-405.

Hudson, L.C. and Money, D.W. 1995. Symmetric Bilateral Brachymetacarpalia of a Dog. Vet. Pathol. 32, 187-189.

Jezyk, P.F. 1985. Constitutional disorders of the skeleton in dogs and cats. In Textbook of Small Animal Orthopaedics, Eds., Newton C.D. and Nunamaker D.M.: International Veterinary Information Service, Ithaca, NY, USA, chapter 57.

Innes, J.F., McKee, W.M., Mitchell, R.A.S., Lascelles, B.D.X. and Johnson, K.A. 2001. Surgical reconstruction of ectrodactyly deformity in four dogs. Vet. Comp. Orthop. Traumatol. 14, 201-209.

Lockwood, A., Montgomery, R. and McEwen, V. 2009. Bilateral radial hemimelia, polydactyly and cardiomegaly in two cats. Vet. Comp. Orthop. Traumatol. 22, 511-513.

Macrì, F., Ciotola, F., Rapisarda, G., Lanteri, G., Albarella, S., Aiudi, G., Liotta, L. and Marino, F. 2014. A rare case of simple syndactyly in a puppy. J. Small Anim. Pract. 55, 170-173.

Macrì, F., Lanteri, G., Rapisarda, G. and Marini, F. 2012. Unilateral forelimb partial aphalangia in a kitten. J. Feline Med. Surg. 14, 272-275.

Macrì, F., Marino, F., Rapisarda, G., Lanteri, G. and Mazzullo, G. 2011. A case of unilateral pelvic limb adactyly in a puppy dog. Anat. Histol. Embryol. 40, 104-106.

Noden, D.M. and de Lahunta, A. 1985. The embryology of domestic animals. Developmental Mechanisms and Malformations. Williams and Wilkins, Baltimore, MD, USA, pp: 196-210.

Nomina Embryologica Veterinaria. 2006. (Second Edition). World Association of Veterinary Anatomists. Available at: (http://www.wava-amav.org/Downloads/nev_2006.pdf).

Ogino, T. 2007. Clinical features and teratogenic mechanisms of congenital absence of digits. Dev. Growth Differ. 49, 523-531.

Pisoni, L., Cinti, F., Del Magno, S. and Joechler, M. 2012. Bilateral radial hemimelia and multiple malformations in a kitten. J. Feline Med. Surg. 14, 598-602.

Pisoni, L., Del Magno, S., Cinti, F., Dalpozzo, B., Bellei, E., Cloriti, E. and Joechler, M. 2014. Surgical induction of metacarpal synostosis for treatment of ectrodactyly in a dog. Vet. Comp. Orthop. Traumatol. 27, 166-171.

Pratschke, K. 1996. A case of ectrodactyly in a dog. Irish Vet. J. 49, 412-413.

Schwabe, G.C. and Mundlos, S. 2004. Genetics of congenital hand anomalies. Handchir. Mikrochir. Plast. Chir. 36, 85-97.

Temtamy, S.A. and Aglan, M.S. 2008. Brachydactyly. Orphanet J. Rare Dis. 3, 15.

Towle, H.A. and Breur, G.J. 2004. Dysostoses of the canine and feline appendicular skeleton. J. Am. Vet. Med. Assoc. 225, 1685-1692.

Towle, H., Friedlander, K., Ko, R., Aper, R. and Breur, G. 2007. Surgical treatment of simple syndactylism with secondary deep digital flexor tendon contracture in a Basset Hound. Vet. Comp. Orthop. Traumatol. 20, 219-223.

PERMISSIONS

All chapters in this book were first published in OVJ, by Tripoli University; hereby published with permission under the Creative Commons Attribution License or equivalent. Every chapter published in this book has been scrutinized by our experts. Their significance has been extensively debated. The topics covered herein carry significant findings which will fuel the growth of the discipline. They may even be implemented as practical applications or may be referred to as a beginning point for another development.

The contributors of this book come from diverse backgrounds, making this book a truly international effort. This book will bring forth new frontiers with its revolutionizing research information and detailed analysis of the nascent developments around the world.

We would like to thank all the contributing authors for lending their expertise to make the book truly unique. They have played a crucial role in the development of this book. Without their invaluable contributions this book wouldn't have been possible. They have made vital efforts to compile up to date information on the varied aspects of this subject to make this book a valuable addition to the collection of many professionals and students.

This book was conceptualized with the vision of imparting up-to-date information and advanced data in this field. To ensure the same, a matchless editorial board was set up. Every individual on the board went through rigorous rounds of assessment to prove their worth. After which they invested a large part of their time researching and compiling the most relevant data for our readers.

The editorial board has been involved in producing this book since its inception. They have spent rigorous hours researching and exploring the diverse topics which have resulted in the successful publishing of this book. They have passed on their knowledge of decades through this book. To expedite this challenging task, the publisher supported the team at every step. A small team of assistant editors was also appointed to further simplify the editing procedure and attain best results for the readers.

Apart from the editorial board, the designing team has also invested a significant amount of their time in understanding the subject and creating the most relevant covers. They scrutinized every image to scout for the most suitable representation of the subject and create an appropriate cover for the book.

The publishing team has been an ardent support to the editorial, designing and production team. Their endless efforts to recruit the best for this project, has resulted in the accomplishment of this book. They are a veteran in the field of academics and their pool of knowledge is as vast as their experience in printing. Their expertise and guidance has proved useful at every step. Their uncompromising quality standards have made this book an exceptional effort. Their encouragement from time to time has been an inspiration for everyone.

The publisher and the editorial board hope that this book will prove to be a valuable piece of knowledge for researchers, students, practitioners and scholars across the globe.

LIST OF CONTRIBUTORS

J. Bondeson
Department of Rheumatology, School of Medicine, Cardiff University, Cardiff, CF14 4XN, UK

A. Cirla and G. Bertolini
San Marco Veterinary Clinic, via Sorio 114/c – 35141 Padova, Italy

M. Rondena
San Marco Veterinary Laboratory, via Sorio 114/c – 35141 Padova, Italy

A. Giuliano, R. Salgüero and J. Dobson
Queen's Veterinary School Hospital, University of Cambridge, Madingley Road, Cambridge, CB3 0ES,United Kingdom

A. Zatelli and P. D'Ippolito
Medical Consultancy Services, G. Calì Street 60, TBX1424 TàXbiex, Malta

X. Roura
Hospital Clínic Veterinari, Universitat Autònoma de Barcelona, Spain

M. Berlanda
Department of Animal Medicine, Production and Health, viale dell'Università 16, 35020 Legnaro (PD), University of Padova, Italy

E. Zini
Department of Animal Medicine, Production and Health, viale dell'Università 16, 35020 Legnaro (PD), University of Padova, Italy
Clinic for Small Animal Internal Medicine, Vetsuisse Faculty, University of Zurich, Winterthurerstrasse 260, 8057 Zurich, Switzerland
Istituto Veterinario di Novara, Strada Provinciale 9, 28060 Granozzo con Monticello (NO), Italy

Liga Kovalcuka and Agris Ilgazs
Latvia University of Agriculture, Faculty of Veterinary Medicine, Clinical Institute, K. Helmaņa iela 8, Jelgava,LV-3004, Latvia

Dace Bandere
Riga Stradiņš University, Faculty of Pharmacy, Department of Pharmaceutical Chemistry, Dzirciema iela 16, Rīga, LV-1007, Latvia

David L. Williams
University of Cambridge, Department of Veterinary medicine, United Kingdom

Angel Bhathal
Faculty of Pharmacy and Pharmaceutical Sciences, University of Alberta, Edmonton, Alberta T6G 2H7, Canada

Meredith Spryszak, Christopher Louizos and Grace Frankel
College of Pharmacy, Faculty of Health Sciences, University of Manitoba, Winnipeg, Manitoba R3E 0T5, Canada

P. Pessina, I. Sartore and A. Meikle
Laboratorio de Técnicas Nucleares, Facultad de Veterinaria, Universidad de la República, Lasplaces 1550, Montevideo, Uruguay

V.A. Castillo
Cat. Clin. Méd. Peq. An. and U. Endocrinología, Escuela Medicina Veterinaria, Facultad de Ciencias Veterinarias, Universidad de Buenos Aires. Av. Chorroarín 280, C. Autónoma de Buenos Aires, Argentina

D. César
Instituto Plan Agropecuario, Br. Artigas 3802, Montevideo, Uruguay

David L. Williams and Philippa Burg
Department of Veterinary Medicine, University of Cambridge, Madingley Road, Cambridge, CB3 0ES, UK

M. Ricciardi
"Pingry" Veterinary Hospital, via Medaglie d'Oro 5, Bari Italy

E.A. Soler Arias and V.A. Castillo
Hospital Escuela, Unidad de Endocrinología, Area de Clínica Médica de Pequeños Animales, Fac. de Ciencias Veterinarias, UBA, Av. Chorroarín 280, Ciudad Autónoma de Buenos Aires, Argentina

M.E. Caneda Aristarain
Alumna de Programa de Investigación. Fac. de Ciencias Veterinarias, UBA, Chorroarín 280, Ciudad Autónoma de Buenos Aires, Argentina

Laura Nordio and Chiara Giudice
Department of Veterinary Medicine, Università di Milano, via Celoria 10, 20133, Milano (MI), Italy

Sabina Fattori
Studio veterinario associato di Fattori Sabina e Gasparini Emanuele, Via Gabrielli Gabrielangelo 85, 61032, Fano (PU), Italy

T. Iwanaga
Veterinary Teaching Hospital, Joint Faculty of Veterinary Medicine, Kagoshima University, Korimoto 1-21-24, Kagoshima 890-0065, Japan

S. Tokunaga
Veterinary Teaching Hospital, Joint Faculty of Veterinary Medicine, Kagoshima University, Korimoto 1-21-24, Kagoshima 890-0065, Japan
Department of Environmental and Radiological Health Sciences, College of Veterinary Medicine and Biomedical Sciences, Colorado State University, Fort Collins, CO, 80523, USA

Y. Momoi
Department of Clinical Medical Science, Joint Faculty of Veterinary Medicine, Kagoshima University, Korimoto 1-21-24, Kagoshima 890-0065, Japan

Stephan Neumann, Julia Schüttler and Sonja Gaedke
Institute of Veterinary Medicine, University of Goettingen, Burckhardtweg 2, D-37077 Goettingen, Germany

Jens Linek
Veterinary specialists, Hamburg, Germany

Gerhard Loesenbeck
Laboklin GmbH&CO.KG, Bad Kissingen, Germany

F. Di Dona, G. Della Valle, C. Balestriere, B. Lamagna, G. Napoleone, F. Lamagna and G. Fatone
Department of Veterinary Medicine and Animal Productions, University of Napoli "Federico II", Italy

L. Meomartino
Interdepartmental Center of Veterinary Radiology, University of Napoli "Federico II", Italy

V. Castillo, M.F. Cabrera Blatter, D. Miceli, E. Soler Arias and P. Vidal
Cat. Clin. Méd. Peq. An. and U. Endocrinología, Escuela Medicina Veterinaria, Facultad de Ciencias Veterinarias, Universidad de Buenos Aires. Av.Chorroarín 280, C. Autónoma de Buenos Aires, Argentina

P. Pessina
Laboratorio de Técnicas Nucleares, Facultad de Veterinaria, Universidad de la República, Lasplaces 1550, Montevideo, Uruguay

P. Hall
Cat. Cirugía and U. Cirugía, Hosp., Escuela Medicina Veterinaria, Facultad de Ciencias Veterinarias, Universidad de Buenos Aires. Av.Chorroarín 280, C. Autónoma de Buenos Aires, Argentina

Harumichi Itoh, Kazuhito Itamoto, Tomoya Haraguchi and Shimpei Nishikawa
Department of Small Animal Clinical Science, Joint Faculty of Veterinary Medicine, Yamaguchi University, 1677-1 Yoshida, Yamaguchi City, Yamaguchi, 753-8511, Japan

Shotaro Eto, Kenji Tani, Masato Hiyama and Yasuho Taura
Department of Veterinary Surgery, Joint Faculty of Veterinary Medicine, Yamaguchi University, 1677-1 Yoshida, Yamaguchi City, Yamaguchi, 753-8511, Japan

Yoshiki Itoh, Toshie Iseri and Munekazu Nakaichi
Laboratory of Veterinary Radiology Yamaguchi University, 1677-1 Yoshida, Yamaguchi City, Yamaguchi, 753-8511, Japan

Raquel de Araújo Cantarella, Juliana Kravetz de Oliveira and Fabiano Montiani-Ferreira
Universidade Federal do Paraná (UFPR), Departamento de Medicina Veterinária, Rua dos Funcionários, 1540, Bairro Juvevê, 80035-050, Curitiba – PR, Brazil

Daniel M. Dorbandt
Department of Veterinary Clinical Medicine, College of Veterinary Medicine, University of Illinois at Urbana-Champaign, 1008, West Hazelwood Drive, Urbana, Illinois 61802, USA
Central Hospital for Veterinary Medicine, North Haven, Connecticut 06473, USA

Alessio Pierini, Filippo Cinti and Guido Pisani
Centro Veterinario Luni Mare, Ortonovo (SP), 19034, Italy

Diana Binanti
AbLab, Laboratorio di Analisi Veterinarie, Sarzana (SP), 19038, Italy

Caroline Constantino and Rafael Felipe da Costa Vieira
Department of Veterinary Medicine, Federal University of Paraná, Curitiba, PR, 80035-050, Brazil

Edson Ferraz Evaristo de Paula
Animal Protection Section, City Secretary of Environment, Curitiba, PR, 80020-290, Brazil

Ana Pérola Drulla Brandão and Fernando Ferreira
Department of Preventive Veterinary Medicine, University of São Paulo, São Paulo, SP, 05508-270, Brazil

Alexander Welker Biondo
Department of Veterinary Medicine, Federal University of Paraná, Curitiba, PR, 80035-050, Brazil
Animal Protection Section, City Secretary of Environment, Curitiba, PR, 80020-290, Brazil

Jonathan D. Pucket
Department of Veterinary Clinical Sciences, College of Veterinary Health Sciences, Oklahoma State University, Stillwater, OK 74078, USA

Rachel A. Allbaugh
Department of Veterinary Clinical Sciences, College of Veterinary Medicine, Iowa State University, Ames, IA 50011, USA

Mary L. Higginbotham and Amy J. Rankin
Department of Clinical Science, College of Veterinary Medicine, Kansas State University, Manhattan, KS 66506, USA

Leandro Teixeira
Department of Pathological Sciences, College of Veterinary Medicine, University of Wisconsin-Madison, WI 53706, USA

Francesca Rizzo, Cecilia Benetti and Consuelo Ballatori
Clinica Veterinaria Colombo, Viale Colombo 153, 55041, Lido di Camaiore (LU), Italy

Diana Binanti
AbLab, Laboratorio di Analisi Veterinarie, Sarzana (SP), 19038, Italy

Mahir A.G. Kubba
Department of Pathology and Clinical Pathology, Faculty of Veterinary Medicine, University of Tripoli, Libya

Donna M. White, Alastair R. Mair and Fernando Martinez-Taboada
Department of Anaesthesia and Analgesia, Veterinary Teaching Hospital, University of Sydney, Evelyn Williams Building B10, 65 Parramatta Road, Camperdown, NSW. 2050. Australia

E.A. Soler Arias and V.A. Castillo
Hospital Escuela, Unidad de Endocrinología, Area de Clínica Médica de Pequeños Animales, Fac. de Ciencias Veterinarias, UBA, Av. Chorroarín 280, Ciudad Autónoma de Buenos Aires, Argentina

R.H. Trigo
Catedra de Patología, Fac. de Ciencias Veterinarias, UBA, Av. Chorroarín 280, Ciudad Autónoma de Buenos Aires, Argentina

M.E. Caneda Aristarain
Alumna de Programa de Investigación. Fac. de Ciencias Veterinarias, UBA, Chorroarín 280, Ciudad Autónoma de Buenos Aires, Argentina

Izumi Ando
Cooperative Major in Advanced Health Science, Graduate School of Bio-Applications and System Engineering, Tokyo University of Agriculture and Technology, Tokyo 183-8509, Japan

Kaoru Karasawa and Akane Tanaka
Cooperative Major in Advanced Health Science, Graduate School of Bio-Applications and System Engineering, Tokyo University of Agriculture and Technology, Tokyo 183-8509, Japan
Laboratory of Comparative Animal Medicine, Division of Animal Life Science, Institute of Agriculture, Tokyo University of Agriculture and Technology, Tokyo 183-8509, Japan

Shinichi Yokota
Laboratory of Veterinary Molecular Pathology and Therapeutics, Division of Animal Life Science, Institute of Agriculture, Tokyo University of Agriculture and Technology, Tokyo 183-8509, Japan

Takao Shioya
The Eye Mate Inc., Tokyo 177-0051, Japan

Hiroshi Matsuda
Cooperative Major in Advanced Health Science, Graduate School of Bio-Applications and System Engineering, Tokyo University of Agriculture and Technology, Tokyo 183-8509, Japan
Laboratory of Veterinary Molecular Pathology and Therapeutics, Division of Animal Life Science, Institute of Agriculture, Tokyo University of Agriculture and Technology, Tokyo 183-8509, Japan

Karla Dzul-Rosado, Cesar Lugo-Caballero, Raul Tello-Martin, Karina López-Avila and Jorge Zavala-Castro
Center of Research and Regional Studies Dr Hideyo Noguchi, Autonomous University of Yucatan. Av. Itzáes and 59th street, number490, Mérida, Yucatán. Postal code 97000, Mexico

Thomas Rohwedder and Peter Böttcher
Department of Small Animal Medicine, University of Leipzig, An den Tierkliniken 23, 04103 Leipzig, Germany

Martin Fischer
Institute of Systematic Zoology and Evolutionary Biology with Phyletic Museum, Friedrich-Schiller-University, Jena, Germany

Marisa da Fonseca Ferreira, Arielle Elizabeth Ann Aylor, Richard John Mellanby, Susan Mary Campbell and Adam George Gow
Hospital for Small Animals, The Royal (Dick) School of Veterinary Studies, The University of Edinburgh, UK

Erika Fernanda V. Garcia, Catherine A. Loughin, Dominic J. Marino and Joseph Sackman
Department of Surgery, Long Island Veterinary Specialists, 163 South Service Road, Plainview, NY 11803, USA

Scott E. Umbaugh, Jiyuan Fu and Samrut Subedi
Computer Vision and Image Processing Laboratory, Electrical and Computer Engineering Department, Southern Illinois University at Edwardsville, Edwardsville, IL 62026-1801, USA

Martin L. Lesser and Meredith Akerman
North Shore - LIJ Health System Feinstein Institute for Medical Research, Biostatistics Unit, Manhasset, NY 11030, USA

João Eduardo W. Schossler
Universidade Federal de Santa Maria, Santa Maria, Brazil

Anna Suñol and Joan Mascort
Hospital Ars Veterinaria, carrer Cavallers n°37, 08034, Barcelona, Spain

Cristina Font
Hospital Ars Veterinaria, carrer Cavallers n°37, 08034, Barcelona, Spain
Hospital Canis Girona. Carrer Can Pau Birol, 38. 17006 Girona, Spain

Alicia Rami Bastante
Neuroscience Institute of Barcelona. Universitat Autònoma de Barcelona, edifici M1, campus de Bellaterra E-98193, Cerdanyola del Vallès, Spain

Martí Pumarola
Department of Animal Medicine and Surgery, Veterinary Faculty, Universitat Autonoma de Barcelona, 08193 Bellaterra (Cerdanyola del Vallès), Barcelona, Spain

Alejandro Lujan Feliu-Pascual
Hospital Ars Veterinaria, carrer Cavallers n°37, 08034, Barcelona, Spain
AÚNA Especialidades Veterinarias, Calle Algepser 22-1, 46980 Paterna, Valencia, Spain

David Williams and Heather Hewitt
Department of Veterinary Medicine, University of Cambridge, Madingley Road, Cambridge CB3 0ES, UK

M. Longo
Dipartimento di Medicina Veterinaria (DIMEVET), Università degli Studi di Milano, Az.Polo Veterinario di Lodi, Lodi, Italy
Centro Traumatologico Ortopedico Veterinario, Arenzano (GE), Italy

D. Binanti
AbLab, Veterinary Diagnostic Laboratory, Sarzana (SP), Italy

P.G. Zagarella and F. Iocca
Centro Traumatologico Ortopedico Veterinario, Arenzano (GE), Italy

D. De Zani, G. Ravasio, M. Di Giancamillo and D.D. Zani
Dipartimento di Medicina Veterinaria (DIMEVET), Università degli Studi di Milano, Az.Polo Veterinario di Lodi, Lodi, Italy

Index